Clinical and Surgical Aspects of Congenital Heart Diseases

Georgios Tagarakis • Ahmed Gheni Sarfan
Hashim Talib Hashim • Joseph Varney
Editors

Clinical and Surgical Aspects of Congenital Heart Diseases

Text and Study Guide

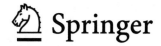
Springer

Editors
Georgios Tagarakis
Aristotle University of Thessaloniki
Thessaloniki, Greece

Ahmed Gheni Sarfan
Aarhus University
Aarhus, Denmark

Hashim Talib Hashim (iD)
University of Baghdad
Baghdad, Iraq

Joseph Varney
American University of the Caribbean School
Cupecoy, Sint Maarten (Dutch part)

ISBN 978-3-031-23064-6   ISBN 978-3-031-23062-2   (eBook)
https://doi.org/10.1007/978-3-031-23062-2

This Springer imprint is published by the registered company Springer Nature Switzerland AG
The registered company address is: Gewerbestrasse 11, 6330 Cham, Switzerland

I want to dedicate this work:

To the most brilliant people I have ever seen, those who taught me how to be on the right way, how to dream, how to think outside the box, and how to believe in myself. Those who have spent their lives to put me on the top. To my great father (Talib Hashim Manea) and my great mother (Jawaher Mutar Mohammed).

To my brothers, sisters, and friends and to everyone who helped me and encouraged me even with a word.

To myself, who went through a lot of difficulties, issues, problems, downs and ups, and hard times but still strong and stepping on all these tough times to create my own times and happiness till the end of my life, In Shaa Allah.

Hashim
19-20/11/2021
H.T.H

Preface

This book talks about congenital heart diseases in both adult and children from all aspects. It describes the disease, pathology, treatment, complications, and follow-up with details depending on the novel research and literature review. The book not only talks about the surgical and medical treatment, but it also talks about the laparoscopic techniques that can help in the treatment. Also, it talks about the epidemiology of each disease of them and its prevalence. It describes the genetic basis of medicine in cardiology and the diagnostic criteria for the heart disease during pregnancy. All these topics are discussed in a scientific medical language with appropriate illustrations and charts that make the understanding of the whole procedure easy for all the medical doctors and healthcare workers.

This book is—to our knowledge—the first book that vastly focuses on cardiosurgical and medical aspects of the congenital heart diseases, emerging from the significant need to fill a defect in the related cardiology and surgical resource map and incorporate meaningful updates regarding all aspects of the congenital heart diseases. Many books were dedicated to the subject over the years, but those were rather superficial, genetic, or pathological.

Clinical and Surgical Aspects of Congenital Heart Diseases: Text and Study Guide is composed of 30 chapters, containing concise and up-to-date information.

The book contains a lot of diagrams, tables, illustrations, and figures attempting to make it more interesting and easier to memorize by readers.

More than 200 single best answer multiple choice questions (MCQs), distributed along the chapters, covering important aspects of the congenital heart surgery and medicine, from embryology, epidemiology, medicine, pathology, and ultimately surgery.

There are many books that the literature currently holds books discussing congenital heart disease in detail. But these books either talk about these topics in general or are from the aspect of internal medicine. What we have done in our book is to talk about these topics from the surgical perspective and cover the details of congenital heart disease in a step-by-step fashion. Moreover, we have discussed laparoscopic surgeries in treating congenital heart disease, which has not been covered by other books or guidelines in a range of knowledge and experience as vast as our teams. We touch on the perfusion in congenital heart surgeries, which has not been mentioned independently in any other book that currently exists. In this book, we are presenting new, unique, and sequenced surgical guidelines in treating congenital heart disease either in childhood or adulthood with pros and cons. Detailed ways with highly organized, attractive graphs and photos will make this book easily understandable for medical students, surgical residents, and surgeons alike.

Thessaloniki, Greece

Aarhus, Denmark

Baghdad, Iraq

Cupecoy, Sint Maarten

1 September 2021

Georgios Tagarakis

Ahmed Gheni Sarfan

Hashim Talib Hashim

Joseph Varney

Contents

Genetic Basis of Congenital Heart Disease

Hashir Ali Awan and Irfan Ullah

Abstract

Most cases of congenital heart diseases (CHDs) are sporadic in nature and the exact causal mechanism is unknown, but a genetic underpinning is strongly implicated. Genetic variations occur spontaneously, but evidence of familial diseases passing as recessive alleles is well-documented. With advances in genetic analyses, copy number variations (CNVs), which changed thousands of bases consisting of coding and noncoding sequences, were suspected as causes behind CHD. Disruption in gene dosage leads to altered levels of crucial proteins in heart development that are part of transcription factor families, signaling pathways, or structural proteins.

Keywords

Congenital heart defects · Genetic variations · Morphological defects · Congenital anomalies · Aneuploidy · Copy number variations · Microdeletion

Introduction

Approximately one-third of all major congenital anomalies in newborns are *congenital heart diseases* (CHDs, also referred to as congenital heart anomalies), making them the most commonly occurring congenital disorder [1].

Some form of CHD in 2019, representing an incidence of 2305 per 100,000 live births [2]. The incidence of CHD in the last three decades has been relatively stable, but the mortality (in both infants and adults) due to CHD has declined by 60.4% to 2.8 per 100,000 population in 2019 [2]. Due to the development of medical and surgical methods to alleviate the condition, there is a great proportion of children who are able to survive to adulthood. Consequently, as of now, there are more adults with CHD than children [3]. Unlike other cardiovascular disorders, no well-established preventive measures reduce the incidence (and in turn the mortality) of CHD, and deaths can only be reduced via immediate diagnosis and surgical treatment. Therefore, owing to their weak healthcare infrastructures, a relatively higher death rate due to CHD is seen in countries with a low sociodemographic index (SDI) [2].

The classification of CHDs is accomplished in various ways. The subdivision into two broad categories of cyanotic and non-cyanotic is based on whether right-to-left shunting occurs and if the baby turns blue or not [4]. Another way to divide it into major categories is to check for extracardiac anomalies and conclude whether the CHD is isolated or syndromic (complex) [5]. However, the *International Congenital Heart Surgery Nomenclature* divided CHD into four major defects: hypoplastic, obstructive, cyanotic, and septal [5].

Starting soon after fertilization, the development of the heart and the associated great vessels has an intricate progression consisting of different stages closely regulated by embryonic signaling systems on a molecular level [5, 6]. While differing in severity, congenital anomalies can occur as a result of errors at any step that adversely impact the developmental process. Causes of these errors are manifold. The etiology of CHD can be broadly divided into genetic and nongenetic in nature. However, the causes behind CHD are considered to be largely multifactorial, occurring via a contribution of both genetic vulnerabilities and environmental influences [3, 5]. Exposure of the mother to teratogenic substances and agents is considered a nongenetic and environmental factor in increasing the risk of infants to be born with heart defects. While nonsyndromic presentation of CHD without any extracardiac involvement has been associated with a teratogenic etiology, confirmation of a genetic origin behind some isolated heart defects

H. A. Awan
Dow Medical College, Dow University of Health Sciences, Karachi, Pakistan

I. Ullah (✉)
Kabir Medical College, Gandhara University, Peshawar, Pakistan

© The Author(s), under exclusive license to Springer Nature Switzerland AG 2023
G. Tagarakis et al. (eds.), *Clinical and Surgical Aspects of Congenital Heart Diseases*,
https://doi.org/10.1007/978-3-031-23062-2_1

elucidates the possibility of genetic reasons behind both syndromic and nonsyndromic CHD [6]. In addition, an interesting confluence of environmental factors and the underlying genetic makeup of a person is now increasingly being appreciated as "epigenetics" [6].

In contrast to environmental effects, multiple epidemiological studies conclude that the key involvement in the etiology of CHD is genetic in nature [5]. Genetic causes have been implicated after recent advances in our understanding of genomes and variations among them [7]. Whole exome sequencing (WES) and next-generation sequencing (NGS) have allowed valuable insight to be gained regarding pathogenic variants causing (or associated with) CHD [3]. Various models have been employed to illustrate the exact nature of CHD as a genetic phenomenon. One of the earliest recognized causes behind CHD was aneuploidy, usually having a syndromic, multisystem presentation and occurring sporadically [8]. Further studies have illustrated subchromosomal differences in the number of copies of specific genetic sequences, called copy number variations (CNVs), that may sometimes be pathogenic and lead to isolated or complex CHDs [5, 6]. CNVs can be insertions or deletions of a large number of nucleotides and are sometimes called microdeletions or microduplications [8]. In addition, certain monogenic mutations, both inherited and occurring de novo, may lead to congenital defects as well. These may be a result of single nucleotide polymorphisms (SNPs) or part of an insertion or deletion (INDEL) of nucleotides [8]. Approximately 400 genes have been linked to the occurrence of CHD. Alteration in these genes disturbs transcription factors, signaling mechanisms, and multiple other biological processes in the body [9]. While some mutations, mostly monogenic variations, are rare familial defects that are inherited in a mendelian fashion, a vast majority of genetic events leading to CHD are sporadic in nature [5, 8].

In addition to sporadic genetic events leading to CHDs, the presence of rare familial genetic variations is tantamount to the presence of a genetic source of CHD [5]. Autosomal dominant, autosomal recessive, and X-linked inheritance patterns of monogenic mutations have all been identified in families with recurring isolated or complex cardiac defects [6]. Furthermore, the relatively greater incidence of identified familial CHDs in regions with high consanguinity explains the presence of recessive alleles that have more chances of manifesting in such settings. Most studies on consanguineous unions have indicated a greater likelihood of children developing nonsyndromic CHDs [10]. Consequently, the risk and incidence of CHDs increase with how closely related the parents are to each other [11]. Moreover, there is nearly three times greater chance of both monozygotic twins (with identical genetic makeup) having CHD than the chance of both dizygotic (non-identical) twins [11], further showcasing the presence of recessive alleles and a genetic contri-

bution to CHD. On the other hand, the existence of dominant alleles due to CHD has also been described. Most of the cases occur sporadically, and mutations are hypothesized to arise de novo without a mendelian inheritance pattern. Dominant mutations of certain genes are generally considered to impart a more deleterious effect, and affected individuals are prone to negative evolutionary selection [5]. Since the severe phenotypic effect of these dominant alleles may affect the viability of the fetus and also, to some extent, dictate the probability of individuals surviving until the reproductive age, a lower incidence of such traits is seen recurring consecutively in offspring and running in families in an extended pedigree [6, 8]. Therefore, it can be concluded that a major subset of the reported cases of CHDs caused by dominant alleles are not due to inherited mutations but rather caused by de novo alterations in the specific genes [5, 6]. In fact, an NGS study revealed that the prevalence of de novo autosomal dominant variants is four times higher (8%) than the prevalence of inherited recessive variants [3].

A challenge in accurately ascertaining the role of each genetic variation and correlating them with one subdivision of heart defects is the heterogeneity observed in cases of CHD. The same genetic variant in different subjects leads to widely varying phenotypes, depicting differing expressivity of specific mutations even among families [6, 9]. Furthermore, a variable penetrance of known disease-associated genetic variants presents as individuals carrying those variants with no defect [9]. This heterogeneity indicates the possible role of other genetic and nongenetic factors that result in vast diversity in disease presentation.

Aneuploidy

Aneuploidy is an abnormality in the total number of chromosomes. Aneuploidies were one of the earliest recognized causal factors that formed a genetic basis for CHD [8]. Fetal aneuploidy is associated with nearly one-third (33%) of all CHD [12]. Another study estimates that one out of eight children with CHD has a chromosomal abnormality, including aneuploidies [13]. The addition or removal of an entire chromosome causes a "bulk" gain or loss of genes [5] that invariably exerts a wide range of cardiac and extracardiac effects. This is shown by an overwhelming 98% of fetuses with CHD and aneuploidy showing at least one extracardiac irregularity [12]. Furthermore, aneuploidy presumably affects viability of fetuses as the prevalence of aneuploidy is considerably higher in fetuses with prenatally diagnosed CHD than in neonates born with CHD [8]. In addition, due to the relatively large size of the genetic change in aneuploidies, a targeted gene or sequence of genes cannot be accurately determined to be responsible for cardiac anomalies [5]. Similarly, a wide range of phenotypical presentations are associated with each aneuploidy, and virtually any anomaly can result from each aneuploidy [8, 14]. Nevertheless, specific phenotypes of CHD are notably linked with certain aneuploidies [8].

Multiple aneuploidies are associated with CHD. These include Down syndrome (trisomy 21), Turner syndrome (monosomy X), Patau syndrome (trisomy 13), and Edwards syndrome (trisomy 18). Up to half of all cases of Down and Turner syndromes and nearly all cases of Patau and Edwards syndromes will show a cardiac anomaly at birth [5]. Down syndrome and Turner syndrome have the greatest incidence among aneuploidies that cause CHD [6].

Trisomy 21 (Down Syndrome)

Down syndrome (DS) (trisomy 21) is the most common aneuploidy overall and the most commonly associated aneuploidy with CHD [3]. It is caused by a child having an extra copy of the 21st chromosome. Also, 62% of the diagnosed CHD cases with an aneuploidy were children with DS [15]. An estimated 44% of all DS cases are predicted to have cardiac anomalies [16]. A population-based study in Atlanta revealed that atrioventricular septal defects (AVSDs) were the most commonly occurring defect in DS infants [17]. Similarly, a Moroccan retrospective study also asserted that the most common phenotype of CHD found in children with DS was AVSD [18]. Genetic analyses have identified various genes on chromosome 21 that may have a pathogenic role to play in causing CHD in DS. Some of the most important genes are DSCAM and COL6A2 [8, 19]. Interestingly, experimental studies revealed that overexpression of DSCAM and COL6A2 together is responsible for defects in cardiac morphology, and each gene when overexpressed individually fails to elicit a reaction.

Monosomy X (Turner Syndrome)

"Turner syndrome (TS) is characterized by a partial or complete absence of one X chromosome and is often referred to as Monosomy X," and 23–50% of children with TS may have a cardiac anomaly [20]. Like DS, TS also has a predominant association with certain phenotypes, most notably left-sided obstructive heart defects and aortic anomalies. As many as 30% of all CHDs in TS may be bicuspid aortic valve (BAV) [20]. In fact, an individual with TS is 30–60 times more likely to have a BAV than a female with no aneuploidy [20]. It is theorized that the reason behind the majority of cardiac defects in TS being aortic in nature are possibly due to genes present on the short arm of the X chromosome that regulate the formation of the aortic valve or the aorta [21].

Copy Number Variations

CNVs are *en masse* insertions or deletions (microdeletions) of more than 1000 bases (1 kb) up to several million bases (several Mbs). The number of copies of each gene sequence differs between individuals, and CNVs may alter their quantity [5, 22]. These subchromosomal aberrations can be harmless or harmful, depending on whether they alter gene dosage, consist of coding or noncoding regions, or have been associated with a syndrome [5, 23]. Some CNVs, however, have been identified to have a pathogenic effect and contributing to cardiac anomalies at birth [8, 24]. While CNVs can be inherited, most occur de novo as demonstrated by genetic trio studies [22, 25]. Multiple cohort studies investigating particular heart defects have shown affected individuals having considerably higher CNVs than healthy controls [8]. A study involving 422 subjects with CHD found that CNVs are more frequently found in children with CHD than in children without any anomaly [26]. Despite the genetic diversity of the human population, new technologies like WES and advanced cytogenetic analysis methods have allowed rapid progress in identifying variations in the number of copies of each sequence [8], and CNVs are now increasingly being recognized as an important contributor to the incidence of CHD [27]. Subsequently, several clinical syndromes involving cardiac anomalies have now been related to CNVs. Additionally, CNVs are linked with a considerably greater risk of nonsyndromic CHDs [28]. In line with this, it is estimated that children with pathogenic CNVs have a 2.55 times greater risk of having an isolated CHD than unaffected children [26]. Similarly, affected children with CNVs are 3.43 times more vulnerable to death or transplant [26].

Microdeletions are traditionally believed to be more damaging as alterations in gene dosage would cause haploinsufficiency in relation to genes that are known to be involved in cardiac development [3, 14]. Consequently, morphological defects may result due to perturbation in the developmental process. However, in microdeletions that result in a syndromic or multisystemic presentation, it is unclear whether the loss of a particular gene in the CNV has pleiotropic effects on the phenotype or the resultant pathology is due to a collective and contiguous loss of multiple genes with altered gene dosage of each causing a certain component of the phenotype [3, 14].

22q11.2 Deletion Syndrome

One of the most common microdeletions (~3 Mb) is the 22q11.2 deletion syndrome (22q11.2DS), causing cardiac and extracardiac defects [22, 29], and 90–95% of 22q11.2DS cases occur sporadically, with deletions occurring de novo in the proband without either parent showing the CNV [21]. While 22q11.2DS is a distinct entity, a vast majority of its features overlap with DiGeorge syndrome and velocardiofacial syndrome [3]. It is estimated that a 22q11.2 deletion is found in 1.9% of all children with cardiac malformations at birth [30]. On the other hand, among those with a 22q11.2 deletion, a vast majority (81%) have CHD [21]. Phenotypically, 22q11.2DS is highly correlated with conotruncal abnormalities in the heart, most commonly presenting as tetralogy of Fallot [30]. Moreover, a considerable proportion of individuals with aortic arch defects show a 22q11.2 deletion. Up to 48% of patients with an interruption of the aortic arch (IAA) and 35% of patients with a truncus arteriosus (TA) have an underlying 22q11.2 deletion [8]. Out of 30 genes impacted by the 22q11.2 deletion, one of the most crucial genes is TBX1, encoding for a T-box transcription factor that plays an important role in the development of the second heart field (concerned with the formation of the right ventricle and the outflow tract) [9, 14]. Mouse models investigating mutations that lead to loss of function or total loss of the TBX1 gene have depicted serious cardiac problems comprising conotruncal defects [31]. Other genes of interest that are lost in 22q11.2DS are CRKL and DGCR8 [29, 32].

Other Common CNVs

The 7q11.23 deletion causing the Williams syndrome leads to the haploinsufficiency of nearly 25 genes, including the ELN gene that codes for elastin [5, 14]. The deleterious effect of the ELN gene has been implicated as the causal factor behind the appearance of cardiac anomalies such as supravalvular aortic and pulmonary stenosis as a component of the syndrome [3, 33]. Nevertheless, due to a contiguous loss of genes, Williams syndrome also exhibits phenotypic variability [3]. Furthermore, terminal deletion in the long arm of chromosome 11 causing Jacobsen syndrome [34] has been associated with multiple phenotypic presentations. Importantly, the frequency of individuals with Jacobsen syndrome that show hypoplastic left heart syndrome (HLHS) is considerably greater than the general public [35]. Additionally, other CNVs have also been implicated in syndromic and nonsyndromic CHDs such as 8p23.1 deletion (affecting GATA4 gene), 1p36 deletion, 15q11.2 deletion, 1q21.1 deletion (affecting GJA5 gene), and 1q21.1 duplication (affecting GJA5 gene) [3, 5, 22].

Single-Gene Variations

Most commonly, SNPs and INDELs cause point mutations, or single-gene variations, in the genome [3, 5]. Some of these mutations have a loss of function (LOF) or inactivating impact, leading to haploinsufficiency [5]. As a result, the gene dosage and the subsequent protein dosage are lowered, disrupting the normal processes involved in heart development [8]. Point mutations of different genes may lead to either syndromic or nonsyndromic phenotypes.

Syndromic Single-Gene Variations

Several mutations have been implicated in the causation of CHD that occurs as a component of a larger syndrome. While many syndromes have been described, some of the important and more prevalent syndromes include Alagille syndrome, Holt–Oram syndrome, and Noonan syndrome.

Alagille Syndrome

"Alagille syndrome (AS) is a multisystemic autosomal dominant disorder that exhibits cardiac and extracardiac abnormalities" [36]. Different subsets of CHD are found in 90–97% of all patients with AS. Arterial stenoses are overrepresented in individuals with AS, but other morphological defects like TOF are also common [3]. Pathogenic mutations in the JAG1 gene constitute the largest proportion of genetic changes responsible for AS, followed by the NOTCH2 gene [3]. A study in Philadelphia investigated genetic variants in clinically diagnosed AS patients and reported that 94.3% of their cohort had a mutation in JAG1 and only 2.5% had a mutation in the NOTCH2 gene [37]. Both genes encode ligands in the NOTCH signaling pathway that plays a vital role in lineage differentiation [14].

Holt–Oram Syndrome

"Holt–Oram syndrome (HOS) is an autosomal dominant disorder characterized by congenital defects in heart morphology along with upper limb anomalies and is sometimes also referred to as the 'heart-hand' syndrome" [38]. Associated with a wide range of cardiac phenotypes, HOS typically presents as a septal defect. A retrospective study of 212 patients of HOS to ascertain the genotype-phenotype correlation documented atrial septal defects (ASDs) as the most common cardiac phenotype of the disorder, occurring in 61.5% of the patients [39]. From a molecular perspective, HOS most commonly arises from a LOF mutation in the TBX5 gene [8, 39]. TBX5 (like TBX1 in 22q11.2DS) is a transcription factor belonging to the T-box family [14]. A cross-sectional study found that 74% of all patients with HOS had a mutation of the TBX5 gene [40]. TBX5 is especially important for the development of limbs, the cardiac septum, and the heart's conduction system [3, 8].

Noonan Syndrome

Noonan syndrome (NS) is also an autosomal dominant disorder that has a multiorgan presentation with cardiac, neurodevelopment, and other abnormalities. It is considered to be the second most common syndrome causing CHD after DS [41]. More than 80% of individuals with NS have at least one form of cardiac anomaly [42]. Like other genetic syndromes, NS also exhibits inconsistent expressivity in terms of the phenotype, but the most common congenital heart defect recorded is pulmonary valve stenosis [42, 43]. On a genetic level, NS is most commonly associated with rare gain-of-function (GOF) mutations in the PTPN11 gene, accounting for half the cases [44]. PTPN11 encodes for proteins that, via a series of reactions, affect the RAS/MAPK (mitogen-activated protein kinase) signaling pathways that are vital for cell differentiation and survival [14]. This is also the reason why NS is sometimes referred to as a "RASopathy" [3, 21]. Apart from PTPN11, mutations in 12 other genes playing a crucial role in the RAS/MAPK pathway are linked to the causality of NS [45].

Nonsyndromic Single-Gene Variations

Functional alteration of specific genes via mutations may also present in an isolated manner without any extracardiac anomalies. Three categories of single-gene variations have been highlighted by observing which functional process or protein they alter: transcription factors, signaling pathways, or structural proteins [5]. Several gene families have been implicated in each category. In transcription factors most commonly affected by mutations, the GATA family of zinc-finger factors, T-Box transcription factors, NKX2-5 genes for homeobox transcription factors, and FOX family encoding for Forkhead box factors have been considered most important in organogenesis including the heart [7, 9]. Signaling pathways such as the Wnt/β-catenin, NOTCH, Nodal, Sonic Hedgehog, and the RAS-MAPK channels have been known to play a crucial role in the development of the heart, especially looping and cell differentiation, and have been frequently associated with mutations that result in congenital defects [8, 21]. While research on structural proteins is still limited, genes encoding for elastin (ELN), myosin heavy chains (MYH6 and MYH7), and cardiac actin (ACTC) have been studied, and known mutations in these genes have caused cardiac anomalies at birth.

Multiple Choice Questions (MCQs)

1. Among the following, which cardiovascular disease has no well-established preventative measures?
   A. Ischemic heart disease
   B. Peripheral artery disease
   C. Congenital heart disease
   D. Cardiomyopathy

2. According to the International Congenital Heart Surgery Nomenclature, how many major subdivisions of heart defects exist?
   A. One
   B. Two
   C. Three
   D. Four

3. Which one of the following is not part of the subtypes defined by the International Congenital Heart Surgery Nomenclature?
   A. Hypoplastic
   B. Conotruncal
   C. Cyanotic
   D. Obstructive

4. Term describing the confluence of environmental factors and the underlying genetic makeup of a person is:
   A. Ectogenetics
   B. Envirogenetics
   C. Metagenetics
   D. Epigenetics

5. Which of the following is not a subchromosomal genetic basis for congenital heart disease?
   A. Insertion
   B. Deletion
   C. Aneuploidy
   D. Copy number variation

6. Approximately how many genes have been linked to occurrence of congenital heart disease?
   A. 400
   B. 800
   C. 1200
   D. 1600

7. Aneuploidy can be defined as:
   A. Abnormality in the quality of chromosomes
   B. Abnormality in the quantity of chromosomes
   C. Abnormality in the quality of sex chromosomes
   D. Normal number of chromosomes

8. Down syndrome is caused by an individual having an extra copy of which chromosome?
   A. 17
   B. 35
   C. 21
   D. 8

9. Monosomy X caused which syndromic disease?
   A. Patau syndrome
   B. Edwards syndrome
   C. Turner syndrome
   D. Klinefelter Syndrome

10. Most common type of heart defect associated with Down syndrome is:
    A. Conotruncal abnormalities
    B. Hypoplastic defects

C. Tetralogy of Fallot

D. Atrioventricular septal defects

11. Disruptions in which gene(s) have been implicated in the occurrence of heart defects in Down syndrome?

A. DSCAM

B. COL6A2

C. Both DSCAM and COL6A2 together

D. Neither DSCAM nor COL6A2

12. Bicuspid aortic valve (BAV) is associated with which aneuploidy?

A. Patau syndrome

B. Down syndrome

C. Edwards syndrome

D. Turner syndrome

13. Copy number variations (CNVs) include deletions or insertions of at least how many bases?

A. 10

B. 100

C. 1000

D. 10,000

14. What is the size of microdeletion leading to 22q11.2 deletion syndrome?

A. ~3 Kb

B. ~3 Mb

C. ~30 Kb

D. ~30 Mb

15. TBX1 gene is impacted in which of the following CNVs?

A. 22q11.2 deletion

B. 8p23.1 deletion

C. 1q21.1 deletion

D. 7q11.23 deletion

16. TBX1 gene plays an important role in the development of the:

A. Cardiac valves

B. Primary heart field

C. Secondary heart field

D. Cardiac septum

17. 7q11.23 deletion causing Williams syndrome causes disruption in which of the following gene sequences?

A. CRKL

B. GATA4

C. TBX1

D. ELN

18. Alagille syndrome is mostly caused by a single-gene variation in which gene?

A. NOTCH5

B. ELN

C. TBX5

D. JAG1

19. The actual name of the "heart-hand syndrome" is:

A. Noonan syndrome

B. Alagille syndrome

C. DiGeorge syndrome

D. Holt–Oram syndrome

20. The "heart-hand syndrome" is caused by a mutation in the TBX5 gene. What type of protein does it encode for?

A. Signaling pathway protein

B. Cardiac structural protein

C. Transcription factor

D. Cardiac enzyme

21. Noonan syndrome is also referred to as a:

A. Cardiopathy

B. Cardiomyopathy

C. RASopathy

D. Neuropathy

22. What kind of mutation in the PTPN11 gene leads to Noonan syndrome?

A. Gain-of-function (GOF)

B. Loss-of-function (LOF)

C. Inactivation

D. Switch-of-function (SOF)

23. Which of the following does not encode for a cardiac structural protein?

A. ACTC

B. MYH6

C. ELN

D. GATA4

24. Which of the following is not a family of transcription factors associated with congenital heart disease?

A. T-Box

B. RAS/MAPK

C. GATA

D. FOX

25. A vast variety of single-gene variations and genetic events leading to congenital heart disease are of what nature?

A. Inherited

B. Familial

C. Sporadic

D. Environmental

Answers

1. C

2. D

3. B

4. D

5. A

6. A

7. B

8. C

9. C

10. D

11. C

12. D

13. C
14. B
15. A
16. C
17. D
18. D
19. D
20. B
21. C
22. A
23. D
24. A
25. A

References

1. van der Linde D, Konings EE, Slager MA, et al. Birth prevalence of congenital heart disease worldwide: a systematic review and meta-analysis. J Am Coll Cardiol. 2011;58(21):2241–7. https://doi.org/10.1016/j.jacc.2011.08.025.

2. Roth GA, Mensah GA, Johnson CO, et al. Global burden of cardiovascular diseases and risk factors, 1990–2019: update from the GBD 2019 study [published correction appears in J Am Coll Cardiol. 2021;77(15):1958–1959]. J Am Coll Cardiol. 2020;76(25):2982–3021. https://doi.org/10.1016/j.jacc.2020.11.010.

3. Pierpont ME, Brueckner M, Chung WK, et al. Genetic basis for congenital heart disease: revisited: a scientific statement from the American Heart Association [published correction appears in circulation. 2018;138(21):e713]. Circulation. 2018;138(21):e653–711. https://doi.org/10.1161/CIR.0000000000000606.

4. Ossa Galvis MM, Bhakta RT, Tarmahomed A, et al. Cyanotic heart disease. In: StatPearls [Internet]. Treasure Island: StatPearls. 2021 [cited 2021 Sep 8]. https://www.ncbi.nlm.nih.gov/books/NBK500001/.

5. Shabana NA, Shahid SU, Irfan U. Genetic contribution to congenital heart disease (CHD). Pediatr Cardiol. 2020;41(1):12–23. https://doi.org/10.1007/s00246-019-02271-4.

6. Cowan JR, Ware SM. Genetics and genetic testing in congenital heart disease. Clin Perinatol. 2015;42(2):373–93, ix. https://doi.org/10.1016/j.clp.2015.02.009.

7. Sun R, Liu M, Lu L, Zheng Y, Zhang P. Congenital heart disease: causes, diagnosis, symptoms, and treatments. Cell Biochem Biophys. 2015;72(3):857–60. https://doi.org/10.1007/s12013-015-0551-6.

8. Zaidi S, Brueckner M. Genetics and genomics of congenital heart disease. Circ Res. 2017;120(6):923–40. https://doi.org/10.1161/CIRCRESAHA.116.309140.

9. Williams K, Carson J, Lo C. Genetics of congenital heart disease. Biomolecules. 2019;9(12):879. https://doi.org/10.3390/biom9120879.

10. Shieh JT, Bittles AH, Hudgins L. Consanguinity and the risk of congenital heart disease. Am J Med Genet A. 2012;158A(5):1236–41. https://doi.org/10.1002/ajmg.a.35272.

11. Wang X, Li P, Chen S, et al. Influence of genes and the environment in familial congenital heart defects. Mol Med Rep. 2014;9(2):695–700. https://doi.org/10.3892/mmr.2013.1847.

12. Wimalasundera RC, Gardiner HM. Congenital heart disease and aneuploidy. Prenat Diagn. 2004;24(13):1116–22. https://doi.org/10.1002/pd.1068.

13. Hartman RJ, Rasmussen SA, Botto LD, et al. The contribution of chromosomal abnormalities to congenital heart defects: a population-based study. Pediatr Cardiol. 2011;32(8):1147–57. https://doi.org/10.1007/s00246-011-0034-5.

14. Fahed AC, Gelb BD, Seidman JG, Seidman CE. Genetics of congenital heart disease: the glass half empty [published correction appears in Circ Res. 2013;112(12):e182]. Circ Res. 2013;112(4):707–20. https://doi.org/10.1161/CIRCRESAHA.112.300853.

15. Geddes GC, Earing MG. Genetic evaluation of patients with congenital heart disease. Curr Opin Pediatr. 2018;30(6):707–13. https://doi.org/10.1097/MOP.0000000000000682.

16. Bull MJ. Down syndrome. N Engl J Med. 2020;382(24):2344–52. https://doi.org/10.1056/NEJMra1706537.

17. Freeman SB, Taft LF, Dooley KJ, et al. Population-based study of congenital heart defects in Down syndrome. Am J Med Genet. 1998;80(3):213–7.

18. Benhaourech S, Drighil A, Hammiri AE. Congenital heart disease and Down syndrome: various aspects of a confirmed association. Cardiovasc J Afr. 2016;27(5):287–90. https://doi.org/10.5830/CVJA-2016-019.

19. Calcagni G, Unolt M, Digilio MC, et al. Congenital heart disease and genetic syndromes: new insights into molecular mechanisms. Expert Rev Mol Diagn. 2017;17(9):861–70. https://doi.org/10.1080/14737159.2017.1360766.

20. Silberbach M, Roos-Hesselink JW, Andersen NH, et al. Cardiovascular health in Turner syndrome: a scientific statement from the American Heart Association. Circ Genom Precis Med. 2018;11(10):e000048. https://doi.org/10.1161/HCG.0000000000000048.

21. Hopkins MK, Dugoff L, Kuller JA. Congenital heart disease: prenatal diagnosis and genetic associations. Obstet Gynecol Surv. 2019;74(8):497–503. https://doi.org/10.1097/OGX.0000000000000702.

22. Costain G, Silversides CK, Bassett AS. The importance of copy number variation in congenital heart disease. NPJ Genom Med. 2016;1:16031. https://doi.org/10.1038/npjgenmed.2016.31.

23. Lee TM, Bacha EA. Copy number variants in congenital heart disease: a new risk factor impacting outcomes? J Thorac Cardiovasc Surg. 2016;151(4):1152–3. https://doi.org/10.1016/j.jtcvs.2015.10.002.

24. Soemedi R, Wilson IJ, Bentham J, et al. Contribution of global rare copy-number variants to the risk of sporadic congenital heart disease. Am J Hum Genet. 2012;91(3):489–501. https://doi.org/10.1016/j.ajhg.2012.08.003.

25. Glessner JT, Bick AG, Ito K, et al. Increased frequency of de novo copy number variants in congenital heart disease by integrative analysis of single nucleotide polymorphism array and exome sequence data. Circ Res. 2014;115(10):884–96. https://doi.org/10.1161/CIRCRESAHA.115.304458.

26. Kim DS, Kim JH, Burt AA, et al. Burden of potentially pathologic copy number variants is higher in children with isolated congenital heart disease and significantly impairs covariate-adjusted transplant-free survival. J Thorac Cardiovasc Surg. 2016;151(4):1147–51.e4. https://doi.org/10.1016/j.jtcvs.2015.09.136.

27. Liu Y, Chang X, Glessner J, et al. Association of rare recurrent copy number variants with congenital heart defects based on next-generation sequencing data from family trios. Front Genet. 2019;10:819. https://doi.org/10.3389/fgene.2019.00819.

28. Southard AE, Edelmann LJ, Gelb BD. Role of copy number variants in structural birth defects. Pediatrics. 2012;129(4):755–63. https://doi.org/10.1542/peds.2011-2337.

29. Goldmuntz E. 22q11.2 deletion syndrome and congenital heart disease. Am J Med Genet C Semin Med Genet. 2020;184(1):64–72. https://doi.org/10.1002/ajmg.c.31774.

30. Agergaard P, Olesen C, Østergaard JR, Christiansen M, Sørensen KM. The prevalence of chromosome 22q11.2 deletions in 2,478 children with cardiovascular malformations. A population-based study. Am J Med Genet A. 2012;158A(3):498–508. https://doi.org/10.1002/ajmg.a.34250.

31. McDonald-McGinn DM, Sullivan KE, Marino B, et al. 22q11.2 deletion syndrome. Nat Rev Dis Primers. 2015;1:15071. https://doi.org/10.1038/nrdp.2015.71.

32. Morrow BE, McDonald-McGinn DM, Emanuel BS, Vermeesch JR, Scambler PJ. Molecular genetics of 22q11.2 deletion syndrome. Am J Med Genet A. 2018;176(10):2070–81. https://doi.org/10.1002/ajmg.a.40504.

33. Yuan SM. Congenital heart defects in Williams syndrome. Turk J Pediatr. 2017;59(3):225–32. https://doi.org/10.24953/turkjped.2017.03.001.

34. Favier R, Akshoomoff N, Mattson S, Grossfeld P. Jacobsen syndrome: advances in our knowledge of phenotype and genotype. Am J Med Genet C Semin Med Genet. 2015;169(3):239–50. https://doi.org/10.1002/ajmg.c.31448.

35. Ye M, Coldren C, Liang X, et al. Deletion of ETS-1, a gene in the Jacobsen syndrome critical region, causes ventricular septal defects and abnormal ventricular morphology in mice. Hum Mol Genet. 2010;19(4):648–56. https://doi.org/10.1093/hmg/ddp532.

36. Mitchell E, Gilbert M, Loomes KM. Alagille Syndrome. Clin Liver Dis. 2018;22(4):625–41. https://doi.org/10.1016/j.cld.2018.06.001.

37. Gilbert MA, Bauer RC, Rajagopalan R, et al. Alagille syndrome mutation update: comprehensive overview of JAG1 and NOTCH2 mutation frequencies and insight into missense variant classification. Hum Mutat. 2019;40(12):2197–220. https://doi.org/10.1002/humu.23879.

38. Krauser AF, Ponnarasu S, Schury MP. Holt Oram syndrome. In: StatPearls. Treasure Island: StatPearls Publishing; 2021.

39. Vanlerberghe C, Jourdain AS, Ghoumid J, et al. Holt-Oram syndrome: clinical and molecular description of 78 patients with TBX5 variants. Eur J Hum Genet. 2019;27(3):360–8. https://doi.org/10.1038/s41431-018-0303-3.

40. McDermott DA, Bressan MC, He J, et al. TBX5 genetic testing validates strict clinical criteria for Holt-Oram syndrome. Pediatr Res. 2005;58(5):981–6. https://doi.org/10.1203/01.PDR.0000182593.95441.64.

41. Roberts AE, Allanson JE, Tartaglia M, Gelb BD. Noonan syndrome. Lancet. 2013;381(9863):333–42. https://doi.org/10.1016/S0140-6736(12)61023-X.

42. Linglart L, Gelb BD. Congenital heart defects in Noonan syndrome: diagnosis, management, and treatment. Am J Med Genet C Semin Med Genet. 2020;184(1):73–80. https://doi.org/10.1002/ajmg.c.31765.

43. Tartaglia M, Kalidas K, Shaw A, et al. PTPN11 mutations in Noonan syndrome: molecular spectrum, genotype-phenotype correlation, and phenotypic heterogeneity. Am J Hum Genet. 2002;70(6):1555–63. https://doi.org/10.1086/340847.

44. Tartaglia M, Mehler EL, Goldberg R, et al. Mutations in PTPN11, encoding the protein tyrosine phosphatase SHP-2, cause Noonan syndrome [published correction appears in Nat Genet 2001;29(4):491] [published correction appears in Nat Genet 2002;30(1):123]. Nat Genet. 2001;29(4):465–8. https://doi.org/10.1038/ng77.

45. Saliba A, Figueiredo ACV, Baroneza JE, et al. Genetic and genomics in congenital heart disease: a clinical review. J Pediatr (Rio J). 2020;96(3):279–88. https://doi.org/10.1016/j.jped.2019.07.004.

Epidemiology of Congenital Heart Diseases

Mustafa Hussein Ajlan Al-Jarshawi, Ahmed Hamid Jabbar,
Haitham Albadree, Ameen Abdul Hasan Manea Al Alwany,
Yousif Ali Madlul, Hiba Hussein Shaker,
and Ali Tarik Abdulwahid

Abstract

Understanding the epidemiology of congenital heart defects is crucial because of their high prevalence, their effect on the healthcare system, and the fact that better health policy recommendations can be derived from this knowledge. Despite recent improvements in surgical techniques and diagnostic tools, this major health issue continues to account for a high percentage of deaths and hospitalizations. It is possible that the varying prevalence of congenital heart defects across the globe is due to regional variations in multifactorial risk factors or to the unequal availability of healthcare services in some parts of the world. It is worth noting that there is substantial variation regarding the occurrence of the various major types of heart defects between different studies.

Keywords

Congenital heart diseases · Epidemiology · Prevalence Incidence · Mortality · Risk factors · Ventricular septal defect · Atrial septal defect · Tetralogy of Fallot

M. H. A. Al-Jarshawi (✉)
Leicester Medical School, University of Leicester, Leicester, UK

A. H. Jabbar
Al-Kindy Teaching Hospital, Baghdad, Iraq

H. Albadree
Internal Medicine Department, College of Medicine, University of Baghdad, Baghdad, Iraq
e-mail: haitham.nabeel1500d@comed.uobaghdad.edu.iq

A. A. H. M. Al Alwany · Y. A. Madlul · H. H. Shaker · A. T. Abdulwahid
College of Medicine, University of Baghdad, Baghdad, Iraq
e-mail: ameen.a@comed.uobaghdad.edu.iq;
youssef.ali1800d@comed.uobaghdad.edu.iq;
heba.hussein1800d@comed.uobaghdad.edu.iq;
Alitarik@comed.uobaghdad.edu.iq

Introduction

"Congenital heart disease (CHD) refers to a group of congenital malformations that affect the heart and/or the great vessels and are apparent at birth but not always obvious from a clinical perspective." In the past, only a small fraction of patients with extreme cases of these diseases made it to adulthood [1].

"It is the most prevalent form of congenital anomaly in newborns." Due to the severity of its comorbidities and the extensive medical care it necessitates, CHD is a global health concern. In 2004, well over 46,000 people of varying ages were admitted to hospitals in the United States due to heart defects, and these conditions were responsible for a substantial $1.4 billion in medical spending [2].

In recent decades, there has been a shift in the mortality rate and prevalence of heart defects, which has been accompanied by the development of new and better diagnostic techniques, improved management, and a deeper understanding of cardiac physiology and pathology [3].

Among all forms of congenital abnormalities, heart defects are by far the most fatal to infants [4]. As they account for 30–50% of all birth defect-related deaths in young children and infants, heart defects are among the most common birth defects that result in fatalities [5–8]. Two-fifths of all CHD cases are considered "critical" [9]. Infants with critical congenital heart defects (CHDs) need immediate medical attention in the form of either surgery or a catheter-based intervention [10]. When it comes to infants who have a critical heart defect, any delay in the diagnosis of a critical heart defect in infants can increase not only the risk of mortality but also the likelihood of developing future complications [11].

Prevalence

The number of living patients who are diagnosed with a particular illness or condition during a given time period is the primary factor that determines a disease's prevalence. In terms of statistics, it is possible to determine it by using the formula which is as follows [3]:

$$\text{Prevalence} = \frac{\text{No.of cases with specific disease / condition}}{\text{Total no.of population}} \times 10^n$$

The birth prevalence of heart defects has increased dramatically over the past few decades, as it is now 9 for every 1000 live births, whereas previous reports indicated that there was only 1 for every 1000 births in 1930 [12]. Because the yearly number of births across the globe is approximately 150 million births, this equates to 1.35 million live births each year that are affected by CHD [13]. In light of this, it is the duty of the health system to work toward minimizing the incidence of heart defects. This emergence in birth prevalence might not actually represent a true upsurge; rather, it might be the result of advances in diagnostic and screening technology. Additionally, advancements in the field of surgery have contributed significantly to the dramatic rise in the patient survival rate and life expectancy [14, 15]. Due to the variety of approaches taken by epidemiologists, it is challenging to access and evaluate data on birth prevalence by region [16]. In developing nations in particular, there may be a substantial sampling bias due to regional variations in healthcare availability and quality [17].

Although CHD is on the rise across all age groups, from children to adults, more adults are affected by the disease because a more severe form of CHD is more common in adults [18, 19]. A new phenomenon, adult congenital heart disease, has emerged as a direct result of the improved care given to CHD patients from birth (discussed further on in this chapter) [12].

Etiology

Large epidemiological studies have allocated data concerning the risk factors attributable to CHD in order to better understand the underlying cause and the likely factors involved in preventing the development of CHD to some extent or to be able to implement preventative health measures to reduce the incidences of CHD as it puts a major strain on the healthcare system and the families as well [20].

The predominant etiological factor responsible for CHD is not clear, as it is caused by multiple factors [21]. Only about 15% of children born with heart defects have chromosomal abnormalities that can be identified, like Down syndrome [22, 23]. It is estimated that 3–5% of all heart defect cases are induced by single-gene defects, which are also often linked to multiple other types of birth defects [24–26].

It is likely that nonsyndromic heart defects, which account for the vast majority of cases, are brought on by the interaction of a number of environmental and genetic factors [21, 27, 28].

Mortality and Survival Rate

Numerous CHD patients have been able to live longer due to medical advancements, but despite such achievements, CHD persists as the major cause of death among birth defects [29].

Major improvements have been made in the past decades regarding the survival of patients with severe defects due to CHD [30]. Furthermore, the majority of deaths caused by CHD occurred in younger children; this highlights the importance of early detection and prevention policies [31].

Patients with isolated noncritical CHDs have a markedly increased chance of surviving for at least a year, especially in comparison to those with isolated critical CHDs; furthermore, their chances of living into adulthood (i.e., beyond the age of 18) are much higher. It is important to note that a series of major prognostic factors, such as birth era and weight at birth, have a considerable influence on the survival of patients who have critical congenital heart disease [32].

When compared to the past, the relative contributions of various causes to patients' deaths from congenital heart disease have also shifted [3]. Even though there was a comparative rise in the number of deaths that were caused by myocardial infarction over the course of the past few decades, arrhythmia continues to be the primary contributory cause of death in patients who have CHD [30].

Classification of Congenital Heart Disease

The research on CHD has supported a wide variety of different classification schemes over the years. In spite of this, we will divide CHD into two categories in this chapter, cyanotic and acyanotic, depending on whether or not a blood shunt is present [33–36].

Acyanotic Congenital Heart Disease

Ventricular Septal Defects

With an approximate prevalence of 1 in every 250–300 live births, ventricular septal defects are among the most common forms of heart defects in children [12, 37, 38]. VSDs are less common in adults because 75% of them either heal on their own by the time a child enters school or are surgically repaired by then [39].

The clinical manifestations of ventricular septal defects can differ among individuals based on the size of the defect and the impact of the shunting [38].

Small VSDs typically exhibit no symptoms and are discovered coincidently during a clinical examination, while patients with large-sized defects have a greater risk of developing heart failure at a young age [40].

Atrial Septal Defects

Nearly 10% of heart defect cases are due to atrial septal defects, and their prevalence at birth ranges from about 1–2 in every 1000 live births [12, 37, 41, 42]. Also, 7–10% of all CHD and 20–40% of all recently diagnosed adult CHD are attributable to ASD, making it one of the more commonly detected acyanotic congenital heart defects detected in adults [43, 44]. Earlier incidence studies relied on surgical methods or autopsy to diagnose ASD; this has likely changed since the widespread adoption of echocardiography to diagnose cardiac defects in the last few decades [45].

Depending on the size of the defect and any related congenital defects, the clinical manifestations can extend from asymptomatic to cases with serious cardiac comorbidities [46].

Patent Ductus Arteriosus

Approximately 10% of all people born with heart defects have PDA, and approximately twice as many females as males are affected by the condition [12, 37].

Within 48 h of birth, the ductus arteriosus will have actively constricted and obliterated itself, a process that seems to be reliant on the levels of prostaglandins and oxygen [47, 48].

The clinical manifestations of patient populations with PDA are determined by the size of the defect in addition to the intensity of blood shunting, as newborns with small PDAs are frequently asymptomatic and PDAs are coincidentally discovered. However, in patients with larger PDAs, more severe symptoms can occur [49].

Cyanotic Congenital Heart Disease

Tetralogy of Fallot

"Tetralogy of Fallot (TOF) is the most common cyanotic congenital heart disease following infancy, with an incidence of 4 to 5 per 10,000 live births" [12, 50]. TOF accounts for 1/3 of heart defect cases in patients under 15 years old, while the estimated prevalence of the condition in adults is somewhere between 1 in 3000 and 1 in 4300 people [51].

Genomic research has shown that 22q11.2 deletions may be present in some people with TOF [52].

Transposition of the Great Arteries

"TGA can be recognized by the fact that the aorta and the pulmonary arteries originate from the right ventricle and the left ventricle of the heart, respectively" [53].

The prevalence rate of TGA, which is anticipated to be between 2.3 and 4.7 per 10,000 live births, places it among the most common cyanotic heart defects in newborns [37, 54]. Around 20% of cyanotic heart defects are caused by it, and it accounts for nearly 3% of all CHD cases [37].

The mortality rate for TGA is high; 90% of cases are potentially lethal within the first year [55]. However, this rate has been falling in the past few years due to the development of effective surgical intervention; today, the survival rate for patients who received arterial switch operation is almost 90% after 20 years [56].

Adult Congenital Heart Disease

The burden of congenital heart disease (CHD) has transitioned from children to adults as a result of recent advancements in diagnostic techniques and management of the condition. In the past, CHD was regarded as a condition of children because most newborns who were born with a severe type of condition did not live to become adults [57]. The adult population with heart defects is expanding at a faster rate than the pediatric population, which has important implications for the treatment of adults [58].

In 2010, 1.4 million adults with CHD were living in the United States, with 160,000 having a severe form of the disease [59].

References

1. Šamánek M. Children with congenital heart disease: probability of natural survival. Pediatr Cardiol. 1992;13(3):152–8.
2. Russo CA, Elixhauser A. Hospitalizations for birth defects, 2004. In: Healthcare cost and utilization project (HCUP) statistical briefs [Internet]. Agency for Healthcare Research and Quality (US); 2007.
3. van der Bom T, Zomer AC, Zwinderman AH, Meijboom FJ, Bouma BJ, Mulder BJ. The changing epidemiology of congenital heart disease. Nat Rev Cardiol. 2011;8(1):50–60.
4. Smitha R, Karat SC, Narayanappa D, Krishnamurthy B, Prasanth SN, Ramachandra NB. Prevalence of congenital heart diseases in Mysore. Indian J Hum Genet. 2006;12(1):11–6.
5. Petrini J, Damus K, Johnston RB Jr. An overview of infant mortality and birth defects in the United States. Teratology. 1997;56(1–2):8–10.

6. Petrini J, Damus K, Russell R, Poschman K, Davidoff MJ, Mattison D. Contribution of birth defects to infant mortality in the United States. Teratology. 2002;66(S1 Suppl 1):S3–6.

7. Yang Q, Khoury MJ, Mannino D. Trends and patterns of mortality associated with birth defects and genetic diseases in the United States, 1979-1992: an analysis of multiple-cause mortality data. Genet Epidemiol. 1997;14(5):493–505.

8. Yang Q, Chen H, Correa A, Devine O, Mathews TJ, Honein MA. Racial differences in infant mortality attributable to birth defects in the United States, 1989-2002. Birth Defects Res A Clin Mol Teratol. 2006;76(10):706–13.

9. Botto LD, Correa A, Erickson JD. Racial and temporal variations in the prevalence of heart defects. Pediatrics. 2001;107(3):e32.

10. Zeng Z, Zhang H, Liu F, Zhang N. Current diagnosis and treatments for critical congenital heart defects. Exp Ther Med. 2016;11(5):1550–4.

11. Kuehl KS, Loffredo CA, Ferencz C. Failure to diagnose congenital heart disease in infancy. Pediatrics. 1999;103(4 Pt 1):743–7.

12. van der Linde D, Konings EE, Slager MA, Witsenburg M, Helbing WA, Takkenberg JJ, et al. Birth prevalence of congenital heart disease worldwide: a systematic review and meta-analysis. J Am Coll Cardiol. 2011;58(21):2241–7.

13. Hoffman JI. Incidence of congenital heart disease: I. Postnatal incidence. Pediatr Cardiol. 1995;16(3):103–13.

14. Somerville J. The Denolin lecture: the woman with congenital heart disease. Eur Heart J. 1998;19(12):1766–75.

15. Engelfriet P, Mulder BJ. Gender differences in adult congenital heart disease. Neth Heart J. 2009;17(11):414–7.

16. Bernier PL, Stefanescu A, Samoukovic G, Tchervenkov CI. The challenge of congenital heart disease worldwide: epidemiologic and demographic facts. In: Seminars in thoracic and cardiovascular surgery: pediatric cardiac surgery annual, vol. 13, no. 1. WB Saunders; 2010. pp. 26–34.

17. Pradat P, Francannet C, Harris JA, Robert E. The epidemiology of cardiovascular defects, part I: a study based on data from three large registries of congenital malformations. Pediatr Cardiol. 2003;24(3):195–221.

18. Marelli AJ, Mackie AS, Ionescu-Ittu R, Rahme E, Pilote L. Congenital heart disease in the general population: changing prevalence and age distribution. Circulation. 2007;115(2):163–72.

19. Shiina Y, Toyoda T, Kawasoe Y, Tateno S, Shirai T, Wakisaka Y, et al. Prevalence of adult patients with congenital heart disease in Japan. Int J Cardiol. 2011;146(1):13–6.

20. Zimmerman MS, Smith AG, Sable CA, Echko MM, Wilner LB, Olsen HE, et al.; GBD 2017 Congenital Heart Disease Collaborators. Global, regional, and national burden of congenital heart disease, 1990-2017: a systematic analysis for the global burden of disease study 2017. Lancet Child Adolesc Health. 2020;4(3):185–200.

21. Nora JJ. Multifactorial inheritance hypothesis for the etiology of congenital heart diseases. The genetic-environmental interaction. Circulation. 1968;38(3):604–17.

22. Kerstjens-Frederikse W. Congenital heart defects and pulmonary arterial hypertension: genes, environment and heredity. University of Groningen; 2014. 199 p.

23. Nora JJ, Berg K, Nora AH. Cardiovascular diseases: genetics, epidemiology, and prevention. Oxford: Oxford University Press; 1991.

24. van Engelen K, Topf A, Keavney BD, Goodship JA, van der Velde ET, Baars MJ, et al. 22q11.2 deletion syndrome is under-recognised in adult patients with tetralogy of Fallot and pulmonary atresia. Heart. 2010;96(8):621–4.

25. Joziasse IC, van de Smagt JJ, Smith K, Bakkers J, Sieswerda GJ, Mulder BJ, et al. Genes in congenital heart disease: atrioventricular valve formation. Basic Res Cardiol. 2008;103(3):216–27.

26. Botto LD, Correa A. Decreasing the burden of congenital heart anomalies: an epidemiologic evaluation of risk factors and survival. Prog Pediatr Cardiol. 2003;18(2):111–21.

27. Smith KA, Joziasse IC, Chocron S, van Dinther M, Guryev V, Verhoeven MC, et al. Dominant-negative ALK2 allele associates with congenital heart defects. Circulation. 2009;119(24):3062–9.

28. Joziasse IC, van der Smagt JJ, Poot M, Hochstenbach R, Nelen MR, van Gijn M, et al. A duplication including GATA4 does not co-segregate with congenital heart defects. Am J Med Genet A. 2009;149A(5):1062–6.

29. Bouma BJ, Mulder BJ. Changing landscape of congenital heart disease. Circ Res. 2017;120(6):908–22.

30. Pillutla P, Shetty KD, Foster E. Mortality associated with adult congenital heart disease: trends in the US population from 1979 to 2005. Am Heart J. 2009;158(5):874–9.

31. Billett J, Majeed A, Gatzoulis M, Cowie M. Trends in hospital admissions, in-hospital case fatality and population mortality from congenital heart disease in England, 1994 to 2004. Heart. 2008;94(3):342–8.

32. Oster ME, Lee KA, Honein MA, Riehle-Colarusso T, Shin M, Correa A. Temporal trends in survival among infants with critical congenital heart defects. Pediatrics. 2013;131(5):e1502–8.

33. Warnes CA, Liberthson R, Danielson GK, Dore A, Harris L, Hoffman JI, Somerville J, Williams RG, Webb GD. Task force 1: the changing profile of congenital heart disease in adult life. J Am Coll Cardiol. 2001;37(5):1170–5.

34. Stout KK, Daniels CJ, Aboulhosn JA, Bozkurt B, Broberg CS, Colman JM, Crumb SR, Dearani JA, Fuller S, Gurvitz M, Khairy P. 2018 AHA/ACC guideline for the management of adults with congenital heart disease: a report of the American College of Cardiology/American Heart Association Task Force on clinical practice guidelines. J Am Coll Cardiol. 2019;73(12):e81–e192.

35. Miller MR, Forrest CB, Kan JS. Parental preferences for primary and specialty care collaboration in the management of teenagers with congenital heart disease. Pediatrics. 2000;106(2):264–9.

36. Flocco SF, Lillo A, Dellafiore F, Goossens E, editors. Congenital heart disease: the nursing care handbook. Springer; 2018.

37. Reller MD, Strickland MJ, Riehle-Colarusso T, Mahle WT, Correa A. Prevalence of congenital heart defects in metropolitan Atlanta, 1998-2005. J Pediatr. 2008;153(6):807–13.

38. Dakkak W, Oliver TI. Ventricular septal defect [Updated 2021 Jun 8]. In: StatPearls [Internet]. Treasure Island: StatPearls Publishing; 2021. https://www.ncbi.nlm.nih.gov/books/NBK470330/.

39. Du ZD, Roguin N, Wu XJ. Spontaneous closure of muscular ventricular septal defect identified by echocardiography in neonates. Cardiol Young. 1998;8(4):500–5.

40. Fulton DR, Saleeb S. Isolated ventricular septal defects in infants and children: anatomy, clinical features, and diagnosis. UpToDate. 2019.

41. Schwedler G, Lindinger A, Lange PE, Sax U, Olchvary J, Peters B, et al. Frequency and spectrum of congenital heart defects among live births in Germany: a study of the competence network for congenital heart defects. Clin Res Cardiol. 2011;100(12):1111–7.

42. Wu MH, Chen HC, Lu CW, Wang JK, Huang SC, Huang SK. Prevalence of congenital heart disease at live birth in Taiwan. J Pediatr. 2010;156(5):782–5.

43. Bissessor N. Current perspectives in percutaneous atrial septal defect closure devices. Med Devices (Auckl). 2015;8:297–303.

44. Suradi HS, Hijazi ZM. Adult congenital interventions in heart failure. Interv Cardiol Clin. 2017;6(3):427–43.

45. Constantinescu T, Magda SL, Niculescu R, et al. New echocardiographic techniques in pulmonary arterial hypertension vs. right heart catheterization—a pilot study. Maedica (Buchar). 2013;8(2):116–23.

46. De Faria Yeh D, Bhatt A, editors. Chapter 4. Atrial septal defects and sinus venosus defects. Adult congenital heart disease in clinical practice. Springer; 2018. p. 35.

47. Loftin CD, Trivedi DB, Langenbach R. Cyclooxygenase-1-selective inhibition prolongs gestation in mice without adverse effects on the ductus arteriosus. J Clin Invest. 2002;110(4):549–57.

48. Coggins KG, Latour A, Nguyen MS, Audoly L, Coffman TM, Koller BH. Metabolism of PGE2 by prostaglandin dehydrogenase is essential for remodeling the ductus arteriosus. Nat Med. 2002;8(2):91–2.

49. Gillam-Krakauer M, Mahajan K. Patent ductus arteriosus [Updated 2021 Aug 11]. In: StatPearls [Internet]. Treasure Island: StatPearls Publishing; 2021. https://www.ncbi.nlm.nih.gov/books/NBK430758/.

50. Hoffman JI, Kaplan S. The incidence of congenital heart disease. J Am Coll Cardiol. 2002;39(12):1890–900.

51. Maury P, Sacher F, Rollin A, Mondoly P, Duparc A, Zeppenfeld K, et al.; Réseau francophone de rythmologie pédiatrique et congénitale. Ventricular arrhythmias and sudden death in tetralogy of Fallot. Arch Cardiovasc Dis. 2017;110(5):354–362.

52. Rauch R, Hofbeck M, Zweier C, Koch A, Zink S, Trautmann U, et al. Comprehensive genotype-phenotype analysis in 230 patients with tetralogy of Fallot. J Med Genet. 2010;47(5):321–31.

53. Szymanski MW, Moore SM, Kritzmire SM, et al. Transposition of the great arteries [Updated 2021 Aug 11]. In: StatPearls [Internet]. Treasure Island: StatPearls Publishing; 2021. https://www.ncbi.nlm.nih.gov/books/NBK538434/.

54. Centers for Disease Control and Prevention (CDC). Improved national prevalence estimates for 18 selected major birth defects—United States, 1999-2001. MMWR Morb Mortal Wkly Rep. 2006;54(51):1301–5.

55. Wernovsky G. Transposition of the great arteries. In: Allen HD, Shaddy RE, Driscoll DJ, Feltes TF, editors. Moss and Adams' heart disease in infants, children, and adolescents: including the Fetus and young adult. 7th ed. Philadelphia: Wolters Kluwer Health/ Lipincott Williams & Wilkins; 2008. p. 1039.

56. Villafañe J, Lantin-Hermoso MR, Bhatt AB, Tweddell JS, Geva T, Nathan M, et al.; American College of Cardiology's Adult Congenital and Pediatric Cardiology Council. D-transposition of the great arteries: the current era of the arterial switch operation. J Am Coll Cardiol. 2014;64(5):498–511.

57. Ntiloudi D, Giannakoulas G, Parcharidou D, Panagiotidis T, Gatzoulis MA, Karvounis H. Adult congenital heart disease: a paradigm of epidemiological change. Int J Cardiol. 2016;218:269–74.

58. Gatzoulis MA, Swan L, Therrien J, Pantely GA. Chapter 1. Epidemiology of congenital heart disease. In: Adult congenital heart disease: a practical guide. Blackwell Publishing; 2005. p. 3.

59. Gilboa SM, Devine OJ, Kucik JE, Oster ME, Riehle-Colarusso T, Nembhard WN, et al. Congenital heart defects in the United States: estimating the magnitude of the affected population in 2010. Circulation. 2016;134(2):101–9.

Diagnosis of CHD During Perinatal Life

Shoaib Ahmad, Ahmed Dheyaa Al-Obaidi,
Abeer Mundher Ali, and Sara Shihab Ahmad

Abstract

The purpose of this chapter is to discuss the essentials of using ultrasound in screening for cardiac diseases prenatally, so we can detect them earlier and take action. All pregnancies (low and high risk) go through standard obstetric ultrasonography; nevertheless, diagnosing structural heart problems remains challenging and requires collaboration among teams of cardiologists and specialists in fetal ultrasonography. This chapter provides an overview of fetal ultrasonography and the views required to make a perinatal CHD diagnosis. Furthermore, the characteristics of each defect on fetal ultrasonography have been discussed.

Keywords

Diagnosis · Congenital heart diseases · Ultrasound Prenatal · Screening tests · Amniotic fluid Ultrasonography

Introduction

The anatomical or functional abnormality of the heart or other major arteries at birth is known as congenital heart disease (CHD). It is the most frequent congenital anomaly that affects roughly 8–10 out of every 1000 living births and full-term birth. It may be even ten times greater in pre-term babies amounting to 8.3% [1]. In such a situation, survival, morbidity, and the medical care required depends on the time of diagnosis, treatment delay, and the severity of the CHD. As a result, it has been proven that diagnosing a curable CHD in the womb reduces the risk of perinatal morbidity and mortality. Routine obstetric ultrasounds can give suspicion of a congenital cardiovascular defect which can later be confirmed by a fetal echocardiogram. However, CHD has a varying range of detection rates, and the examiner's experience, maternal weight, the effect of the presence of scars in the abdomen, age of gestation, transducer frequency, AFI (amniotic fluid index), and position of the fetus can all contribute to this variation.

General Considerations for a Fetal Cardiac Scan

A cardiac exam of the developing fetus is most effective in the period of 18–22 weeks of pregnancy. Several defects can be detected during the end of the first and the beginning of the second trimesters of pregnancy, particularly when there is high nuchal translucency. Despite the highly recognized utility of the "four-chamber view," it should be kept in mind that early detection of CHD is not always possible with this single scanning plane. Hence, a thorough cardiac examination should be performed. The diseases not detectable by this single scanning plane include "transposition of great arteries" (TGA) and "coarctation of aorta."

Views of a Fetal Cardiac Scan

A basic fetal cardiac scan should include some recommended views that include

1. Four chamber views
2. Right ventricular outflow tract view (RVOT)
3. Left ventricular outflow tract view (LVOT)

S. Ahmad (✉)
Department of Pediatrics, District Head Quarters Teaching Hospital, Faisalabad, Pakistan

A. D. Al-Obaidi · A. M. Ali · S. S. Ahmad
College of Medicine, University of Baghdad, Baghdad, Iraq

Additional views can be performed if a complex fetal cardiac scan is required. These views include the following:

1. Bicaval view
2. Aortic arch view
3. Three-vessel trachea view
4. Three-vessel view
5. Diaphragmatic view

Basic Fetal Cardiac Scan

The basic fetal cardiac scan includes a general overview of the whole fetal heart and involves checking the following characteristics [2].

General View
1. Normal cardiac situs, position, and axis
2. Four cardiac chambers
3. Position and location of the heart in the chest (should be most toward left)
4. Presence of pericardial effusion or hypertrophy

Atria
1. Atria that are approximately the exact same size
2. Presence of flap of foramen ovale in the left atrium
3. Presence of "atrial septum primum"

Ventricles
1. Ventricles that are approximately the exact same size
2. Intact ventricular septum
3. Right ventricular apex moderator band
4. No cardiac wall hypertrophies

Atrioventricular Walls
1. Both valves have free movements and are open.
2. The leaflet of the tricuspid valve enters closer to the apex of the heart than to the mitral valve at the ventricular septum.

Four-Chamber View of the Heart

It is one of the most important and basic planes of the heart. It is a part of the basic cardiac fetal scan and involves the assessment of the principal structures of the heart, its contractility, and its size in addition to its rhythm. The assessment of cardiomegaly is done by measuring the cardiothoracic ratio in small fetuses.

The shape, size, and function of each chamber should also be assessed. **RA** has an appendage that is pyramidal in shape with a broad base. The inferior vena cava opens into the RA. **LA** is more to the posterior side and is known by its "finger-like" appendage. Foramen ovale and the pulmonary veins further help identify the left atrium. The foramen ovale moves toward the LA from the RA in the case of normal fetal circulation as the blood that has been fully oxygenated moves from the RA after being received from the ductus venosus into the inferior vena cava.

The ventricles, on the other hand, are separated by an inter-ventricular septum, which should be evaluated for any defects, such as "ventricular septal defects" (VSDs). The ventricle septum is twice the length of an atrial septum, and additional scans or planes should be used to properly assess for a VSD. The continuity of the aorta with the septum should be looked for in the LVOT view [3].

The right ventricle appears trabeculated due to a moderator band in the retro-sternal location. Moreover, the lumen of the RV is also shorter than the LV.

Heart rhythm and rate are also to be assessed, with the normal heart rate being 120–160 bpm. However, there are a few exceptions as the age of the fetus varies. For example, a mild bradycardia can be observed in normal second trimester fetuses. Some fetuses may suffer from fixed bradycardia i.e., below 110 bpm, and they need a thorough evaluation for heart block. Various conditions can also result in tachycardia, so the fetus should always be evaluated for fetal distress or any other tachyarrhythmia [3].

Left Ventricular Outflow Tract View

In general, views of the outflow tract could be approached by first identifying the origin of the major arteries, which is accomplished by sliding the transducer cephally (toward the fetal head). The aortic root and the trunk make up the LV outflow tract. The "LVOT view" helps in

- Confirming the morphological origin of aorta from the Lt ventricle as a continuation of septum
- Performing a detailed evaluation of the aortic valve for its mobility and size
- Thickness of the inter-ventricular septum (normal size ranging from 2 to 4 mm)
- Tracing the aortic arch and the three branches that arise from it
- Identifying the conotruncal abnormalities
- Identifying ventricular septal defects

In the LVOT view, the following points should be ensured:

- A smooth ventricular contour
- Origin of the head and neck vessels from the aortic arch
- Anterior aortic wall and septal continuation
- Aortic angle with the septum
- Septal thickness

Right Ventricular Outflow Tract View

The main pulmonary artery (PA) and the pulmonary conus make up the RV outflow tract (RVOT). The PA normally crosses the ascending aorta, but in the case of TGA, they run alongside each other. The pulmonary trunk should also be confirmed arising from the right ventricle. This can be done by "the great arteries short-axis view" that also shows right and left pulmonary artery bifurcation.

Fetal Congenital Heart Diseases

Conotruncal Anomalies

1. **Teratology of Fallot**

   It is the most common cyanotic congenital heart disease in children. The four main characteristics of TOF include
   - An "overriding" aorta
   - Infundibular stenosis of the pulmonary valve
   - RVH
   - VSD
     Prenatally, in the case of TOF on USG:
   - The "five-chamber view" and the "basal short-axis view" can help identify the defect as it can show the overriding of the aorta and a possible VSD at the outlet.
   - Prenatally, the "four-chamber view" is normal.
   - In the 3VT view, a larger aorta and a smaller pulmonary artery can be noticed.
   - Prenatally, hypertrophy of the right ventricle cannot be identified.

2. **The Transposition of Great Arteries (TGA)**

   The transposition of great arteries is characterized by anomalous origin of both the pulmonary artery from the left ventricle and subsequently the aorta from the right ventricle.

   It is mostly associated with a VSD. The TGA is classified into two main classes:
   - D-TGA (Dextro-TGA)
   - L-TGA (Levo-TGA)
     In the **D-TGA** case, on USG prenatally:
   - Normal view of the four chambers.
   - The view of the five chambers shows the abnormal origin of the pulmonary artery from the left ventricle and an abnormal origin of the aorta from the right ventricle.
   - In 3VT viewing, a left pulmonary artery posteriorly and right aorta anteriorly can be detected.

In the case of L-TGA, on prenatal USG:
- On view of the four chambers, a moderator band is seen on the left-sided ventricle.
- The aorta is located anteriorly and in the same time to the left of the pulmonary artery.

Right Heart Defects

1. **Pulmonary Atresia**

   Based on fetal ultrasonography,
   - On view of the five chambers, an immobile and a thickened pulmonary valve could be recognized.
   - By color Doppler, an opposite flowing from the ductus arteriosus into the pulmonary artery also signifies pulmonary atresia.
   - On a 3V view, the pulmonary artery is always smaller than the aorta.
     The features of the right ventricle vary according to the type of changes in the tricuspid valve:
   - The RV can be hypoplastic in the case of PA and TV stenosis.
   - The RV will be enlarged in the case of an incompetent tricuspid valve.

2. **Pulmonary Stenosis**

   Based on fetal ultrasonography,
   - Normal view of the four chambers.
   - On view of the five chambers, an abnormal echogenicity of the pulmonary valve can be appreciated.
     For such high-risk patients that show echogenic abnormalities of the pulmonary valve or are suffering from rubella syndrome, a referral for further flow investigation by Doppler should be done.

3. **Tricuspid Atresia**

   Based on fetal ultrasonography,
   - On view of four chambers, an immovable and hyperechoic tricuspid valve can be identified.
   - On color Doppler, during diastole a lack of flow is detected across the tricuspid valve.
     Tricuspid stenosis can easily be identified prenatally, but serial ultrasounds are required to establish the LV function and to rule out any other RV flow obstruction.

4. **Tricuspid Stenosis**

   Based on fetal ultrasonography,
   - On the four-chamber view, thick cusps and restrictive diastolic openings are the main characteristics.
   - On color Doppler, detection of any lack of flowing across the valve signifies tricuspid stenosis.

Anomalies of the Left Heart

1. **Aortic Stenosis**

    In 30% of the cases, aortic stenosis exists as an associated anomaly. It can also present as Shone syndrome, which is an obstructive left-sided lesion.

    On the basis of fetal ultrasonography,

    - On a five-chamber view, an abnormal aortic valve can be seen. It is usually thickened and less mobile.
    - On color Doppler, reduced flow can be observed.
    - On a 3V view, the small size of the transverse aorta and reversed flow can be observed.
    - On a four-chamber view, a dilated left ventricle with fibroelastosis of the endocardium can be seen.

2. **Mitral Stenosis**

    In the case of mitral stenosis, there is a difference between the size of the ventricles and the atrioventricular valves. Moreover, a less mobile and thickened mitral valve can be seen on ultrasonography.

Septal Defects

1. **Atrial Septal Defect**

    The atrial septal defect is due to abnormal embryologic development. It can be associated with syndromes that include

    - Noonan syndrome
    - Treacher–Collins syndrome
    - Holt–Oram syndrome

    Atrial septal defects are generally well-tolerated in fetal life. They can either exist separately or be associated with other congenital heart diseases. ASD can be of the following types:

    - ASD secundum
    - Coronary sinus ASD
    - ASD primum
    - Sinus venosus ASD

    ASD secundum is an atrial septum defect located in the middle. During the life of the fetus, this is considered normal communication since the two atria are already communicating through the foramen ovale. Hence, prenatally, it is almost impossible to detect secundum ASD as there is good compensation.

    On fetal ultrasonography,

    - On a four-chamber view, a foramen ovale of diameter greater than the aortic diameter is suggestive of secundum ASD.
    - *Sinus venosus ASD and primum ASD* have not been reported yet in fetal life.

2. **Ventricular Septal Defect**

    The ventricular septal defect occurs in 30% of the neonates with a CHD and is hence the most common heart defect in neonates. Defects in the ventricular septum are mainly determined according to the site of the septal defect [3].

    (a) Muscular
    (b) Supracristal
    (c) Membranous

    The least common of the three is supracristal VSD. In most of the cases, a VSD can spontaneously close, but it depends on the size and location of the VSD.

    On fetal ultrasonography,

    - Bidirectional shunt can be seen using the lateral view of the four-chamber view to confirm a VSD.
    - On a five-chamber view, outlet defects can be identified including a membranous VSD.
    - A misaligned VSD can lead to suspicion of other associated heart defects.

MCQs

1. The ideal duration of performing a fetal cardiac examination is
    A. Between 10 and 14 weeks
    B. Between 14 and 18 weeks
    C. Between 18 and 22 weeks
    D. Between 22 and 24 weeks
    Answer: C

2. The left atrium is identified as a
    A. Trabeculated shape
    B. Complex part
    C. Finger-like appendage
    D. None
    Answer: C

3. The normal heart rate on fetal cardiac ultrasonography is
    A. 140–180 bpm
    B. 120–160 bpm
    C. 180–200 bpm
    D. 70–80 bpm
    Answer: B

4. On fetal ultrasonography, the right ventricle appears
    A. Trabeculated
    B. Complex
    C. Finger-like appendage
    D. None
    Answer: A

5. An ASD can be associated with
    A. Noonan syndrome
    B. Treacher–Collins syndrome
    C. Holt–Oram syndrome
    D. All
    Answer: D

6. Which of the following is impossible to detect on fetal ultrasonography?
    A. Secundum ASD
    B. Sinus venosus ASD

C. Primum ASD

D. Coronary sinus ASD

Answer: A

7. The right ventricle is _____ in the case of pulmonary atresia

A. Hypoplastic

B. Hypertrophic

C. Dilated

D. None

Answer: A

8. The most common congenital CHD in neonates is

A. TOF

B. VSD

C. ASD

D. TGA

Answer: B

9. Aortic root and the trunk make up the

A. LVOT

B. RVOT

C. Atrial septum

D. Ventricular septum

Answer: A

10. In the case of aortic stenosis, the LV will be

A. Hypoplastic

B. Hypertrophic

C. Dilated

D. None

Answer: C

References

1. Moons P, Sluysmans T, de Wolf D, Massin M, Suys B, Benatar A, Gewillig M. Congenital heart disease in 111 225 births in Belgium: birth prevalence, treatment and survival in the 21st century. Acta Paediatr. 2009;98:472–7.

2. Cardiac screening examination of the fetus: guidelines for performing the 'basic' and 'extended basic' cardiac scan. Ultrasound Obstet Gynecol. 2006;27:107–113.

3. Bravo-valenzuela NJ, Peixoto AB, Araujo Júnior E. Prenatal diagnosis of congenital heart disease: a review of current knowledge. Indian Heart J. 2018;70:150–64.

Ventricular Septal Defect

Yassen Ayad and Ameer Almamoury

Abstract

"Ventricular septal defect (VSD) is one of the most common congenital heart lesions." The most common type of clinically significant VSD is a membranous VSD. Small VSD can be detected by the presence of holosystolic high-pitched systolic murmur. The management of ventricular septal defects (VSDs) is dependent on the size of the defect and degree of shunting. Patients with moderate to large defects who are diagnosed as infants must be continuously monitored in their first weeks of life. Patients who look to be in a good health are scheduled for a follow-up with a pediatric cardiologist 3–4 weeks after the delivery. Monitors growth and change in the cardiac examination can provide to a patient in primary care. The choice of treatment approach is based on the clinical findings and size of the defect. For asymptomatic patients who typically have a small defect, we suggest no intervention. For symptomatic patients, medical therapy for heart failure is generally warranted. Symptoms typically occur in patients with moderate to large defects. For patients who are not adequately managed by medical therapy and/or have evidence of elevated pulmonary artery pressure (PAP) or valvular involvement, we suggest surgical closure of the VS. Medical therapy is focused on reducing the symptoms and complications of heart failure.

Keywords

Bicuspid aortic valve · Heart failure · Pulmonary hypertension · Interventricular septum Immunoprophylaxis · Ventricular septal defect Subaortic stenosis

Y. Ayad (✉)
Al-Zahraa Medical College, Basra, Iraq

A. Almamoury
Al Qadisiyah College of Medicine, Al Diwaniyah, Iraq
e-mail: med-16.13@qu.edu.iq

Introduction

"One of the most common congenital heart defects is a ventricular septal defect (VSD) (second only to bicuspid aortic valve)" [1].

Pathophysiology

VSD in the fetus has little effect on the hemodynamic state, resistance equal through the chamber of the heart. Extrauterine like the PVR drop and close of ductus arteriosus lead to change in resistance through the chamber, direction of flow depends mainly on difference of resistance of each circulation, high systemic resistance, and low pulmonary resistance, typically left to right shunt. Small VSD if does not close by own will cause a mild increase in resistance and redirection shunt in reverse of large VSD, depending mainly on the pressure difference between the right ventricle and left ventricle [2–5].

Left to right shunt due to large VSD lead to equal pressure on each side of the ventricle. This effect increases pulmonary blood flow leading to congestion and edema. Pulmonary hypertension due to pulmonary vascular alteration and remodeling. To maintain normal systemic blood flow in patients with considerable left to right shunting left ventricle output must be increased. Increased alpha-adrenergic, increased circulating catecholamine concentrations, and increased angiotensin II and vasopressin concentrations exacerbate cardiac failure [6–10].

Clinical Features

Presentation

VSDs of moderate to large size can be discovered in the womb early whichcan happen on their own or in combination with other heart problems. Depending on the size and location of isolated VSDs, some will close during pregnancy [11]. Small to moderate VSDs can be missed by fetal echocardiography due to the physiology of equal ventricular pressure in the fetus. The discovery of an in utero VSD or other structural cardiac abnormalities should prompt discussion about possible chromosomal problems and the need for additional testing [12–14].

Patients with VSD present mostly during the neonatal period. Depending on the magnitude of the lesion, the clinical presentation can range from an isolated murmur discovered by chance at a health monitoring visit to acute cardiac failure [15]. Small, restricted VSDs in infants are frequently asymptomatic. Infants with moderate to large VSDs, on the other hand, frequently show indications of heart failure. Small VSD diagnosis by accident with murmur without clinical symptoms can be detected in the first day of life of the neonate. Symptoms appear in moderate and large VSD infants within first weeks of life, with signs and symptoms of heart failure resemble by poor feeding, tachypnea, failure to thrive, hepatomegaly, cardiomegaly, and pulmonary rales [16]. Thrill can palpate in the third and fourth left sternal border. Blowing holosystolic murmur is classically seen in the patient with VSD heard on the left sternal border, moderate and large VSD heard louder than small, rumbling sounds may be heard if the VSD is big enough to cause mitral valve defect. Diastole rumbling sound usually indicates left to right shunt, heard at the apex. A decrescendo murmur in the left sternal border indicates aortic regurgitation and degree splitting of S2 indicates the size of defect [17–20].

Diagnosis

VSD diagnosis by Echocardiogram, to make the diagnosis, locate the defect, and estimate the size of the shunt, two-dimensional Doppler echocardiography is usually sufficient. Echo is used to confirm the diagnosis that is made typically by holosystolic murmur, locate the defect and measure the size. Chest radiograph if obtained is not that useful and varies depending on the size of the defect also may show signs of heart failure if developed in a baby. ECG is typically normal in most of the cases but also shows left ventricle hypertrophy. Now a days cardiac catheterization is rarely used for diagnosis [21, 22].

Differential Diagnosis

Usually, VSD can be distinguished from non-cardiac causes of respiratory distress by the presence of systolic murmur on physical exam and diagnostic test. Other anomalies like acyanotic congenital heart disease also can distinguish by ECHO [21, 22].

Management

Overview

The extent of the defect and degree of shunting are determined by the clinical examination and echocardiography. Patient with small VSD does not require surgical intervention, these patients are usually asymptomatic, with a good chance of spontaneous closure or a reduction in the extent of the defect over time. Medical therapy patients with heart failure symptoms must receive medical treatment [23]. Medical care may be sufficient to meet the needs of people with moderate defects. Surgical correction is frequently required for people with more severe symptoms, and medication care is used to alleviate symptoms in the meanwhile. Patients with a risk for long-term sequelae and failed medical therapy are recommended to the closure of the defect surgically [24].

Neonates

Ongoing neonatal surveillance is critical for determining which infants will remain asymptomatic and require no intervention versus those who will develop heart failure and require intervention.

Small VSD

Small VSD asymptomatic also good chance of spontaneous closure. Patients should have a follow-up assessment by a pediatric cardiologist at 3–4 weeks of age to detect any indications or symptoms of increased left ventricular volume overload. A follow-up evaluation with the cardiologist is scheduled for those patients who remain asymptomatic at roughly 6 months of age. Primary care provides routine care in between visits with the cardiologist. If the patient develops symptoms (e.g., poor weight gain, tachypnea), he or she should be referred to a specialist for a cardiac evaluation as soon as possible. If the murmur is no longer present at the 6-month visit, a repeat echocardiogram is not required unless clinical concerns occur. If the murmur is still present at the 12-month cardiology visit and the patient is asymptomatic and clinically stable, there is no need for additional treatment. Patients with membranous defects usually have an echocardiographic follow-up at 3 years of age. If a patient with a muscular defect stays asymptomatic, no echocardiogram is required. In any symptomatic patient, medical therapy is started. However, because heart failure is not commonly associated with small VSDs, the emergence of new symptoms, especially late in the course of the disease, should prompt a reevaluation of the original diagnosis and a search for other sources of the symptoms [25, 26].

Moderate to Large VSD

Pulmonary vascular resistance (PVR) diminishes, and infants with moderate to large VSDs frequently become symptomatic within the first few months of life. During the first weeks of life, the primary care provider should keep an eye on the baby for signs of heart failure. Because of the projected decrease in PVR resulting in increased left ventricular (LV) flow. If symptoms arise, medical treatment is recommended, as described in the sections below. Infants who remain asymptomatic should be followed up on and monitored on a regular basis [11, 27].

Asymptomatic patients—all infants with moderate to large VSDs should have regular follow-up during their first year of life, even if symptoms are absent. It is critical to look for signs of pulmonary hypertension in these people. Echocardiography is conducted to determine pulmonary artery pressure if the murmur is diminished but the pulmonic component of the second heart sound (S2) is increased in strength [15]. Symptomatic patient may avoid surgical intervention through medical ways and management, including nutritional support and pharmacological treatment. Nutritional support may help infants with moderate to large VSDs gain weight. Because of the higher metabolic demand, these infants may require a caloric intake of more than 150 kcal/kg per day [28]. Feeding fatigue is common in infants with heart failure, and their intake may be reduced. Providing more frequent feedings is one way to enhance daily calorie intake; however, parents may find this difficult. These infants typically take a long time to eat, and the time required to ensure optimal intake might be significant. To increase caloric intake, nasogastric feedings may be required. Bolus or continuous feeds, which can be administered at any time of day or night, are examples of this. When these procedures are used, it usually means that the VSD will need to be closed. Fluid restriction is often ineffective in the therapy of infants with VSD-related heart failure because it leads to insufficient calorie intake. Although fluid restriction is commonly used to treat adults and older children with heart failure, it is ineffective in infants who are completely reliant on liquids. As stated in the following section, diuretic therapy rather than fluid restriction should be utilized to minimize and avoid volume excess. Supplemental iron should be given to infants with iron deficiency anemia to boost their hematocrit and oxygen-carrying capacity. Medical care for heart failure differs based on the severity of the symptoms of heart failure [29]. The mainstay of treatment is diuretics. Angiotensin-converting enzyme inhibitors have been utilized in the past, but their efficacy appears to be low therefore they are no longer used consistently. Intravenous (IV) inotropic drugs may be administered as a temporary strategy in extreme situations. We rarely prescribe oral digoxin because of the risk of side effects [30–32].

Closure Interventions

The severity of heart failure, vascular disease (PHVD) progression, pulmonary hypertension or other complications, the likelihood of defect reduction or spontaneous closure, the morbidity and mortality of the procedure in young infants in the center where surgery to be performed, and the likelihood of successful surgical closure are all factors to consider [33–35]. Because infants with Down syndrome are more likely to have PHVD, early surgical intervention in children with moderate to large defects may be necessary. In most cases, primary patch surgical closure is the recommended method. Transcatheter closure is often reserved for patients with defects that are difficult to close operatively (e.g., remote apical muscular defect, multiple muscular defects ["Swiss cheese" septum]) or who are unable to undergo cardiopulmonary bypass for a variety of reasons. Indications if symptoms are persistent with the option of medical management, pulmonary hypertension is established, and reversible shunt (left to right). VSD closure is generally not recommended if pulmonary vascular resistance (PVR) is greater than 12 Wood units (WU). Closure of the defect may result in decreased cardiac output and increased peri-operative mortality in these patients with severe pulmonary hypertension, as previously mentioned [35]. Method of choice for most children with VSD required surgical intervention is direct patch closer under cardiopulmonary bypass. Transcatheter closure several series have documented successful transcatheter closure for muscular, peri-membranous, and residual VSDs following surgical repair. Though the technique has gained favor in some countries, transcatheter closure of VSD remains technically demanding and has a greater complication rate than surgery [36–40].

References

1. [Internet]. 2022 [cited 14 August 2022]. https://www.oakbaynews.com/national-marketplace/vsd-surgery-how-much-does-it-cost/.
2. Van Praagh R, Geva T, Kreutzer J. Ventricular septal defects: how shall we describe, name and classify them? J Am Coll Cardiol. 1989;14:1298.
3. Moe DG, Guntheroth WG. Spontaneous closure of uncomplicated ventricular septal defect. Am J Cardiol. 1987;60:674.
4. Du ZD, Roguin N, Wu XJ. Spontaneous closure of muscular ventricular septal defect identified by echocardiography in neonates. Cardiol Young. 1998;8:500.
5. Varghese PJ, Izukawa T, Celermajer J, et al. Aneurysm of the membranous ventricular septum. A method of spontaneous closure of small ventricular septal defect. Am J Cardiol. 1969;24:531.
6. Freedom RM, White RD, Pieroni DR, et al. The natural history of the so-called aneurysm of the membranous ventricular septum in childhood. Circulation. 1974;49:375.
7. Misra KP, Hildner FJ, Cohen LS, et al. Aneurysm of the membranous ventricular septum. A mechanism for spontaneous closure of ventricular septal defect. N Engl J Med. 1970;283:58.

8. Ramaciotti C, Keren A, Silverman NH. Importance of (perimembranous) ventricular septal aneurysm in the natural history of isolated perimembranous ventricular septal defect. Am J Cardiol. 1986;57:268.
9. Anderson RH, Lenox CC, Zuberbuhler JR. Mechanisms of closure of perimembranous ventricular septal defect. Am J Cardiol. 1983;52:341.
10. Titus JL, Daugherty GW, Edwards JE. Anatomy of the atrioventricular conduction system in ventricular septal defect. Circulation. 1963;28:72.
11. Gómez O, Martínez JM, Olivella A, et al. Isolated ventricular septal defects in the era of advanced fetal echocardiography: risk of chromosomal anomalies and spontaneous closure rate from diagnosis to age of 1 year. Ultrasound Obstet Gynecol. 2014;43:65.
12. Roguin N, Du ZD, Barak M, et al. High prevalence of muscular ventricular septal defect in neonates. J Am Coll Cardiol. 1995;26:1545.
13. Miyake T, Shinohara T, Inoue T, et al. Spontaneous closure of muscular trabecular ventricular septal defect: comparison of defect positions. Acta Paediatr. 2011;100:e158.
14. Perloff JK. Ventricular septal defect. In: The clinical recognition of congenital heart disease, 5th ed. Philadelphia: W.B. Saunders Company; 2003. p. 311.
15. Gumbiner CH, Takao A. Ventricular septal defect. In: Garson A, Bricker JT, Fisher DJ, Neish SR, editors. The science and practice of pediatric cardiology. 2nd ed. Baltimore: Williams & Wilkins; 1998. p. 1119.
16. Kidd L, Driscoll DJ, Gersony WM, et al. Second natural history study of congenital heart defects. Results of treatment of patients with ventricular septal defects. Circulation. 1993;87:I38.
17. Soto B, Becker AE, Moulaert AJ, et al. Classification of ventricular septal defects. Br Heart J. 1980;43:332.
18. Ando M, Takao A. Pathological anatomy of ventricular septal defect associated with aortic valve prolapse and regurgitation. Heart Vessel. 1986;2:117.
19. Zhao QM, Niu C, Liu F, et al. Spontaneous closure rates of ventricular septal defects (6,750 consecutive neonates). Am J Cardiol. 2019;124:613.
20. Zhang J, Ko JM, Guileyardo JM, Roberts WC. A review of spontaneous closure of ventricular septal defect. Proc (Bayl Univ Med Cent). 2015;28:516.
21. Gabriel HM, Heger M, Innerhofer P, et al. Long-term outcome of patients with ventricular septal defect considered not to require surgical closure during childhood. J Am Coll Cardiol. 2002;39:1066.
22. Neumayer U, Stone S, Somerville J. Small ventricular septal defects in adults. Eur Heart J. 1998;19:1573.
23. Stout KK, Daniels CJ, Aboulhosn JA, et al. 2018 AHA/ACC guideline for the management of adults with congenital heart disease: a report of the American College of Cardiology/American Heart Association task force on clinical practice guidelines. J Am Coll Cardiol. 2019;73:e81.
24. Shirali GS, Smith EO, Geva T. Quantitation of echocardiographic predictors of outcome in infants with isolated ventricular septal defect. Am Heart J. 1995;130:1228.
25. Onat T, Ahunbay G, Batmaz G, Celebi A. The natural course of isolated ventricular septal defect during adolescence. Pediatr Cardiol. 1998;19:230.
26. Kleinman CS, Tabibian M, Starc TJ, et al. Spontaneous regression of left ventricular dilation in children with restrictive ventricular septal defects. J Pediatr. 2007;150:583.
27. Lin MT, Chen YS, Huang SC, et al. Alternative approach for selected severe pulmonary hypertension of congenital heart defect without initial correction—palliative surgical treatment. Int J Cardiol. 2011;151:313.
28. Miller RH, Schiebler GL, Grumbar P, Krovetz LJ. Relation of hemodynamics to height and weight percentiles in children with ventricular septal defects. Am Heart J. 1969;78:523.
29. Levy RJ, Rosenthal A, Miettinen OS, Nadas AS. Determinants of growth in patients with ventricular septal defect. Circulation. 1978;57:793.
30. Fyler DC, Rudolph AM, Wittenborg MH, Nadas AS. Ventricular septal defect in infants and children; a correlation of clinical, physiologic, and autopsy data. Circulation. 1958;18:833.
31. Evans JR, Rowe RD, Keith JD. Spontaneous closure of ventricular septal defects. Circulation. 1960;22:1044.
32. Nadas AS, Ellison RC. Phonocardiographic analysis of diastolic flow murmurs in secundum atrial septal defect and ventricular septal defect. Br Heart J. 1967;29:684.
33. Gersony WM, Hayes CJ, Driscoll DJ, et al. Bacterial endocarditis in patients with aortic stenosis, pulmonary stenosis, or ventricular septal defect. Circulation. 1993;87:I121.
34. Frontera-Izquierdo P, Cabezuelo-Huerta G. Natural and modified history of isolated ventricular septal defect: a 17-year study. Pediatr Cardiol. 1992;13:193.
35. Johnson DH, Rosenthal A, Nadas AS. A forty-year review of bacterial endocarditis in infancy and childhood. Circulation. 1975;51:581.
36. Otterstad JE, Nitter-Hauge S, Myhre E. Isolated ventricular septal defect in adults. Clinical and haemodynamic findings. Br Heart J. 1983;50:343.
37. Shah P, Singh WS, Rose V, Keith JD. Incidence of bacterial endocarditis in ventricular septal defects. Circulation. 1966;34:127.
38. Kaplan S, Daoud GI, Benzing G 3rd, et al. Natural history of ventricular septal defect. Am J Dis Child. 1963;105:581.
39. Moller JH, Patton C, Varco RL, Lillehei CW. Late results (30 to 35 years) after operative closure of isolated ventricular septal defect from 1954 to 1960. Am J Cardiol. 1991;68:1491.
40. Kirklin JW, Dushane JW. Indications for repair of ventricular septal defects. Am J Cardiol. 1963;12:75.

Atrial Septal Defect

Dimitrios V. Moysidis, Eleftherios Gemousakakis,
Alexandros Liatsos, Christos Tsagkaris,
and Andreas S. Papazoglou

Abstract

"Atrial septal defects (ASDs) are a frequent type of congenital heart disease characterized by an abnormal communication between the two atria of the heart, which leads to a left-to-right shunt." They are formed during embryological development due to disorders in atrial septation. Most ASDs are of small size and therefore are asymptomatic during infancy and childhood. However, most of them, except for some patients who have mild or nonspecific symptoms, become obvious by the age of 40 years, when they cause clinical manifestations, such as fatigue, exercise intolerance, and dyspnea. In childhood, the vast majority of isolated ASDs close spontaneously. Large and persistently symptomatic moderate-sized defects should be repaired. Intervention is also required in adulthood in symptomatic patients, right ventricular overload, left-to-right shunt, or paradoxical embolism. Transcatheter device closure is always preferred against surgical repair.

Keywords

Congenital heart disease · Atrial septal defects · Atrial septation · Ostium secundum · Crochetage sign Left-to-right shunt · Eisenmenger syndrome Spontaneous closure · Paradoxical embolism Transcatheter device closure

Introduction

"Atrial septal defects (ASDs) constitute a frequent type of congenital heart disease characterized by an abnormal communication between the two atria of the heart through an insufficient interatrial septal tissue" [1] (Fig. 1). The prevalence of ASD is estimated to be approximately 1.6 per 1000 live births and 0.88 per 1000 adults while ASDs account for 7–10% of all congenital heart defects (CHDs). During the last two decades, an increase in the incidence of new ASD cases has been observed, which however is probably attributed to the widespread use of echocardiography. The prevalence of ASD is also higher in females [2]. In a large database of European patients with CHDs, conducted in the Netherlands, 67% of patients suffering from ASD were females [3].

Geographic distribution seems to be unequal too, with the highest ASD birth prevalence found in Asia, North America, and Europe [4]. Familial history of congenital heart anomalies increases the risk of a secundum ASD, which is further increased when at least one sibling has an ASD [5]. ASDs, in most cases, present as isolated defects, but they might also complicate other diseases or be a part of a syndrome, such as Down syndrome, Hurler syndrome, Noonan syndrome, chondroectodermal dysplasia, congenital rubella, and others [6].

Isolated ASDs are most commonly diagnosed in asymptomatic patients during their first two decades of life. Therefore, many patients get diagnosed incidentally during an echocardiographic investigation of a murmur. The age in which symptoms may occur depends on the size of the defect. Patients with smaller ASDs (less than 5 mm) might never present with clinically significant symptomatology. These defects are most likely to close spontaneously. Bigger defects (5–10 mm) usually lead to symptoms during the fourth or fifth decade, while defects with a diameter of more than 10 mm can become clinically obvious during the third decade of life [6].

D. V. Moysidis (✉) · E. Gemousakakis · A. Liatsos · A. S. Papazoglou
School of Medicine, Aristotle University of Thessaloniki (AUTh), Thessaloniki, Greece

C. Tsagkaris
School of Medicine, University of Crete (UoC), Heraklion, Greece

© The Author(s), under exclusive license to Springer Nature Switzerland AG 2023
G. Tagarakis et al. (eds.), *Clinical and Surgical Aspects of Congenital Heart Diseases*,
https://doi.org/10.1007/978-3-031-23062-2_5

**Atrial Septal Defect
(ASD)**

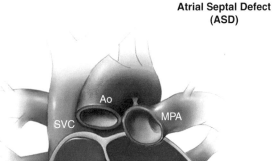

RA. Right Atrium   SVC. Superior Vena Cava   TV. Tricuspid Valve
RV. Right Ventricle   IVC. Inferior Vena Cava   MV. Mitral Valve
LA. Left Atrium   MPA. Main Pulmonary Artery
LV. Left Ventricle   Ao. Aorta

Fig. 1 Atrial septal defect illustration (*Adapted from Wikipedia commons (free copyright license)*)

Patients often present with fatigue, shortness of breath, palpitations, exercise intolerance, and syncope. If left undiagnosed and untreated, ASDs could eventually cause right-sided heart failure, manifestations of thromboembolism, and cyanosis associated with Eisenmenger syndrome. Infants with significant defects might rarely present with tachypnea, recurrent respiratory infections, and failure to thrive [7]. The most common cause of death in patients with unrepaired defects is heart failure [8]. Untreated patients and even patients, who do not receive early diagnosis and appropriate management, may experience higher rates of mortality and morbidity. On the contrary, an early and proper management approach increases event-free survival rates. However, the risk of atrial arrhythmias and thromboembolism seems to remain higher in comparison to the general population [9].

Pathophysiology

Lack of sufficient tissue to completely septate the atria is the causing factor of ASDs. Foramen ovale is vital for fetal circulation, as flow through this lesion is essential for systemic circulation perfusion. Atrial septal embryonic development is depicted in Fig. 2. Defects in any stage of this process can lead to the occurrence of ASDs. The predisposing risk factors and associated conditions (i.e., maternal exposure to chemicals, alcohol consumption during the first trimester, and gestational diabetes) have been long studied; however, their relationship has not yet been established [10, 11].

Based on the location of the defect and, by extension, of the liable embryogenetic abnormality, ASDs are classified into four types (Fig. 3):

1. Ostium secundum, which is located in fossa ovalis, represents the majority of ASDs, accounting for about 70% of all cases. It is the result of either poor growth of the secundum septum or its excessive absorption [12]. It is usually an isolated congenital heart disorder, but it might also be associated with other congenital cardiac and extra-cardiac abnormalities. Holt–Oram syndrome, which is also known as the heart-hand syndrome, is the most well-described disorder frequently accompanied by a secundum ASD [13].
2. Ostium primum type, which accounts for 15–20% of ASDs, is formed when primum septum fails to fuse with the endocardial cushions at the base of the interatrial septum [12]. It can be either isolated or, most commonly, associated with atrioventricular (AV) valve anomalies, particularly a cleft in the anterior mitral valve leaflet [13, 14]. This comorbidity can also be accompanied by a contiguous defect in the inlet ventricular septum. This combination of primum ASD, cleft mitral valve, and an inlet ventricular septal defect, is known as a partial AV septal defect (AVSD), whose most severe form is the complete AV septal (or canal) defect [15].
3. Superior and inferior sinus venosus defects, which account for approximately 5–10% of all ASDs, are located in the venoatrial part of the atrial septum [13]. They represent an abnormality in the insertion of the superior or inferior vena cava, which overrides the interatrial septum. These defects are technically not considered to be ASDs since the defect is within the sinus venosus septum.
4. Coronary sinus defects, which is the most uncommon type of ASD, account for less than 1% of ASD patients.

ASDs in adults can give birth to a left-to-right shunt which generates volume overload of the right heart chambers. The severity of this shunt, as well as the direction and magnitude of blood, is determined by the size of the defect and the relative atrial pressures, which are linked to the compliances of the ventricles. These parameters also determine the natural course of isolated ASDs, which varies from spontaneous closure to asymptomatic right ventricular (RV) enlargement leading to the gradual development of symptoms with age [16].

Fig. 2 Formation of atrial septum

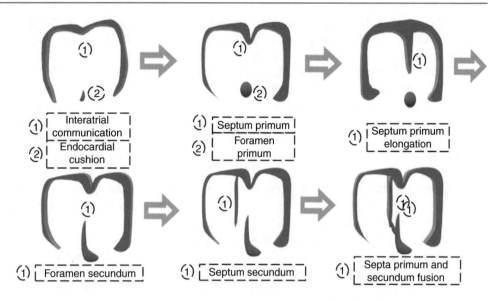

Fig. 3 Types of ASD

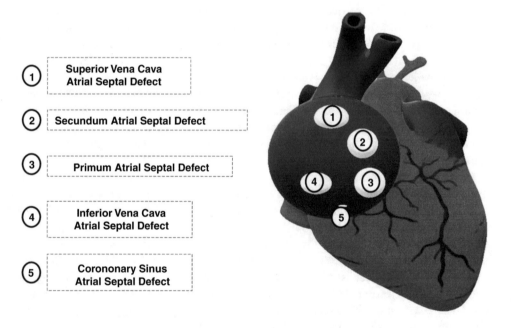

1. Superior Vena Cava Atrial Septal Defect

2. Secundum Atrial Septal Defect

3. Primum Atrial Septal Defect

4. Inferior Vena Cava Atrial Septal Defect

5. Corononary Sinus Atrial Septal Defect

Spontaneous closure of ASDs has been described in approximately 40% of secundum ASDs. These small intra-atrial defects (usually less than 8 mm in diameter) limit the size of the shunt by their own resistance (pressure-separating effect) and do not cause major hemodynamic disturbances [17]. On the other hand, secundum ASDs of diameter greater than 8 mm, primum ASDs, sinus venosus defects, and coronary sinus defects do not seem to spontaneously close. On the contrary, they create size-dependent volume overload of the right heart and pulmonary arteries, which can lead later to the progressive development of pulmonary vascular obstructive disease and eventually pulmonary hypertension. This mainly occurs when the degree of shunting is significant. After years of pulmonary vascular injury, an irreversibly high pulmonary vascular resistance can gradually occur,

creating a right-heart hypertrophy and consequently establishing a paradoxical right-to-left shunt (Eisenmenger syndrome).

The pressure difference between the left and right atrium can be significantly altered under several conditions. The presence of additional mitral stenosis entails a major increase in the pressure difference between the left and right atrium (Lutembacher's syndrome), which increases the left-to-right shunt with the same defect size. Furthermore, in adult patients, especially in those older than 50 years, age-induced increases in left-to-right shunting (due to relative increases in the left versus right ventricular end-diastolic pressures), systematic hypertension, and other acquired heart disease might lead to increased left ventricular (LV) end-diastolic and/or left atrial pressure, particularly in patients with moderate and large ASDs [18]. These conditions might lead to ventricular diastolic dysfunction and left atrial enlargement, thereby providing fertile ground for mitral regurgitation and atrial fibrillation. These alterations in the heart's physiology increase the likelihood of developing symptoms and complications as described in the next section [17].

Diagnosis

Clinical Manifestations and Physical Findings

Most ASDs are of small size and therefore are asymptomatic during infancy and childhood. A murmur detected on physical examination or an incidental finding on an echocardiogram obtained for other reasons can lead to their evaluation and diagnosis. On the other hand, children with large ASDs occasionally suffer from heart failure (relative signs: tachypnea, rales, failure to thrive, hepatomegaly), recurrent respiratory infections, or failure to thrive. Symptoms and signs of pulmonary hypertension are uncommon in pediatric patients with ASDs but can occasionally occur.

In adult patients, ASD diagnosis should be established as soon as possible to increase the possibility of a timely repair. Even though most of these young patients have no or few symptoms on physical examination (right-sided volume overload is usually well tolerated for a long time), there is a number of findings that may give rise to clinical suspicion of an underlying ASD. Most patients with a significant shunt flow (i.e., pulmonary to systemic blood flow ratio [Qp:Qs] ≥1.5:1) will become symptomatic by the age of 40 years, except for some patients who have mild or nonspecific symptoms, and others who adapt to their limitations. Fatigue, exercise intolerance, and dyspnea are common clinical manifestations of ASDs in adults, while some patients develop heart failure. ASD repair reduces the severity of these symptoms. The classic physical findings of an isolated ASD in adults are typically similar to those observed in children [19–21].

Complications in patients with ASDs involve atrial arrhythmias, pulmonary hypertension (including Eisenmenger syndrome), cyanosis, and paradoxical embolism. Atrial arrhythmias (particularly atrial fibrillation, but also atrial flutter and other supraventricular tachycardias) are common in patients with ASDs after the third decade. The risk increases with age and pulmonary hypertension. Patients usually suffer from palpitations, dyspnea, and an increased risk of cardio-embolic events. The development of pulmonary vascular injury is related to the degree and duration of right heart volume overload. Pulmonary vascular damage acts as the pathogenetic substrate of pulmonary hypertension. As the disease progresses, right heart failure can be developed, and its features (elevated jugular venous pressure, hepatic congestion, tricuspid regurgitation, and pedal edema) might become obvious [16–19].

Furthermore, right heart failure might lead to elevated right heart pressures, and thus inversed (right-to-left) shunt, which is called Eisenmenger syndrome. Eisenmenger syndrome is accompanied by cyanosis and clubbing in addition to clinical signs of pulmonary hypertension. Last but not least, patients with an ASD are at risk for stroke, transient ischemic attack, or peripheral emboli due to paradoxical embolization (embolus carried from the venous side of circulation to the arterial side) [22, 23].

Electrocardiogram

An electrocardiogram (ECG) is a crucial part of the primary diagnostic evaluation of suspected heart conditions. Nevertheless, it is neither necessary nor sufficient to diagnose an ASD. Patients with small shunt or uncomplicated ASD can have a normal ECG. Sinus rhythm is observed in the majority of the patients, but the presence of atrial arrhythmias can complicate the clinical course of some patients and lead to relevant ECG evaluation and findings [13].

Right axis deviation and a "crochetage" sign (R wave notching in II, III, and aVF leads), which is correlated with the left-to-right shunt severity, can be found in secundum ASDs (Fig. 4). "Crochetage" sign involves at least one ECG lead in 73%, and all inferior leads in 27% of the ASD patients. Presence in all three inferior leads or co-occurrence with the right bundle branch block (RBBB) increases both the sensitivity and specificity of the sign [24]. Interestingly, "crochetage" sign disappears in approximately 50% of the patients within 2 weeks after ASD closure [14, 25].

Right ventricular hypertrophy and RBBB can also be observed. Left axis deviation and incomplete RBBB typically suggest the presence of a primum ASD.

Chest Radiograph

Chest radiograph findings depend on the degree of shunting. Normal chest radiograph is frequent—if not typical—in patients with small defects. Larger ASDs leading to significant left-to-right shunt often appear with right heart enlargement and prominent pulmonary vascularity (eventual signs of pulmonary arterial hypertension [PAH]). Dilation of the left atrium can also be marked, especially due to mitral regurgitation. The heart shadow often obtains a characteristic triangular appearance as the enlarged pulmonary arteries prevent the normal aortic arch from forming the heart border (Fig. 5) [19, 25, 27].

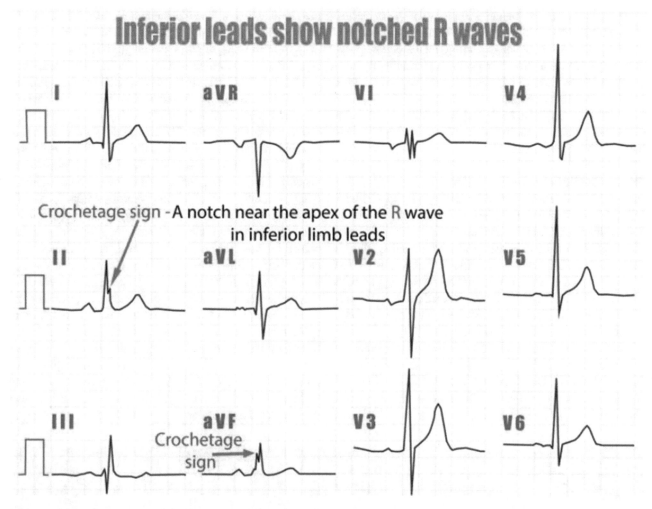

Fig. 4 Crochetage sign in ECG (*Jason Winter 2016-The ECG Educator Blog*)

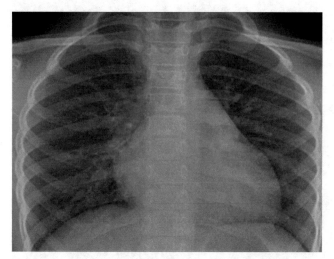

Fig. 5 Chest X-ray of a child with large ASD and hemodynamically significant left-to-right shunt (*Reprinted with permission from Arun Gopalakrishnan and Kerala Journal of Cardiology* [26])

Imaging-Based Diagnosis

Imaging is necessary to confirm the diagnosis of ASD. Echocardiography is the imaging modality of choice, utilized ante- or/and postnatally to establish the specific type, location, and size of ASD, and to identify associated abnormalities or complications.

In particular, the antenatal detection of an ASD depends on both disease type and operator. When performed by an experienced fetal echocardiographer, the third-level obstetric ultrasound can establish the diagnosis of a primum ASD at 18–22 weeks of gestation [28]. However, the most frequent ASD type, secundum ASD, cannot be reliably detected prenatally due to the sizable PFO observed in healthy fetuses. This makes the distinction between a small to moderate-size secundum ASD from a PFO with right-to-left shunt almost impossible. Yet, fetal echocardiography may still raise suspicion for a very large secundum ASD, which should be confirmed postnatally, as required for any other suspected prenatal ASD case. With regard to the sinus venosus and coronary sinus ASDs, although a trained fetal echocardiographer may have the ability to detect them prenatally, the sensitivity and specificity of this diagnostic method have not yet been reported for these more unusual types of ASD.

Ultimately, antenatal ASD imaging findings need to be confirmed postnatally through one of the following imaging-based diagnostic approaches:

Transthoracic Echocardiography

In general, the transthoracic echocardiography (TTE) with Doppler is the initial imaging test of choice for the diagnosis and evaluation of primum and secundum ASDs [29], with the diagnoses of the latter being usually definitive (Fig. 6) [30]. A comprehensive TTE includes 2D imaging as well as color-flow, pulsed-wave, and continuous-wave Doppler with multiple echocardiographic views obtained to assess the precise location and size of the ASD, as well as the hemodynamic alterations associated with the shunt [29].

A primum or secundum ASD is suspected in the presence of abrupt discontinuity, hypermobility, or drop out of the interatrial septum. On M-mode, RV dilatation and abnormal septal motion serve as signs of ASD in cases with significant shunting [31]. The subcostal four-chamber view improves the visualization of the atrial septum because the ultrasound beam is generally nearly perpendicular to the atrial septum [32]. Unfortunately, this view is suboptimal in some patients, especially in overweight and obese individuals. Parasternal short-axis and off-axis apical view, as well as other nonstandard views are commonly required to visualize the whole interatrial septum. A recent study aiming to assess the diagnostic sensitivity of the 2D echocardiographic subcostal imaging on patients with a history of ASD (mean age 31 years) demonstrated that the defect could be successfully visualized in 93 out of 105 secundum ASDs, all 32 primum ASDs, and only 7 out of 16 sinus venosus ASDs.

Moreover, it is reported that the operator can usually demonstrate through the pulsewave Doppler a classic triphasic left-to-right shunt at the level of the defect, with characteristic flow waveforms in late systole and diastole and a presystolic accentuation. An experienced echocardiographer is also able to distinguish a physiological venous flow pattern from an ASD flow pattern. In addition, color flow is used to visualize the actual shunt, with a right-to-left or bidirectional flow being developed in patients with RV diastolic dysfunction or significant tricuspid regurgitation. According to Pollick et al., the color jet width may be linked with the left-to-right shunt size [33]. It has been demonstrated that a color flow width of 1.5 cm may suggest

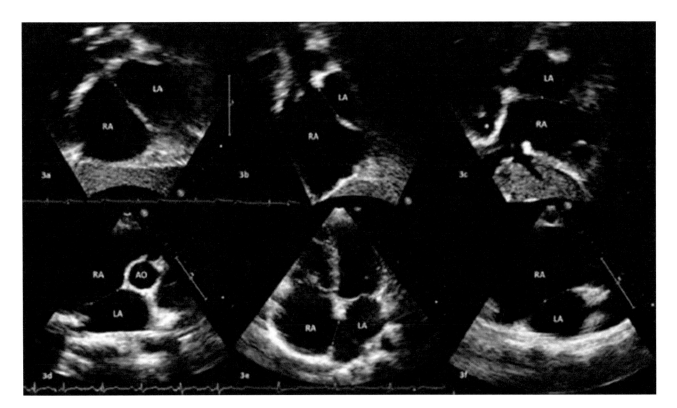

Fig. 6 Transthoracic echocardiographic images of ASD. Panels **3a–3c** are 2D transthoracic echocardiographic images from the subxiphoid window. Panel **3d** is the parasternal short-axis projection showing the aortic rim of the ASD. The mitral rim of the ASD is notable in the apical four-chamber view in panel **3e**. Panel **3f** is the right parasternal window showing the ostium secundum ASD (*Reprinted with permission from Arun Gopalakrishnan and Kerala Journal of Cardiology* [26])

a Qp:Qs ratio greater than 2:1, which has a major prognostic potential as discussed below [33].

Nevertheless, when a defect is not apparent, contrast echocardiography with the administration of agitated saline contrast through a peripheral vein is the primary test used to determine the presence of an ASD, especially for patients with restricted acoustic windows [34]. In the case of an ASD, it shows the extravasation of saline contrast microbubbles from the RA to the LA at the level of the interatrial septum [35]. Furthermore, sinus venosus and coronary sinus ASDs can be diagnosed by the appearance of agitated saline contrast in the left atrium before it appears in the right atrium soon after the injection of contrast saline through the left arm.

Transesophageal Echocardiography

Although 2D TTE (either with Doppler or with peripheral vein injection of agitated saline) is usually adequate to identify the presence of an ASD and assess the cardiac chamber size, one should not discount that the diagnostic sensitivity of the TTE may be subject to the view obtained and operator/ patient factors (i.e., optimal acoustic windows in young patients, but restricted acoustic windows in other patients due to large body habitus, and prior thoracic surgery). Hence, negative suboptimal or noncomprehensive TTEs do not exclude an ASD diagnosis. At the same time, transesophageal echocardiography (TEE) offers an excellent alternative approach in patients with poor imaging quality and is suggested if TTE fails to show an ASD in a patient with suspected ASD (Fig. 7).

TEE is highly accurate for the diagnosis of all types of ASDs in the hands of a trained echocardiographer. TEE further aids in the sizing of secundum ASDs and in detecting the most common forms of anomalous venous connections (PAPVC) [36].

When performed with color flow Doppler or with agitated saline contrast injection, TEE can detect right-to-left and left-to-right shunting with higher sensitivity than via TTE [37]. Furthermore, TEE can also detect flow through multiple ASDs. Finally, TEE imaging prior to planned surgical or percutaneous closure can determine the suitability for transcatheter device closure and prevent unnecessary therapeutic

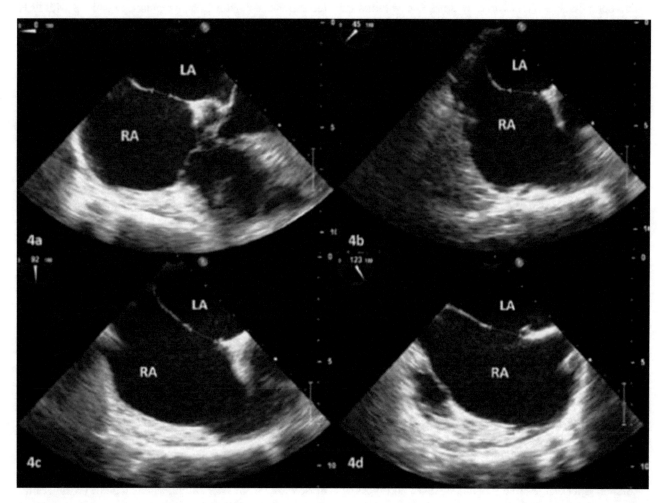

Fig. 7 Transesophageal echocardiographic images of ASD (*Reprinted with permission from Arun Gopalakrishnan and Kerala Journal of Cardiology* [26])

procedures. 3D TEE provides even better sizing and visualization of ASDs and provides important evidence with regard to their shape and their relationship to atrial superior and inferior limbic band tissue, the aortic root, and the AV valves [38–40].

Cardiovascular Magnetic Resonance, Computed Tomography and Cardiac Catheterization

In the presence of nondefinitive TTE and TEE findings with regard to the diagnosis of sinus venosus or unroofed coronary sinus ASDs, the assessment of PAPVC, or the presence of RV volume overload, cardiovascular magnetic resonance (CMR) or computed tomography (CT) imaging can be considered. The CT and CMR procedures require special imaging protocols and should be performed by an experienced cardiac imaging specialist, able to identify, characterize ASDs and abnormal pulmonary venous return, and also estimate shunt flow [41–43].

Additionally, recent advances in CMR and high-resolution contrast CT techniques facilitate the anatomical delineation of ASDs and the quantitative assessment of their hemodynamic complications (ventricular volumes and volumes of pulmonary and systemic flow) [44–46]. The quantification of left-to-right shunt fraction (Qp:Qs ratio) should be performed to determine whether an ASD closure is indicated or not (threshold of 1.5). This is nowadays plausible not only by means of invasive right heart catheterization (invasive oximetry), but also by means of CMR. CMR-based shunt flow calculations do not differ significantly from those of the cardiac catheterization, despite the small overestimation of the Qp:Qs ratio by CMR. Therefore, given that ASDs can be diagnosed and treated with noninvasive imaging assessment (i.e., CMR, CT, TEE, TTE+ Doppler/+saline contrast, 3D echo), cardiac catheterization in the course of the ASD clinical workup is rarely performed nowadays.

Management

Age of the patient, location and size of the defect, presence of pulmonary hypertension, and hemodynamic impact of the shunt are the main factors determining ASD management strategy. In childhood, the vast majority of small isolated secundum ASDs can spontaneously close within the first 2 years of life and in some cases as late as by 5 years of age. Hence, early closure is not indicated for these defects unless there are significant symptoms. Furthermore, there is also no high-quality evidence supporting the closure of a persistent ASD in asymptomatic children older than 2 years old with persistent small defects [47].

Moderate and large-sized secundum ASDs, and types of ASDs other than secundum, are unlikely to close spontaneously. Nevertheless, given the—small—likelihood of spon-

taneous closure during the first 2 years of life, intervention to close these defects tends to be postponed until after the age of 2 years in asymptomatic children. For patients with a persistent moderate or large defect, left-to-right shunting usually deteriorates with age if the defect is not repaired. Hence, the principal indication for ASD closure in children is the presence of a sizable left-to-right shunt leading to a clinically significant right heart overload. The risk of paradoxical embolism through a small ASD is yet to be quantified and the benefit of ASD closure in reducing the cardio-embolic risk has to be compared with the short- and long-term procedural risks. The preferable type of intervention (transcatheter procedure or open surgical repair) depends on the ASD type and the extent of subsequent cardiac dysfunction. Percutaneous closure is generally indicated for secundum ASDs that are not excessively large. In symptomatic infants with primum or sinus venosus or coronary sinus ASDs, surgical repair remains the gold standard [19–21, 30, 47, 48].

In terms of recommendations for intervention in adults, ASD closure in patients with RV overload and no PAH or LV disease is the most well-documented indication and is strongly recommended regardless of symptoms. In patients with PAH, closure should only be considered in the presence of significant left-to-right shunt (Qp:Qs >1.5) and pulmonary vascular resistance (PVR) $\geq$5 WU (persisting after targeted PAH treatment). ASD closure should not be considered as a therapeutic solution in patients with Eisenmenger physiology, and patients with PAH and concomitant PVR $\geq$5 WU, despite targeted PAH treatment, or desaturation on exercise. In patients with (systolic or/and diastolic) LV dysfunction, ASD closure appears to exert a deteriorating effect on heart failure and thus should be carefully evaluated. Balloon pre-interventional testing might be required to carefully weigh the benefit of eliminating left-to-right shunt against the potential negative impact of ASD closure on filling pressures of the LV [49]. In addition, patients with suspected paradoxical embolism should be referred to ASD closure, provided that the presence of PAH or LV dysfunction have been dully excluded [25, 50–53]. Finally, ASD closure is also recommended for patients with documented platypnea-orthodeoxia [48].

ASD closure can be performed either by catheter intervention or by open heart surgery. Percutaneous procedures have reported similar success and mortality rates with lower morbidity (decreased exercise capacity, shortness of breath, right heart failure) and, therefore, transcatheter device closure has become the first choice for secundum defects with a diameter of less than 40 mm, which is the case in 80% of the patients [52, 54–58]. Serious complications have been observed in $\leq$1% of patients [59].

Post-intervention atrial tachyarrhythmias appear to be mostly transient. Other complications include erosion of the atrial wall, anterior mitral leaflet, or the aorta, as well as thromboembolic events, but these are rarely encountered in clinical practice [15, 27]. When this minimally-invasive procedure is not feasible or not suitable for ASD patients, particularly elderly ones, and those with primum, sinus venosus, or coronary sinus ASDs, open heart surgery is required. Nonetheless, mortality rates of surgical repair in isolated ASDs have been reported to be low (<1% in patients without significant concomitant diseases) in experienced centers, with favorable long-term outcomes when performed early (i.e., in childhood, adolescence) and in the absence of PAH [54, 55]. In general, outcomes of an ASD closure seem to be better when the repair is performed until the middle of the third decade of life [54, 55].

Furthermore, patients with either unrepaired or repaired ASDs require further general evaluation and management. First of all, ASDs are a major predisposing factor for atrial arrhythmias, which should be managed according to standard recommendations. Cryo- or radiofrequency ablation (modified maze procedure) can be considered at the time of intervention, as device closure might later restrict electrophysiologists from accessing the left atrium. Additionally, ASDs are frequently associated with pulmonary hypertension, associated with a higher risk of complications (heart failure, cyanosis, pulmonary artery thrombosis). Advanced therapy for PAH hypertension is suitable for patients with pulmonary hypertension secondary to ASD and might improve symptoms or even render the defect operable. Moreover, patients with an ASD are at a substantial risk of infective endocarditis. Thus, appropriate guideline-driven antibiotic prophylaxis should be given when patients undergo procedures with a risk of bacteremia during the first 6 months after ASD closure. On the contrary, no treatment is warranted in isolated ASDs with no residual shunt because they have been correlated with negligible risk of infective endocarditis. All patients and their caregivers should be educated regarding the need to carefully observe oral hygiene and adhere to their medication. Finally, in terms of sports and physical activity, doctors need to provide patients with personalized recommendations based on the defect's size and concomitant symptoms.

Conclusion

ASDs constitute a characteristic type of CHD that remains "silent" and becomes obvious mostly in adulthood as most of them are small in size and therefore asymptomatic during infancy and childhood. Their clinical symptomatology, as well as diagnostic approach, remains the same in children and adults. The age of the patient, the location and the size of the defect, and the presence of pulmonary hypertension along with the hemodynamic impact of created shunts constitute the most significant parts of ASDs' clinical evaluation. Finally,

their management depends on the consideration of the aforementioned parameters and demands a multilevel clinical approach by pediatric cardiologists, adult CHD cardiologists, interventional cardiologists, and cardiac surgeons.

Multiple Choice Questions
1. Which of the following is correct:
   A. The prevalence of atrial septal defects (ASDs) is estimated to be approximately 6 per 1000 live births and 0.88 per 1000 adults while ASDs account for 7–10% of all congenital heart defects.
   B. The prevalence of atrial septal defects (ASDs) is estimated to be approximately 1.6 per 1000 live births and 0.88 per 1000 adults while ASDs account for 27% of all congenital heart defects.
   C. The prevalence of atrial septal defects (ASDs) is estimated to be approximately 1.6 per 1000 live births and 0.88 per 1000 adults while ASDs account for 7–10% of all congenital heart defects.
   D. The prevalence of atrial septal defects is estimated to be approximately 0.16 per 1000 live births and 0.88 per 1000 adults while ASDs account for 27% of all congenital heart defects.
   E. The prevalence of atrial septal defects is estimated to be approximately 1.6 per 1000 live births and 0.88 per 1000 adults while ASDs account for 0.7% of all congenital heart defects.
2. Atrial septal defects are associated with:
   A. Down syndrome
   B. Noonan syndrome
   C. Chondroectodermal dysplasia
   D. Congenital rubella
   E. All the above
3. The most frequent type of atrial septal defect is:
   A. Ostium primum
   B. Ostium secundum
   C. Superior sinus venosus
   D. Inferior sinus venosus
   E. Coronary sinus defect
4. Which of the following is correct:
   A. Atrial septal defects can give birth to a left-to-right shunt, which generates volume overload of the right heart chambers.
   B. Atrial septal defects can give birth to a left-to-right shunt, which generates volume overload of the left heart chambers.
   C. Atrial septal defects can give birth to a left-to-right shunt, which generates pressure overload of the right heart chambers.
   D. Atrial septal defects can give birth to a right-to-left shunt, which generates volume overload of the right heart chambers.

E. Atrial septal defects can give birth to a right-to-left shunt, which generates volume overload of the left heart chambers.

5. Spontaneous closure of ASDs has been described in approximately:
   A. 10% of secundum ASDs
   B. 25% of secundum ASDs
   C. 40% of secundum ASDs
   D. 70% of secundum ASDs
   E. 90% of secundum ASDs

6. Atrial septal defects are not directly associated with:
   A. Arrhythmias
   B. Stroke
   C. Pulmonary hypertension
   D. Mitral stenosis
   E. Dyspnea

7. The "crochetage" sign can be found in patients with atrial septal defect and is characterized by:
   A. R wave notching in V1–V6 leads
   B. R wave notching in II, III, and aVF leads
   C. R wave notching in I, II, and III leads
   D. Q wave notching in V1–V6 leads
   E. Q wave notching in II, III, and aVF leads

8. The gold standard imaging test for the diagnosis of atrial septal defect is:
   A. Cardiovascular magnetic resonance
   B. Transesophageal echocardiograph
   C. Computed tomography
   D. Transthoracic echocardiograph
   E. Cardiac catheterization

9. Which is not an indication for performing an atrial septal defect (ASD) repair:
   A. Large asymptomatic ASDs
   B. Moderate-sized symptomatic ASDs
   C. Pulmonary hypertension with a right-to-left shunt
   D. Pulmonary hypertension with a left-to-right shunt
   E. Paradoxical embolism

10. Which of the following is correct:
    A. Percutaneous procedures have reported higher success rates than surgical repair, with lower morbidity. Serious complications in transcatheter interventions have been observed in ≤1% of patients.
    B. Percutaneous procedures have reported lower success rates than surgical repair, with higher morbidity. Serious complications in transcatheter interventions have been observed in approximately 5% of patients.
    C. Percutaneous procedures have reported similar success and mortality rates compared to surgical repair, with lower morbidity. Serious complications in transcatheter interventions have been observed in ≤0.1% of patients.
    D. Percutaneous procedures have reported lower success rates than surgical repair, with higher morbidity. Serious complications in transcatheter interventions have been observed in ≤1% of patients.
    E. Percutaneous procedures have reported similar success and mortality rates compared to surgical repair, with lower morbidity. Serious complications in transcatheter interventions have been observed in ≤1% of patients.

Answers
1. C
2. E
3. B
4. A
5. C
6. D
7. B
8. D
9. E
10. E

References

1. Geva T, Martins JD, Wald RM. Atrial septal defects. Lancet. 2014;383(9932):1921–32.
2. Engelfriet P, Mulder BJM. Gender differences in adult congenital heart disease. Neth Heart J. 2009;17(11):414–7.
3. Warnes CA. Sex differences in congenital heart disease. Circulation. 2008;118(1):3–5.
4. van der Linde D, Konings EEM, Slager MA, Witsenburg M, Helbing WA, Takkenberg JJM, Roos-Hesselink JW. Birth prevalence of congenital heart disease worldwide: a systematic review and meta-analysis. J Am Coll Cardiol. 2011;58(21):2241–7.
5. Caputo S, Capozzi G, Russo MG, Esposito T, Martina L, Cardaropoli D, Ricci C, Argiento P, Pacileo G, Calabrò R. Familial recurrence of congenital heart disease in patients with ostium secundum atrial septal defect. Eur Heart J. 2005;26(20):2179–84.
6. Menillo AM, Lee LS, Pearson-Shaver AL. Atrial septal defect. [Updated 2021 Aug 11]. In: StatPearls [Internet]. Treasure Island: StatPearls Publishing; 2021. https://www.ncbi.nlm.nih.gov/books/NBK535440/.
7. Lammers A, Hager A, Eicken A, Lange R, Hauser M, Hess J. Need for closure of secundum atrial septal defect in infancy. J Thorac Cardiovasc Surg. 2005;129(6):1353–7.
8. Nyboe C, Karunanithi Z, Nielsen-Kudsk JE, Hjortdal VE. Long-term mortality in patients with atrial septal defect: a nationwide cohort-study. Eur Heart J. 2018;39(12):993–8.
9. Goldberg JF. Long-term follow-up of "simple" lesions—atrial septal defect, ventricular septal defect, and coarctation of the aorta. Congenit Heart Dis. 2015;10(5):466–74.
10. Snyder W. Study: balanced high-fat diet improves body composition, inflammation. https://medschool.vanderbilt.edu/vanderbilt-medicine/study-balanced-high-fat-diet-improves-body-composition-inflammation/.

11. Tsagkaris C, Loudovikou A, Moysidis DV, Papazoglou AS, Kalachanis K. In the footsteps of Scribonius largus, a pioneer of clinical pharmacy in ancient Rome. Borneo J Pharm. 2021;4(3):226–30.
12. UTD-0023—docshare.tips [Internet]. docshare.tips. 2022 [cited 14 August 2022]. https://docshare.tips/utd-0023_5f47e889df891427518b4568.html.
13. Willerson J, Cohn J, Wellens H, Holmes D. Cardiovascular medicine.
14. Hassani C, Saremi F. Comprehensive cross-sectional imaging of the pulmonary veins. Radiographics. 2017;37(7):1928–54.
15. Amin Z, Hijazi ZM, Bass JL, Cheatham JP, Hellenbrand WE, Kleinman CS. Erosion of Amplatzer septal occluder device after closure of secundum atrial septal defects: review of registry of complications and recommendations to minimize future risk. Catheter Cardiovasc Interv. 2004;63(4):496–502.
16. Atrial septal defects. PDF download free [Internet]. docksci.com. 2022 [cited 14 August 2022]. https://docksci.com/atrial-septal-defects_5aea9e92d64ab27b6eb079e2.html.
17. Essentials of pediatric radiology: a multimodality approach—PDF free download [Internet]. epdf.tips. 2022 [cited 14 August 2022]. https://epdf.tips/essentials-of-pediatric-radiology-a-multimodality-approach.html.
18. Butera G, Lucente M, Rosti L, Chessa M, Micheletti A, Giamberti A, et al. A comparison between the early and mid-term results of surgical as opposed to percutaneous closure of defects in the oval fossa in children aged less than 6 years. Cardiol Young. 2007;17(1):35–41. https://doi.org/10.1017/S104795110600134X.
19. Prochownik P, Przewłocki T, Podolec P, Wilkołek P, Sobień B, Gancarczyk U, et al. Improvement of physical capacity in patients undergoing transcatheter closure of atrial septal defects. Adv Interv Cardiol. 2018;14(1):90–4.
20. Holy E, Nietlispach F, Meier B. Transcatheter closure of atrial septal defect and a patent foramen ovale in adults. Emerg Technol Heart Dis. 2020:1009–1024.
21. Ošlaj N. Dijagnostika i liječenje atrijskog septalnog defekta u odraslih [Internet]. Urn.nsk.hr. 2022 [cited 14 August 2022]. https://urn.nsk.hr/urn:nbn:hr:105:203944.
22. Wennevold A. The diastolic murmur of atrial septal defects as detected by intracardiac phonocardiography. Circulation. 1966;34(1):132–8.
23. Perloff JK, Harvey WP. Mechanisms of fixed splitting of the second heart sound. Circulation. 1958;18(5):998–1009.
24. Heller J, Hagège AA, Besse B, Desnos M, Marie F-N, Guerot C. "Crochetage" (Notch) on R wave in inferior limb leads: a new independent electrocardiographic sign of atrial septal defect. J Am Coll Cardiol. 1996;27(4):877–82.
25. Manes A, Palazzini M, Leci E, Bacchi Reggiani ML, Branzi A, Galiè N. Current era survival of patients with pulmonary hypertension associated with congenital heart disease: a comparison between clinical subgroups. Eur Heart J. 2014;35(11):716–24.
26. Gopalakrishnan A. Atrial septal defect—systematic assessment prior to device closure. Kerala J Cardiol. 2017;1:61–8.
27. Krumsdorf U, Ostermayer S, Billinger K, Trepels T, Zadan E, Horvath K, Sievert H. Incidence and clinical course of thrombus formation on atrial septal defect and patient foramen ovale closure devices in 1,000 consecutive patients. J Am Coll Cardiol. 2004;43(2):302–9.
28. Bravo-Valenzuela NJ, Peixoto AB, Araujo Júnior E. Prenatal diagnosis of congenital heart disease: a review of current knowledge. Indian Heart J. 2018;70(1):150–64.
29. Stout KK, Daniels CJ, Aboulhosn JA, Bozkurt B, Broberg CS, Colman JM, Crumb SR, Dearani JA, Fuller S, Gurvitz M, Khairy P, Landzberg MJ, Saidi A, Valente AM, Van Hare GF. 2018 AHA/ACC guideline for the management of adults with congenital heart disease: a report of the American College of Cardiology/American Heart Association task force on clinical practice guidelines. Circulation. 2019;139(14):e698–800.
30. Bricker JT, Omar HA, Merrick J. Adults with childhood illnesses: considerations for practice. Berlin: De Gruyter; 2011. https://doi.org/10.1515/9783110255683.
31. Hari P, Pai RG, Varadarajan P. Echocardiographic evaluation of patent foramen ovale and atrial septal defect. Echocardiography. 2015;32(Suppl 2):S110–24.
32. Shub C, Dimopoulos IN, Seward JB, Callahan JA, Tancredi RG, Schattenberg TT, Reeder GS, Hagler DJ, Tajik AJ. Sensitivity of two-dimensional echocardiography in the direct visualization of atrial septal defect utilizing the subcostal approach: experience with 154 patients. J Am Coll Cardiol. 1983;2(1):127–35.
33. Pollick C, Sullivan H, Cujec B, Wilansky S. Doppler color-flow imaging assessment of shunt size in atrial septal defect. Circulation. 1988;78(3):522–8.
34. Rosenzweig BP, Nayar AC, Varkey MP, Kronzon I. Echo contrast-enhanced diagnosis of atrial septal defect. J Am Soc Echocardiogr. 2001;14(2):155–7.
35. Bradley EA, Zaidi AN. Atrial septal defect. Cardiol Clin. 2020;38(3):317–24.
36. Beerbaum P, Körperich H, Esdorn H, Blanz U, Barth P, Hartmann J, Gieseke J, Meyer H. Atrial septal defects in pediatric patients: noninvasive sizing with cardiovascular MR imaging. Radiology. 2003;228(2):361–9.
37. Konstantinides S, Kasper W, Geibel A, Hofmann T, Köster W, Just H. Detection of left-to-right shunt in atrial septal defect by negative contrast echocardiography: a comparison of transthoracic and transesophageal approach. Am Heart J. 1993;126(4):909–17.
38. Seo J-S, Song J-M, Kim Y-H, Park D-W, Lee S-W, Kim W-J, Kim D-H, Kang D-H, Song J-K. Effect of atrial septal defect shape evaluated using three-dimensional transesophageal echocardiography on size measurements for percutaneous closure. J Am Soc Echocardiogr. 2012;25(10):1031–40.
39. Watanabe N, Taniguchi M, Akagi T, Tanabe Y, Toh N, Kusano K, Ito H, Koide N, Sano S. Usefulness of the right parasternal approach to evaluate the morphology of atrial septal defect for transcatheter closure using two-dimensional and three-dimensional transthoracic echocardiography. J Am Soc Echocardiogr. 2012;25(4):376–82.
40. Roberson DA, Cui W, Patel D, Tsang W, Sugeng L, Weinert L, Bharati S, Lang RM. Three-dimensional transesophageal echocardiography of atrial septal defect: a qualitative and quantitative anatomic study. J Am Soc Echocardiogr. 2011;24(6):600–10.
41. Holmvang G, Palacios IF, Vlahakes GJ, Dinsmore RE, Miller SW, Liberthson RR, Block PC, Ballen B, Brady TJ, Kantor HL. Imaging and sizing of atrial septal defects by magnetic resonance. Circulation. 1995;92(12):3473–80.
42. Brenner LD, Caputo GR, Mostbeck G, Steiman D, Dulce M, Cheitlin MD, O'Sullivan M, Higgins CB. Quantification of left to right atrial shunts with velocity-encoded cine nuclear magnetic resonance imaging. J Am Coll Cardiol. 1992;20(5):1246–50.
43. Powell AJ, Tsai-Goodman B, Prakash A, Greil GF, Geva T. Comparison between phase-velocity cine magnetic resonance imaging and invasive oximetry for quantification of atrial shunts. Am J Cardiol. 2003;91(12):1523–5, A9.
44. Teo KSL, Disney PJ, Dundon BK, Worthley MI, Brown MA, Sanders P, Worthley SG. Assessment of atrial septal defects in adults comparing cardiovascular magnetic resonance with transoesophageal echocardiography. J Cardiovasc Magn Reson. 2010;12(1):44.
45. Valverde I, Simpson J, Schaeffter T, Beerbaum P. 4D phase-contrast flow cardiovascular magnetic resonance: comprehensive quantifi-

cation and visualization of flow dynamics in atrial septal defect and partial anomalous pulmonary venous return. Pediatr Cardiol. 2010;31(8):1244–8.

46. Debl K, Djavidani B, Buchner S, Heinicke N, Poschenrieder F, Feuerbach S, Riegger G, Luchner A. Quantification of left-to-right shunting in adult congenital heart disease: phase-contrast cine MRI compared with invasive oximetry. Br J Radiol. 2009;82(977):386–91.

47. da Cruz E, Ivy D, Hraska V, Jaggers J. Pediatric and congenital cardiology, cardiac surgery and intensive care.

48. Baumgartner H, De Backer J, Babu-Narayan SV, Budts W, Chessa M, Diller GP, Lung B, Kluin J, Lang IM, Meijboom F, Moons P, BJM M, Oechslin E, Roos-Hesselink JW, Schwerzmann M, Sondergaard L, Zeppenfeld K, ESC Scientific Document Group. 2020 ESC guidelines for the management of adult congenital heart disease: the task force for the management of adult congenital heart disease of the European Society of Cardiology (ESC). Endorsed by: Association for European Paediatric and Congenital Cardiology (AEPC), International Society for Adult Congenital Heart Disease (ISACHD). Eur Heart J. 2021;42(6):563–645. https://doi.org/10.1093/eurheartj/ehaa554.

49. Tadros V-X, Asgar AW. Atrial septal defect closure with left ventricular dysfunction. EuroIntervention. 2016;12 Suppl X:X13–7.

50. D'Alto M, Romeo E, Argiento P, Correra A, Santoro G, Gaio G, Sarubbi B, Calabrò R, Russo MG. Hemodynamics of patients developing pulmonary arterial hypertension after shunt closure. Int J Cardiol. 2013;168(4):3797–801.

51. Yong G, Khairy P, De Guise P, Dore A, Marcotte F, Mercier L-A, Noble S, Ibrahim R. Pulmonary arterial hypertension in patients with transcatheter closure of secundum atrial septal defects: a longitudinal study. Circ Cardiovasc Interv. 2009;2(5):455–62.

52. Humenberger M, Rosenhek R, Gabriel H, Rader F, Heger M, Klaar U, Binder T, Probst P, Heinze G, Maurer G, Baumgartner H. Benefit of atrial septal defect closure in adults: impact of age. Eur Heart J. 2011;32(5):553–60.

53. Steele PM, Fuster V, Cohen M, Ritter DG, McGoon DC. Isolated atrial septal defect with pulmonary vascular obstructive disease—long-term follow-up and prediction of outcome after surgical correction. Circulation. 1987;76(5):1037–42.

54. Roos-Hesselink JW, Meijboom FJ, Spitaels SEC, van Domburg R, van Rijen EHM, Utens EMWJ, Bogers AJJC, Simoons ML. Excellent survival and low incidence of arrhythmias, stroke and heart failure long-term after surgical ASD closure at young age. A prospective follow-up study of 21-33 years. Eur Heart J. 2003;24(2):190–7.

55. Murphy JG, Gersh BJ, McGoon MD, Mair DD, Porter CJ, Ilstrup DM, McGoon DC, Puga FJ, Kirklin JW, Danielson GK. Long-term outcome after surgical repair of isolated atrial septal defect. Follow-up at 27 to 32 years. N Engl J Med. 1990;323(24):1645–50.

56. Attie F, Rosas M, Granados N, Zabal C, Buendía A, Calderón J. Surgical treatment for secundum atrial septal defects in patients >40 years old. A randomized clinical trial. J Am Coll Cardiol. 2001;38(7):2035–42.

57. Butera G, Carminati M, Chessa M, Youssef R, Drago M, Giamberti A, Pomè G, Bossone E, Frigiola A. Percutaneous versus surgical closure of secundum atrial septal defect: comparison of early results and complications. Am Heart J. 2006;151(1):228–34.

58. Du ZD, Hijazi ZM, Kleinman CS, Silverman NH, Larntz K. Comparison between transcatheter and surgical closure of secundum atrial septal defect in children and adults: results of a multicenter nonrandomized trial. J Am Coll Cardiol. 2002;39(11):1836–44.

59. Fischer G, Stieh J, Uebing A, Hoffmann U, Morf G, Kramer HH. Experience with transcatheter closure of secundum atrial septal defects using the Amplatzer septal occluder: a single centre study in 236 consecutive patients. Heart. 2003;89(2):199–204.

Patent Ductus Arteriosus

Ahmed Dheyaa Al-Obaidi, Sara Shihab Ahmad,
Abeer Mundher Ali, Ali Talib Hashim, Joseph Varney,
Abbas Kamil sh. Khalaf, and Sara Osama Al-Hasani

Abstract

Patent ductus arteriosus (PDA) is the most prevalent congenital heart defect that is caused by the persistent opening of the ductus arteriosus (DA) after birth. The DA is a connection between the aortic artery and the pulmonary artery that allows oxygenated blood from the placenta to bypass the fetal lung and goes to the systemic circulation during fetal development; this normally closes soon after birth. If normal physiologic closure fails to occur, which happens more commonly in premature neonates, the persistent opening is called patent ductus arteriosus (PDA). This leads to the flow of blood from the aorta to the pulmonary artery. The PDA that is wide enough will cause symptoms of respiratory insufficiency, poor growth, tiring easily, and other respiratory infections; however, if the PDA is not large enough, it may be asymptomatic. Diagnosis is done by (A) physical examination, findings including increased precordial activity, widened pulse pressure, S2 splitting, and a thrill may be presented, and the hallmark physical finding for PDA is a continuous murmur, located at the upper left sternal border, also called "machinery" murmur. There are many differential diagnoses including coronary artery fistula, ventricular septal defect (VSD), and aortic regurgitation. Management of PDA depends on age and other factors. It can be treated by medical treatment including intravenous (IV) indomethacin or ibuprofen, diuretics, and percutaneous catheterization, or by surgical ligation in cases of medical closure failure or it is contraindicated.

Keywords

Patent ductus arteriosus · Congenital defect · Physiologic closure · Premature neonate · Respiratory insufficiency Continuous murmur · Percutaneous catheterization Surgical ligation

Introduction

Patent ductus arteriosus (PDA) is of the most prevalent congenital heart anomalies. It results in persistent contact between the thoracic aorta (descending part) and the pulmonary artery because of improper ductal closure of the fetal circulation. PDA is a medical condition in which, after birth, the ductus arteriosus fails to close. This failure to close enables a portion of oxygenated blood from the aorta to flow back to the lungs through the pulmonary artery due to the elevated aortic pressure. Symptoms are rare at birth and immediately afterward, but sometimes it may manifest at the onset of increased breathing work around the end of the first year and the inability to gain weight at a standard rate.

In newborns with chronic respiratory issues such as hypoxia, PDA is more prevalent, with an increased incidence in premature newborns. Owing to the underdevelopment of the heart and lungs, premature newborns with a PDA are more likely to be hypoxic. PDA has also been shown to occur, and other cardiac abnormalities must be considered at the time of diagnosis. However, treatment varies based on the associated disease. If, in addition to the PDA, the transposition of large vessels is present, the PDA is not surgically closed because it is the only way oxygenated blood into circulation. Prostaglandins are used to maintain the PDA in these situations, while NSAIDs are not given until the surgical repair of the two defects has been completed [1].

A. D. Al-Obaidi · S. S. Ahmad · A. M. Ali · A. K. sh. Khalaf
S. O. Al-Hasani
College of Medicine, University of Baghdad, Baghdad, Iraq
e-mail: abbas.kamel1700b@comed.uobaghdad.edu.iq

A. T. Hashim (✉)
Golestan University of Medical Sciences, Gorgan, Iran

J. Varney
American University of the Caribbean School of Medicine,
St. Maarten, the Netherlands

PDA was initially mentioned by Galen at the start of the first century. However, the first time that an operation was done on the ducturs was in 1888 when Munro dissected and ligated it in an infant corpse. Fifty years later, Robert E. Gross successfully ligated a 7-year-old boy with a PDA. In the history of medicine, this was a pivotal occurrence as it opened the doors for the field of congenital heart surgery [2].

Anatomy

The ductus arteriosus (DA) is an essential structure of fetal circulation during fetal life that enables the blood that leaves the right ventricle to flow into the descending aorta bypassing the pulmonary circulation. It supplies part of the blood that will be delivered to the rest of the systems and organs of the fetus. Usually, the pulmonary vascular bed passes through just about 10% of the correct ventricular output. DA is an embryological remnant of the distal sixth aortic arch, which, near the stem of the left subclavian artery, connects the pulmonary artery to the proximal descending aorta. It travels from the pulmonary artery's anterior aspect to the aorta's posterior aspect [3].

The recurrent laryngeal nerve is an anatomic marker of the DA, which usually emerges anterior and caudal to the ductus, from the vagus nerve. It subsequently loops around the ductus to ascend posterior to the aorta on its way to the larynx. Due to its close approximation, it is the anatomical structure most often damaged in ductal ligation. Other anatomically proximal components less often damaged include the thoracic duct and the phrenic nerve [4].

The normal anatomy of the ductus may not be found in the case of complex congenital heart defects. In combination with complex aortic arch anomalies, anatomical irregularities may differ widely and are prevalent. While performing a surgery, the aorta, the carotid artery, and the pulmonary artery are among the structures that have been confused for the PDA. For this reason, surgeries need to apply a heightened sense of awareness when attempting to locate the PDA. Classification of the DA is determined by its side by using an angiograph. The DA may be right, left, or both. A Lt-DA during fetal development is considered a regular structure. The presence of a Rt-DA, however, is frequently seen with congenital anomalies, such as conotruncal development and aortic arch anomalies. Another classification is the Krichenko classification, which includes five types: "type A (conical), type B (window), type C (tubular), type D (complex), and type E (elongated)" [5].

Pathophysiology

During fetal life, the DA is usually patent. The DA is responsible for much of the Rt ventricular outflow from week 6 of fetal life and onward, leading to 60% of the overall cardiac production in fetal life. In the lungs, just around 5–10% of the outflow passes in. The presence of prostaglandin E2 (PGE2) encourages maintaining the patency of the DA. Before birth, ductal closure may consequently cause the failure of the right side of the fetal heart [6].

Thus, a PDA induces a shunt from left to right as it creates a route for the passage of blood from the systemic to the pulmonary circulation. Therefore, blood will flow in excessive amounts through the lungs (see the image below). The consequence of pulmonary engorgement is diminished pulmonary compliance. The pulmonary vasculature's response to the increased flow of blood is unpredictable.

Relatively few variables depend on the extent of the excess pulmonary blood flow. The greater the internal diameter of the narrowest parts of the DA, the wider the shunt from Lt to Rt. If the DA is restricting, then the magnitude of the shunt also affects the length of the narrowed region. A longer DA is associated with a minor shunt. Finally, the pulmonary vascular resistance relationship to systemic vascular resistance partly regulates the extent of the left-to-right shunt [5, 6].

The flow through the ductus arteriosus is theoretically great if the SVR is high with or without the PVR being low. The direction of blood in a typical PDA is as follows: "PDA, pulmonary arteries, pulmonary capillaries, pulmonary veins, left atrium, left ventricle, and aorta." Therefore, a wide Lt-to-Rt shunt in a PDA can result in Lt-sided cardiomegaly. A sufficiently large PDA can also dilate the pulmonary veins and the ascending aorta [6].

Functional Closure

As the placenta is removed at birth, a significant source of prostaglandin will be lost; furthermore, when the lungs expand, their ability to metabolize prostaglandins will begin. Moreover, oxygen tension in the blood markedly increases with the onset of natural respiration. With this operation, pulmonary vascular resistance decreases. In healthy infants born at term, functional closure of the DA ideally occurs within approximately 15 h. This is caused by a sudden contraction of the DA, which is associated with an increment in (PO_2) coinciding with the first-taken breath. Blood will flow preferentially into the lungs away from the DA [7].

When functional closure of the DA completely occurs and the PVR/SVR < 1, some of the remaining Lt-to-Rt flow will pass in a route starting at the aorta to the DA and eventually into the pulmonary arteries. Despite the fact that the Da of the neonate appears to be majorly responsive to changes in arterial oxygen stress, the exact reasons for closure or persistent patency are complex and include "the autonomic nervous system, ductal musculature manipulation, and chemical mediators." The vascular tone of the ductus is determined by a balance of factors that trigger relaxation and contraction. The high levels of prostaglandin, nitric oxide development, and hypoxemia in the ductus are significant factors that induce relaxation.

Increased PO_2 and endothelin-1, decreased prostaglandin levels and PGE receptors, and increased norepinephrine, bradykinin, and acetylcholine are all factors that favor contraction. Increased prostaglandin sensitivity, combined with hypoxia-causing pulmonary immaturity, leads to increased PDA incidence in premature neonates. Proper anatomical closure can take several weeks to occur, in which the DA can no longer reopen. In 2–3 weeks, the second stage of closure associated with fibrous intima proliferation is complete. PDA typically manifests in infants who are at least 3 months old [8].

In a full-term baby, spontaneous closure after 5 months is uncommon. Patients with a large PDA who are left untreated may develop Eisenmenger syndrome, in which the PVR/SVR > 1, and the usual LT-to-Rt shunting reverses in the Rt-to-Lt direction. The development of this syndrome is considered a contraindication to PDA closure, and the only hope for long-term survival may be lung transplantation. Due to poor prostaglandin metabolism in immature lungs, failure of DA contraction in preterm babies is largely due to high levels of prostaglandins rather than musculature defects. The loss of DA contraction in full-term neonates will most likely be caused by asphyxia or hypoxemia, high pulmonary blood flow, kidney failure, and respiratory disorders [8].

Induction and expression of cyclooxygenase (COX)-2 (an isoform of prostaglandins generating COX) could also prevent ductal closure. Ductal smooth muscle relaxation is caused by activating G protein-coupled EP4 receptors by PGE2. The decrease in prostaglandin levels results in ductus arteriosus constriction during late gestation. The intimate cushions thus come into contact with the ductus lumen and occlude it.

Risk factors include:

- Premature birth
- Genetic conditions such as Down syndrome
- Congenital rubella infections

Epidemiology

In the United States, PDA incidence is approximately

- 0.02–0.005% of live births in **term children**
- 20% in **preterm > 32 weeks** and up **to 60% in those <28 weeks**
- 30% in LBW infants (<2.5 kg)

In addition, the female:male ratio is 2:1 in cases where the PDA is not accompanied by other risk factors. But, in patients with specific teratogenic risk factors (i.e., infection with congenital rubella), the female: male ratio becomes 1:1.

Prognosis

Patients with no additional anomalies other than the ODA tend to follow an excellent prognostic course. Premature infants, however, usually have different sequelae of prematurity that negatively affect their prognosis. Closure of the PDA in those older than 3 months rarely occurs spontaneously. In contrast, this occurs at a rate of 72–75% in premature infants. Generally, after closure, patients' symptoms resolve, and no additional cardiac sequelae develop. On the other hand, premature infants who experience a significant PDA have the risk of the development of bronchopulmonary dysplasia.

Morbidity

Congestive heart failure (CHF) may develop if a large PDA is left untreated. Another concern is the development of pulmonary hypertension [9].

Mortality

Children with large shunts have lower survival rates. Mortality is evidently low in patients with PDA (except in premature infant). Left untreated, mortality for PDA is estimated to be around 20% for patients who are 20 years, 42% for those who are 45 years, and 60% for those who are 60 years. The surgical mortality rate is 20–41% among premature infants [8, 10].

Signs and Symptoms

In the first few days of life, a premature neonate can develop life-threatening pulmonary over-circulation depending mainly on the PDA width, pulmonary vascular resistance (PVR), and gestational age of the neonate. This is different from the presentation in adults, especially for whom PDA is small in size as they may present simply with a newly discovered murmur. Children with PDA are typically asymptomatic. They may experience reduced exercise tolerance (as a result of pulmonary congestion) in addition to a murmur discovered during physical examination. Tachypnea, weakness or feeding difficulty, diaphoresis, and abnormal growth can occur in infants from 3 weeks to 6 weeks old [10].

A moderate-to-large Lt-to-Rt shunt of the DA can be associated with a "hoarse scream, cough," atelectasis, or lower respiratory tract infections such as pneumonia. Failure to prosper may also occur. Apparent symptoms of heart failure may occur; however, these are rare. Adults with undiagnosed PDA may have heart failure-related symptoms, arrhythmia, especially atrial, or even differential cyanosis of the lower limbs, suggesting pulmonary to systemic shunting of non-oxygenated blood. PDA patients can be variable in appearance. Based on physical inspection at birth, typically, patients look healthy and have normal breathing and heart rates. When the blood pressure is collected, a broadened pulse pressure can be noted. There may be prominent suprasternal or carotid pulsations [10].

On examination, these findings exist:

1. Precordial activity is increased if the left-to-right shunt increases as the shunt increases.
2. Apical impulse is displaced, usually laterally. Suprasternal notch or left infraclavicular palpation may reveal a thrill.
3. Usually, there will be an unchanged first heart sound (S1), and the second heart sound (S2) will be distorted by murmur; phonocardiograph evidence from the past indicated that they might be paradoxical S2 splitting and a prolonged duration of ejection through the aortic valve.
4. Ejection systolic murmur is the typical murmur to be expected; nevertheless, a murmur of crescendo/decrescendo character extending to diastole may also occur.
5. Auscultation of the PDA sometimes shows multiple clicks or sounds resembling shaking dice or a bag of rocks.

Bounding of peripheral pulses may be evident. This is linked to the amount of elevated left ventricular stroke volume, which leads to elevated systolic blood pressures. As blood flows away from the aorta into the pulmonary circulation, bounding pulses are caused by low diastolic pressure in the systemic circulation. Diagnosing a PDA on auscultation in a low-birth-weight premature infant can be difficult. Babies with the more serious "hyaline membrane disease (HMD)" may have a greater prevalence of PDA. The exact reason for this is yet unknown. The classic symptoms of a PDA are typically absent in a low-birth-weight premature infant. Rarely is the classic constant murmur heard upon auscultation. There may be a "rough systolic murmur" along the left sternal line. Still, there may be no murmur in a tiny baby with a wide PDA and severe pulmonary over-circulation.

It is essential to differentiate between clinically relevant PDA and non-significant PDAs. PDAs that are clinically relevant are characterized by breathing difficulties, tachycardia, bounding pulses, and metabolic acidosis associated with pulmonary congestion. The shunt from Lt-to-Rt leads to a wide range of possible complications, such as intra-ventricular hemorrhage, chronic lung disease, narcotizing enterocolitis, and even death. Importantly, the symptom of CHF should not be mistaken for upper respiratory infection (URI).

Diagnosis of PDA

PDA diagnosis is majorly based on thorough clinical assessment, including physical examination for murmur, standard electrocardiographic (ECG) anomalies, radiographical findings, and echocardiographic/Doppler performance. The critical diagnostic study used to evaluate PDA is echocardiography. Alternatively, more novel diagnostic methods are magnetic resonance angiography and cardiac computed tomography. Generally, laboratory findings are not beneficial in the workup of a PDA. Yet, to assess the infant's overall health, a complete blood picture (CBP) is obtained. Findings in patients with this condition are, however, usually within reference ranges. If the child has other congenital heart defects, polycythemia may be present. The study of pulse oximetry/arterial blood gas (ABG) typically indicates normal saturation due to pulmonary over-circulation. Hypoxemia and hypercarbia from CHF and air-space disease (pulmonary edema or atelectasis) may be caused by a large ductus arteriosus [9].

Echocardiography

The echocardiographic results for PDA are usually diagnostic. Color flow Doppler imaging can accurately detect high-speed turbulent flow jets in the pulmonary artery; even the tiny PDA is sensitive to this technique. It is rare to rely on alternate imaging methods to make the diagnosis of this disorder. In addition, information on related congenital cardiovascular malformations can be provided. The aortic end of the PDA is first localized by two-dimensional (2D) echocardiography and then traced back to the pulmonary artery. It is challenging to record precisely the scale, form, and direction of the ductus. In the parasternal short-axis perspective and from the suprasternal notch, the PDA can be seen most clearly.

Doppler echocardiography shows steady drainage from the aorta into the main pulmonary artery if no other anomalies are present. If the magnitude of the Lt-to-Rt shunt is high, continued flow around the arch of the aorta to the DA in diastole plus reversal of flow in the descending part of the aorta may be noticed. Higher flow rates in the pulmonary veins are noticeable as the shunt amplitude rises and the left atrium enlarges. The left ventricular size often increases as the shunt magnitude increases.

Chest Radiography

Chest radiograph results vary from normal to showing findings of CHF. Cardiomegaly can be seen. When there is a substantial Lt-to-Rt shunt through the PDA, chest films are widened by the pulmonary veins and arteries in addition to the left atrium and ventricle. The ascending aorta may also be prominent. These will not be seen until the "pulmonary to systemic circulation (QP/QS) ratio" reaches 2:1. A high pulmonary artery pressure may be seen initially as a prominence of the main pulmonary artery. Marked pulmonary overcirculation is seen as pulmonary edema. It is possible to observe accentuated pulmonary vascular markings in the periphery of the lung field and expanded venous markings. The PDA may calcify in elderlies and show on ordinary radiographs [9].

Electrocardiography

The ECG findings are usually normal when the PDA is small. With a larger PDA, hypertrophy of the Lt ventricle may be present. With broad shunts, left atrial enlargement can also be present. There may be proof of right ventricular hypertrophy in the case of severe pulmonary hypertension. Inversion of T-wave and depression of ST-segment may be present in neonates, especially premature neonates with a large PDA, suggesting ischemia or a supply-demand mismatch.

Angiography and Catheterization

Cardiac catheterization and angiography are not usually needed for uncomplicated PDA. In detecting a tiny PDA, the more sensitive method than cardiac catheterization is color flow Doppler mapping. However, if the diagnosis needs to be confirmed in children with other congenital cardiovascular malformations and/or established pulmonary hypertension, cardiac catheterization may be required; pulmonary vasodilator response may be essential in planning surgical intervention.

Catheterization can be used as a therapeutic procedure using coil embolization and as a method to illustrate the following:

- Shunt and its amount
- Pressure in the pulmonary circulation
- Other possible cardiac malformations

Pulmonary artery oxygen saturation is high during a right heart catheterization, except in Eisenmenger syndrome. To assess the occurrence of any vascular pulmonary pathology and the size of the DA, the PVR and shunt (Qp/Qs) can be computed. The definitive method for assessing the presence and scale of the ductus is selective angiography. Angiography, when other abnormalities are suspected, is often used to describe intracardiac anatomy [10].

Managements

The spontaneous closure of a PDA is normal. Therapy is typically prudent if severe respiratory failure or impaired systemic supply of oxygen is present. Intravenous (IV) indomethacin (or newer IV ibuprofen preparation) is also beneficial for the closure of a PDA if given during the first 10–14 days of existence. Catheter closure and surgical ligation, which requires a thoracotomy, are other options. Health management also includes improving the symptoms of CHF. CHF is an indicator that the PDA in infancy is closed. If medical treatment is inadequate, immediate action should be performed to close the system.

Due to the possibility of bacterial endocarditis linked to the open structure, it is suggested that all PDA should eventually be closed. The high pulmonary blood flow hastens the occurrence of obstructive pulmonary vascular disease over time, which is ultimately lethal. The most essential requirement before pharmacological or surgical closure of the PDA is the detection of additional anomalies in the cardiac system such as interrupted aortic arch or aortic-coarctation or pulmonary atresia. Prostaglandin inhibitors (e.g., nonsteroidal anti-inflammatory drugs [NSAIDs]) are one of the ways used to close the DA when surgical ligation is not indicated. A ductal-based lesion necessitates the persistence of a PDA to maintain optimal pulmonary blood flow. Specific interventions for the treatment of a patient with suspected PDA in prehospital and emergency department (ED) consist of oxygen supply via a mask for hypoxia, maintaining adequate respiration in addition to supportive care. Other steps in the form of fluid and sodium restriction as well as the correction of any anemia are also needed. Patients showing signs of florid CHF must be initially stabilized with positive pressure ventilation and diuretics, then transfer to a tertiary care center is mandatory. It may be best to consult a pediatric cardiologist and a pediatric cardiovascular surgeon. Since patients with a PDA are typically asymptomatic, there is no need for acute management. However, before the patency of the ductus is corrected, American Heart Association suggested administering antibiotics in patients for the prevention of bacterial endocarditis during cases of elevated exposure to bacteremia (e.g., instrumentation, dental procedures). Conservative standards require ventilation adjustment by minimizing inspiratory time and providing more supportive expiratory end pressure (PEEP). In addition, fluid limits, which are at most 130 mL/kg/day beyond day three, are also used. This approach has been found to have a high PDA-closure rate.

Standard care with digoxin and diuretic medication generally palliates the condition of CHF-suffering infants. These kids should be treated for ductal closure when they are older (a few years old, for the least) and are successful candidates. Should medical management of CHF fail, patients are essentially referred for early surgical PDA closure. PDA closure is activated by prostaglandin synthesis inhibitor administration, such as indomethacin (0.1 mg/kg body weight) given orally three times per day (every 8 h). This procedure is beneficial in premature infants suffering from "respiratory distress syndrome" exacerbated by Lt-to-Rt shunting through the DA. Intravenous (IV) indomethacin or ibuprofen is typically used to treat premature neonates with severe PDA. In most patients, this has been quite effective. It is unclear if outcomes with indomethacin given by IV route are superior to those with PDA surgical closure, except in premature neonates, where the procedure's safety is a concern. The standard drug treatment was IV indomethacin. The US Food and Drug Association then approved IV ibuprofen (FDA). While ibuprofen and indomethacin are similarly powerful, the occurrence of intraventricular hemorrhage tends to be decreased by indomethacin, but less kidney-related toxicity is seen with ibuprofen [7, 8].

Indomethacin

Indomethacin has proven efficient, leading to the spontaneous closure rate being twice as high. In newborns (4 in number) with a birth weight of 1500–2075 g who were delivered at 35 weeks gestation or more, McCarthy et al. demonstrated the promising effects of indomethacin on PDA. In 13 PDA-suffering patients whose condition was complicated by congenital heart disease, Watanabe et al. evaluated indomethacin therapy and confirmed the closure in 4 of 7 infants with a 2500 g or more birth weight. Indomethacin is effective in both scenarios; the DA can reopen after a few days or weeks. It was also observed that prophylactic indomethacin reduces the occurrence of extreme grades of intracranial hemorrhage. Indomethacin's side effects include vasoconstriction of the blood vessels in the brain.

Ibuprofen

Prophylactic ibuprofen is commonly used as well. The dosage used for ibuprofen is 10 mg/kg of bolus, followed by two additional days of 5 mg/kg/day. Ibuprofen, in preterm infants, carries a relatively lower risk of oliguria as compared with indomethacin. One research, however, observed a higher prevalence of developing pulmonary hypertension. "The Cochrane ibuprofen prophylaxis evaluation" found that while ibuprofen prophylaxis lowers PDA occurrence on day 3, possible adverse effects such as neurodevelopmental problems may develop. The closure of PDA is dependent on gestation, with a 65% cumulative closure rate.

Diuretics

While diuretics and fluid restriction have been suggested to treat symptomatic newborns, this method is not supported by rigorously collected evidence. A systematic review of the use of furosemide in preterm neonates suffering from "respiratory distress syndrome" has demonstrated benefits in the long term that are negligible and a higher rate of symptomatic DA-syndrome development. Infants with signs of failure can be managed at the beginning with diuretics and digoxin, but definitive therapy involves interruption of the ductus.

Catheterization

It is becoming more popular to use the percutaneous route to close the PDA. Transcatheter occlusion is an essential surgical intervention alternative and is now seen as the main treatment for the majority of cases of PDA. In the first few months of life, most patients with PDA alone will have effective catheterization. The most popular treatment for patent ductus arteriosus after the first birthday is occlusion at the time of cardiac catheterization. Additionally, as catheterization procedures advance, the potential to fix abnormalities in smaller newborns has been demonstrated with a high rate of success. For PDA occlusion, many methods and equipment have been used, but conclusive closure rates are not comparable to surgery rates. The patient's size contains contraindications for catheter-based closure [9, 10].

Amplatzer Duct Occluder

More recently, the ability to close PDA during cardiac catheterization has been expanded by the Amplatzer system. This instrument is more stable and more accessible to implant than spring occluding coils in a large PDA. The major downside of the design is that, particularly in children, the aortic portion of the system can project into the aorta and block some of its lumen. Nevertheless, for the treatment of all forms of PDA, the "Amplatzer duct occluder II (ADO II)," a nitinol mesh that is highly flexible and comfortable to use flexible with a symmetrical shape, was approved in Europe.

Rashkind Ductus Occlusion Device

This device consists of either the transvenous or transarterial pathway of a two-umbrella system administered to the ductus. This treatment has an established rate of successful occlusion of 83%.

Surgical Ligation

The standard treatment for large PDA requiring care in infancy remains surgical ligation or surgical ligation and separation. When performed by an experienced pediatric cardiovascular surgeon, this is an incredibly effective, low-risk procedure. This is true even in the tiniest of premature infants. A left posterolateral thoracotomy can be performed by PDA ligation (with or without division) without the need for cardiopulmonary bypass. PDA ligation with "video-assisted thoracoscopic surgery (VATS)" is less invasive, effective, and safe.

The presence of a PDA is, with few exceptions, a sign for surgical closure. The presence of other congenital heart lesions that impede pulmonary blood flow must be paid attention to. In these patients, all possible ways should be tried to maintain ductal flow before a definitive repair can be performed or a permanent shunt can be built. Surgical closure is still needed for very tiny premature infants. In children, repair may be urgent in the case of an asymptomatic patient with evidence of heart or respiratory failure that is not sufficiently managed by medication or may be delayed in an asymptomatic or well-controlled patient receiving medical care.

If a patient is not older than 3 years and PDA closure is done, postoperative outcomes are best. However, for older patients, higher PVR and pulmonary hypertension occurs. Severe pulmonary vascular disease is the main contraindication for repair. Suppose the PDA transient intraoperative occlusion did not lower the high pulmonary arterial pressure with a corresponding increment in aortic pressure. In that case, the closure must be carefully carried out with the possibility of it becoming contraindicated. Ductal closure does not alleviate preexisting pulmonary vascular disease. Surgical ligation problems are often associated with left lateral thoracotomy. Mortality and morbidity caused by surgery are practically nonexistent. However, it is important to note careful approach must be exercised due to the possibility of injuring the pulmonary artery, aorta, and other structures [5, 6].

Hospitalization

Hospitalization is usually minimal. Patients who undergo PDA catheter closure are typically sent home the same day as the operation. Even patients who undergo a regular thoracotomy procedure are rarely hospitalized for more than 2–3 days. Based on defects in other organ systems, the proper treatment and duration of premature neonates' hospitalization are determined.

Multiple Choice Questions

1. The pulse pressure for a newborn with patent ductus arteriosus would be:
   A. Wide
   B. Normal
   C. Fluctuating
   D. Narrow
   Answer is: C.
   The pulse pressure will be widened. Because of left-to-right shunting, the diastolic pressure will be low (due to blood runoff from the aorta into the pulmonary arteries), which will widen the difference between systolic and diastolic pressure.

2. Closure of PDA in a premature infant can be stimulated by administration of:
   A. Indomethacin
   B. Estrogen
   C. Prostaglandin analog
   D. Prostaglandin inhibitors
   Answer is: D.
   Prostaglandin inhibitors. DA normally closes soon after birth. The effect of prostaglandin is what maintains its patency in fetal life. Thus, when there is delayed closure of DA, we can use prostaglandin inhibitors to induce DA closure.

3. Which one is a risk factor for PDA?
   A. Meningococci
   B. Maternal rubella infection
   C. Late-term birth
   D. Male gender
   Answer is: B.

Rubella virus can cross the placenta and then spread through the baby's circulation, causing damage to the blood vessels and heart and other organs.

4. A murmur developed after day 6 of life of a 28-week gestation preterm baby. The physician reported it as a continuous murmur on the left clavicle. What is the appropriate further action?
   A. Measure the JVP
   B. Measure the systolic and diastolic blood pressure
   C. Perform an ECG
   D. Do a complete blood count test
   Answer is: B.
   With these symptoms, a low diastolic BP (wide pulse pressure) is almost diagnostic for PDA.

5. A 7-day-old preterm baby was diagnosed with having a PDA. This defect causes
   A. Diabetes mellitus
   B. Rt-to-Lt shunt
   C. Lt-to-Rt shunt
   D. Aortic stenosis
   Answer is: C.
   Left to right shunt

6. The most common cardiovascular anomaly in the neonatal period is?
   A. Patent ductus arteriosus
   B. Ventricular septal defect
   C. Mitral atresia
   D. Atrial septal defect
   Answer is: A.
   Patent ductus arteriosus is the most common anomaly in neonates.

7. Persistence of a patent ductus arteriosus after birth causes:
   A. Systolic murmur
   B. Right sternal border murmur
   C. Gallop rhythm
   D. Continuous murmur
   Answer is: D.
   PDA causes a continuous murmur that begins in systolic and continuous into diastole through the second heart sound.

8. Which one of the following is not true regarding PDA?
   A. Deoxygenated blood passes to systemic arteries.
   B. The PDA connects the pulmonary artery and the aorta.
   C. Blood is shunted from the aorta to the pulmonary trunk.
   D. It is essential for fetal development.

Answer is: A.
In PDA, the oxygenated blood that is pushed into the aorta during contraction of the heart, part of it crosses into the pulmonary trunk, causing pulmonary circulation overflow.

9. PDA is best diagnosed by:
   A. Echocardiography
   B. Arterial blood gas test
   C. Ultrasonography
   D. CT scan
   Answer is: A.
   Echocardiography is usually diagnostic for PDA. Even tiny PDA are sensitive.

10. A 5-day-old neonate is suspected of having PDA. Which ECG findings will support the diagnosis?
    A. ST-segment elevation
    B. T-wave inversion and ST-segment depression
    C. Wide QRS complex
    D. ST-segment depression
    Answer is: B.
    T-wave inversion and ST-segment depression may be present in neonates, especially premature neonates with a large PDA, suggesting ischemia or a supply–demand mismatch.

References

1. Clyman RI, et al. PDA-TOLERATE trial: an exploratory randomized controlled trial of treatment of moderate-to-large patent ductus arteriosus at 1 week of age. J Pediatr. 2019;205:41–8.
2. Sung SI, et al. Effect of nonintervention vs oral ibuprofen in patent ductus arteriosus in preterm infants: a randomized clinical trial. JAMA Pediatr. 2020;174(8):755–63.
3. Smith A, El-Khuffash AF. Defining "haemodynamic significance" of the patent ductus arteriosus: do we have all the answers? Neonatology. 2020;117(2):225–32.
4. Gillam-Krakauer M, Reese J. Diagnosis and management of patent ductus arteriosus. Neoreviews. 2018;19(7):e394–402.
5. van Laere D, et al. Application of neonatologist performed echocardiography in the assessment of a patent ductus arteriosus. Pediatr Res. 2018;84(1):46–56.
6. Mitra S, McNamara PJ. Patent ductus arteriosus—time for a definitive trial. Clin Perinatol. 2020;47(3):617–39.
7. Clyman RI. Patent ductus arteriosus, its treatments, and the risks of pulmonary morbidity. Semin Perinatol. 2018;42(4):235–42.
8. Deshpande, Poorva, et al. "Patent ductus arteriosus: the physiology of transition." Semin Fetal Neonatal Med. 23(4). 2018:225-231.
9. Härkin P, et al. Morbidities associated with patent ductus arteriosus in preterm infants. Nationwide cohort study. J Matern Fetal Neonatal Med. 2018;31(19):2576–83.
10. Sathanandam SK, et al. Amplatzer piccolo occluder clinical trial for percutaneous closure of the patent ductus arteriosus in patients ≥700 grams. Catheter Cardiovasc Interv. 2020;96(6):1266–76.

The Coarctation of Aorta

Ameer Almamoury

Abstract

Congenital anomaly narrowing of descending aorta is just distal to the subclavian artery typically. Asymptomatic patient present delay by hypertension and headache, also the symptoms appear in adult life. Brachial femoral pulse delay is demonstrated on the physical exam (appearance) . Because of the blood flow through a constricted aorta, the systolic murmur is heard on the left intraclavicular. If the collateral vessels present the murmur, due to the ventricle hypertrophy the fourth heart sound and gallop may be heard and present. Turner syndrome is associated with this anomaly. May be acquired as Takayasu arteritis which is rare. The pseudotype is located typically at the thoracic aorta. There is claudication in the lower limp and hypertensitivity will develop at the upper limp. The ECHO diagnostic confirmation of the disease is also the angiography. The two option for the treatment is balloon angioplasty and stent placement procedure. Also, surgery required for the special case will be discussed later in this chapter.

Keywords

Cardiology · Coarctation · Aorta · Hypertension · Pseudo coarctation · Turner syndrome · Brachio-femoral pulse · Aortic kink · Suprasternal notch · Heart failure · Balloon angioplasty

Introduction

The eccentric narrowness of the aorta on the posterolateral wall is due to internal ridge or shelf and the ridge is composed of similar tissue of the muscular arterial ductus. Common type is the bridge type and less commonly the constriction extends beyond the subclavian artery [1].

Pathophysiology

CoA during the different physiological stages of life has multiple pathological effects on the clinical outcome and hemodynamically change. So in utero does not cause hemodynamic change and problem, by the presence of the PDA the blood will pass and shunt the stenotic and narrowing area but after birth when the opening of the foramen ovale and PDA start to close the blood flow will be affected by presence of constrict area of aorta on the lower extremities [2]. With this change the hemodynamics of the patient will start to decline and range from mild to severe, also the severity of the condition depends mainly on the presence of other congenital defects. During this pathological change and the physiological difference, the heart starts to compensate to estimate the maximum function and restore the physiological mechanism, including myocardial hypertrophy and the development of collateral artery. The collateral blood flow by involving intercostal and internal mammary artery and another close by artery to shunt and circumvents the stenotic area. Time is major effecter to form the collateral vessels, so in neonatal life if the constriction is severe the symptoms will be developed (Figs. 1 and 2).

A. Almamoury (✉)
Al Qadisiyah College of Medicine, Al Diwaniyah, Iraq
e-mail: med-16.13@qu.edu.iq

© The Author(s), under exclusive license to Springer Nature Switzerland AG 2023
G. Tagarakis et al. (eds.), *Clinical and Surgical Aspects of Congenital Heart Diseases*,
https://doi.org/10.1007/978-3-031-23062-2_7

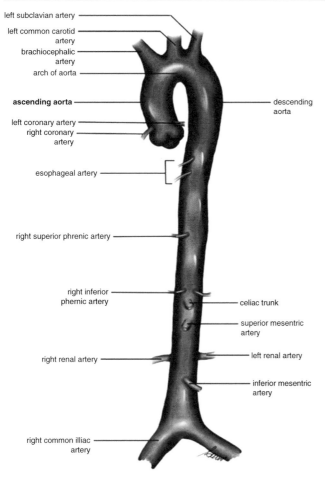

Fig. 1 The normal anatomy of the aorta

Diagnosis

History

More incidence is observed in the male population. Turner syndrome defect X chromosome and because of the sterility in this patient the coarctation cannot be trans [3]. From September to November the peak incidence of the coarctation is found and also from January to March. Produce significant symptoms in early infancy and after the third decade of life. The acute symptoms appear in the infant after the ductus close. More than one-third of the survivors die by the second decade of life and about 50% of them die in the third decade, three-fourth live until the fifth decade. Some report shows survival at 74 years and 76 years [4, 5].

Mild coarctation is always benign but severe cases are always symptomatic. In the early diagnosis, some patient tends to be well clinically so some suspicion required more than measure or get attention to the upper and lower blood pressure. The chief cause of mortality and morbidity is hypertension [6–12]. The incidence of heart failure is high in the infant and less in adult hypertension is verse versa. Ninety percent of infancy with coarctation expire little or no problem. Just in the second of the close of the ductus the blood flows into the lung and the femoral pulse disappears. In Turner syndrome, trisomy 13, 18, 21, 22, 23 XO rupture occurs due to inherent medial abnormality [13–21]. Pseudo coarctation is also reported in this syndrome and gonadal dysgenesis of Turner syndrome is reported that increases atherosclerotic events [22].

Fig. 2 Coarctation of the aorta

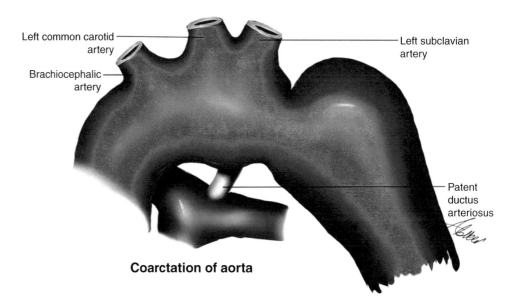

Coarctation of aorta

Physical Examination

Every Turner patient should suspect the coarctation of the aorta and systemic hypertension occurs with or without coarctation and Turner's distinctive appearance [13, 23–29].

In the typical XO phenotype Turner female with short status and neck webbing, scanty pubic and axillary hair, broad chest, inverted nipple, small chin, cubitus valgus, short metacarpal and metatarsal, narrow nail, pigmented cutaneous nevus is also exhibited. The Turner infant exhibit lymphedema of the neck [30–37]. Congenital heart disease on the turner with webbing of the neck more than without webbing! Noonan syndrome is associated only with coarctation of the aorta [22].

Arteril Pulse

Few misdiagnoses can be emerged if we take care of this hallmark and comparison between the upper and lower pressure. Normal arterial blood pressure is based on gender and age. Measurement of blood pressure should be part of regular routine physical examination [30, 38–44]. A pregnant female with coarctation shows a similar fluctuation in blood pressure compared to the uncomplicated pregnant who exhibit toxemia lower than other hypertensive diseases. Pregnant women increase the risk of aortic rupture [22].

Ausculation

The murmur is prominent if the collateral is well-developed. Collateral murmur is crescendo-decrescendo because collateral originating away from the heart has delayed onset. In young children, collateral well-develops without murmur. Adult collateral murmur is conspicuous. The coarctation itself is responsible for systolic murmur size and the location of the coarctation correlates with the murmur. In infant the murmur is absent [45–49]. Heart failure causes the murmur to decrease. Posterior auscultation begins in the midline of the upper thoracic to the mid and lower of the thoracic spine. If the diameter decreases to 2.5 cm the murmur occupies all of the cardiac cycle. Loud brachiocephalic murmur is accompanied by a thrill. The murmur of the abdominal coarctation was heard anteriorly in the epigastrium. Pseudo coarctation creates systolic murmur posterior to the site of the aortic kink [50].

ECG

Electrocardiogram pattern is related to two age groups: the first is symptomatically neonatal coarctation. Coarctation after children is the second group. The mean QRS axis in adult is normal [51–57].

X-Ray

In asymptomatic patient the x-ray is normal [58–62]. X-ray in symptomatic infant discloses pulmonary venous congestion with dilation of the right ventricle. The descending thoracic aorta lining the run parallel to the left edge. One of the classical radiologic signs of the aorta is the notching of the ribs notch which vary from patient to patient and may be single, multiple, shallow, and deep [63]. The notch seldom occurs before 6 years [64]. The notch between the third and the eighth ribs is bilaterally typical for the coarctation distal to the left subclavian artery. In older children and adults with coarctation, the ascending aorta is markedly dilated. In turner syndrome, the ascending aorta may be aneurysmal [65].

Echocardiogram

In order to analyse the ascending aorta segment by segment, transthoracic and transesophageal echo with a doppler scan is used also the brachiocephalic artery, aortic isthmus can be visualized. A long segment of luminal narrowing can be identified as suprasternal notch window with color flow imaging identified as the coarctation. The persistent high-velocity diastolic forward flow indicates the severity [66, 67].

Management

Early Management

The treatment of the coarctation is mainly by surgery or intervention. When arterial hypertension is present the option of the stent is still possible. The main effector on the choice of procedure is stenosis and another associated anomaly [68].

Surgical Treatment

Each surgical technique has its own advantage and disadvantage and long-term problem and must be considered in the follow-up chosen of the procedure depending mainly on the extent of the coarctation and the patient age [69]. There are several operative techniques such as resection and extended end-to-end anastomosis. This is the procedure used in patient older than 1 year and also the main advantage is to remove and excise all abnormal aortic tissue [70, 71]. Tube and jump graft, if the segment of the coarctation is present, use the tube method (interposition) and if the aortic is fragile we use the bypass method. Extra anatomic bypass graft occurs if there are complex cases associated with another CHD and it is a very complex repair (ascending to descending) [72]. Aortaplasty has to be a method with the prosthetic patch or by subclavian flap, the one that is less used in primary repair; in infant surgery usually the subclavian flap is used.

Late Management

There is some warrant situation for intervention or reintervention in any case with a gradient pressure across 20 mmHg or more, Left ventricle hypertrophy, patient with 50% or more aortic narrowing, aortic valve stenosis, aneurysm at the previous coarctation site or aneurysm at the Wills circle [73, 74].

Medical Treatment

Avoidance of obesity and smoking, regulate the lipid profile and cholesterol and limited the risk factor of early coronary artery disease. Renal failure occurs in this patient if the lower arterial pressure is reduced. Antihypertensive drug is used in case of hypertension [75].

Procedure

Balloon angioplasty alternative to surgical repair is preferred in all patients with isolated CoA, also when surgical intervention is not the option. Not recommended in infant less than 4 months, is unlikely to succeed in this setting, and considered also in case of severe ventricle septal defect and heart failure [76, 77]. Stent placement improves luminal diameter, and need to be dilated as the child grow so the adult needs less reintervention. Aortoplasty is avoided in general because of the formation of aneurysm [78–84]. Potential complication of angioplasty includes recoarctation, aortic aneurysm, and aortic dissection. Long-term potential complication of surgical repair of CoA is recoarctation. postoperative complications or early complications include hypertension, nerve injury, and paraplegia because of spinal cord ischemia [85–87].

Follow-Up

Coarctation is one of the complex cardiovascular disorder and complications may appear many years after the initial successful treatment. Arterial hypertension, recurrent obstruction, and aneurysm should be searched well [88]. Using the imaging technique in the following patient is essential to the treatment if necessary and lifesaving should take in Center, the lifelong prophylaxis of infective endocarditis is controversial [89]. The residual gradient should be treated. Pregnant woman with coarctation and gradient hypertension has a high risk of aneurysm and lead to death from aortic rupture or dissection. A fetal echocardiogram is indicated in pregnancies complicated by maternal congenital heart disease or having previous child with CHD [90].

Multiple Choice Questions

1. A 2-year old boy came to the pediatric clinic with his parent complaining difficulty in walking for 2 months. On examination the blood pressure is 140/85 mmHg, systolic murmur in the left parasternal area. What is the most likely finding?
   A. Left ventricle dilated
   B. Ribs shadowing
   C. Prolong QT interval
   D. High respiratory rate
   E. Low oxygen saturation in lower limp

2. An 8 year-old-female came to the emergency department complaining of severe headache and claudication. On the examination of the girl's appearance, short state and webbing of the neck, arterial pulse was checked and the difference in the lower and upper extremity was found.Regarding this finding, the next steps you have to do to confirm the diagnosis is??
   A. Check the blood pressure in the arm
   B. Sent for chest X-ray immediately
   C. Check the blood glucose
   D. Sent for karyogenetic study
   E. Brachio-femoral blood pressure

3. A 34-year-old male came to the emergency department complaining of severe headache and claudication. The patient looked confused and drowsy and after a minute the patient suffered from neurological focal lesion and paraplegia, and stroke symptoms. Afterward the patient passed away and sent for autopsy. The autopsy report showed that the patient has aneurysm in the wills circle that develops acutely on top of chronic infarction that came from reduced perfusion in the brain tissue and hypoxia. The report also shows that the descending aorta looks dilated and hypertrophic thick wall. Regarding the finding, what is the cause of the death in this patient?
   A. Rupture aneurysm
   B. Sever infraction of myocardium
   C. DVT
   D. Sever stroke
   E. Aortic rupture

4. A 2-year-old male child known for the case of CoA was brought by his parent to the pediatric clinic because of the developmental delay of the child. What is the main cause of this delay in this particular patient:
   A. Coarctation itself
   B. The mental and neurological cause
   C. Feeding and nutritional cause
   D. Infection
   E. Heart failure

5. Pediatric department showed a case of the syndrome rare to see, so the syndrome is called Noonan syndrome. What you suspected to see in this patient?
   A. D-TGA

B. Ventricle septal defect
C. Coarctation of aorta
D. Atrial septal defect
E. Patent ductus arteriosus

6. A 9-year-old-girl was referred to the pediatric cardiologist by the gynecological physician, to check her because she suffers from severe claudication and exercise intolerance. On the examination she showed the pulse difference between the brachial and femoral arterial pulse, and development delay. The patient sent for investigation show mild to moderate narrowing in the descending aorta. What is the next step in management of this patient?
   A. Surgery immediately
   B. Beta blocker
   C. Increase the aerobic exercise
   D. Sent for thoracic MRI

7. A 45-year-old male was diagnosed with coarctation aorta. Patient was treated successfully by surgery and he took his medication before 3 days the patient complains from also chest pain. What is the most likely late complication?
   A. Pericarditis
   B. Increase rate of lung cancer
   C. Lower limp paraplegia
   D. Myocardium hypertrophy
   E. Myocarditis

8. A 4-month-old infant child came to the pediatric clinic with his parent because of the failure to thrive and tachypnea. On the examination the pulse rate is high and there is a difference between the brachial and femoral delay. On investigation the patient was sent for a chest X-ray what is the finding that you should find to confirm your diagnosis?
   A. Increase hilar vascularity
   B. Reduce the curve of the left ventricle
   C. Ribs notch
   D. Elevate cardio-lung ratio

9. A 12-year-old African-American boy came to the office because he cannot play with his friend at the school. This problem developed 6 months ago also his limp show cold but not cyanotic. The first thing you do to the patient is check the vital sign that report hypertension 140/85, 18 respiratory rate, also the pulse was 90 per minute in the upper limp and 65 per minute in the lower limp which shows how the patient was misdiagnosed until this age and he is totally normal except for this problem. What is the next step in investigation that gives you more information about this condition?
   A. Chest X-ray
   B. ECG

C. ELISA
D. CBC
E. ECHO
F. RSG

10. An 1-month-old neonate was diagnosed with acyanotic heart disease that is characterized by narrowing of the descending aorta just distal to the patent ductus. What is the hallmark of this disease?
   A. Ribs notching
   B. Ventricle hypertrophy
   C. Brachio-femoral pulse delay
   D. Hilar vascularity

Answers

1. The answer is D.
   This known case of CoA regarding classical finding blood pressure and leg claudication is the most powerful finding in the diagnosis. The decrease in the oxygen saturation in the lower limp is due to the coarctation.

2. The answer is E.
   One of the hallmarks in the diagnosis of CoA is the delay between two pulses and pressure difference in the case of Turner syndrome with the coarctation of the aorta which is the most common congenital anomaly in this patient.

3. The answer is A.
   In this case of the coarctation of the aorta regarding the symptom and autopsy finding, a serious complication is will's circle aneurysm that shows immediately neurological symptoms and death if ruptured.

4. The answer is E.
   The main cause of the growth and development delay in the patient with coarctation is the congestive heart failure

5. The answer is D.
   The most congenital anomaly associated with Noonan syndrome is the coarctation of the aorta

6. The answer is B.
   One of the late managements in the patient of coarctation of the aorta is medical and beta blocker treated the heart failure that causes growth and developmental delay in this patient who complain of it.

7. The answer is D.
   The most common complication of CoA is myocardium hypertrophy of the left ventricle because of the increase in the pressure overload on this side

8. The answer is C.
   One of the most likely diagnostic finding in patient with CoA is ribs notching.

9. The answer is E.
   This is the case of coarctation of the aorta by examination and finding so the most valuable diagnostic

method in congenital heart disease as a whole is echocardiogram

10. The answer is E.

The hallmark of the CoA is the brachio-femoral delay pulse.

References

1. Elzenga NJ, Gittenberger-De Groot AC. Localised coarctation of the aorta. An age dependent spectrum. Br Heart J. 1983;49:317–23.
2. Kappetein AP, Gittenberger-De Groot AC, Zwinderman AH, Rohmer J, Poelmann RE, Huysmans HA. The neural crest as a possible pathogenetic factor in coarctation of the aorta and bicuspid aortic valve. J Thorac Cardiovasc Surg. 1991;102:830–6.
3. Hornberger LK, Weintraub RG, Pesonen E, et al. Echocardiographic study of the morphology and growth of the aortic arch in the human fetus. Observations related to the prenatal diagnosis of coarctation. Circulation. 1992;86:741–7.
4. Morrow WR, Huhta JC, Murphy DJ Jr, Mcnamara DG. Quantitative morphology of the aortic arch in neonatal coarctation. J Am Coll Cardiol. 1986;8:616–20.
5. Allan LD, Chita SK, Anderson RH, Fagg N, Crawford DC, Tynan MJ. Coarctation of the aorta in prenatal life: an echocardiographic, anatomical, and functional study. Br Heart J. 1988;59:356–60.
6. Child JS. Transthoracic and transesophageal echocardiographic imaging: anatomic and hemodynamic assessment. In: Perloff JK, Child JS, editors. Congenital heart disease in adults. Philadelphia: W.B. Saunders; 1998.
7. Simpson IA, Sahn DJ, Valdes-Cruz LM, Chung KJ, Sherman FS, Swensson RE. Color Doppler flow mapping in patients with coarctation of the aorta: new observations and improved evaluation with color flow diameter and proximal acceleration as predictors of severity. Circulation. 1988;77:736–44.
8. Carvalho JS, Redington AN, Shinebourne EA, Rigby ML, Gibson D. Continuous wave Doppler echocardiography and coarctation of the aorta: gradients and flow patterns in the assessment of severity. Br Heart J. 1990;64:133–7.
9. Tacy TA, Baba K, Cape EG. Effect of aortic compliance on Doppler diastolic flow pattern in coarctation of the aorta. J Am Soc Echocardiogr. 1999;12:636–42.
10. Warnes CA, Williams RG, Bashore TM, et al. ACC/AHA 2008 guidelines for the management of adults with congenital heart disease: a report of the American College of Cardiology/American heart association Task Force on Practice guidelines (Writing Committee to Develop guidelines on the management of adults with congenital heart disease). Developed in Collaboration with the American Society of Echocardiography, Heart Rhythm Society, International Society for Adult Congenital Heart Disease, Society for Cardiovascular Angiography and Interventions, and Society of Thoracic Surgeons. J Am Coll Cardiol. 2008;52(23):e143–263.
11. Moltzer E, Mattace Raso FU, Karamermer Y, et al. Comparison of candesartan versus metoprolol for treatment of systemic hypertension after repaired aortic coarctation. Am J Cardiol. 2010;105(2):217–22.
12. Giordano U, Cifra B, Giannico S, et al. Midterm results, and therapeutic management, for patients suffering hypertension after surgical repair of aortic coarctation. Cardiol Young. 2009;19(5):451–5.
13. Boone ML, Swenson BE, Felson B. Rib notching: its many causes. Am J Roentgenol Radium Therapy Nucl Med. 1964;91:1075–88.
14. De Man SA, Andre JL, Bachmann H, et al. Blood pressure in childhood: pooled findings of six European studies. J Hypertens. 1991;9:109–14.
15. Perloff JK. Pregnancy in congenital heart disease: the mother and the fetus. In: Perloff JK, Child JS, editors. Congenital heart disease in adults. 3rd ed. Philadelphia: W.B. Saunders; 2009. p. 144.
16. Vriend JW, Drenthen W, Pieper PG, et al. Outcome of pregnancy in patients after repair of aortic coarctation. Eur Heart J. 2005;26:2173–8.
17. Spencer MP, Johnston FR, Meredith JH. The origin and interpretation of murmurs in coarctation of the aorta. Am Heart J. 1958;56:722–36.
18. Nasser WK, Helmen C. Kinking of the aortic arch (pseudocoarctation). Clinical, radiographic, hemodynamic, and angiographic findings in eight cases. Ann Intern Med. 1966;64:971–8.
19. Garman JE, Hinson RE, Eyler WR. Coarctation of the aorta in infancy: detection on chest radiographs. Radiology. 1965;85:418–22.
20. Bjork L, Friedman R. Routine roentgenographic diagnosis of coarctation of the aorta in the child. Am J Roentgenol Radium Therapy Nucl Med. 1965;95:636–64.
21. Ben-Shoshan M, Rossi NP, Korns ME. Coarctation of the abdominal aorta. Arch Pathol. 1973;95:221–5.
22. Allan LD, Crawford DC, Tynan M. Evolution of coarctation of the aorta in intrauterine life. Br Heart J. 1984;52:471–3.
23. Nora JJ, Torres FG, Sinha AK, Mcnamara DG. Characteristic cardiovascular anomalies of XO Turner syndrome, XX and XY phenotype and XO-XX Turner mosaic. Am J Cardiol. 1970;25:639–41.
24. Mazzanti L, Cacciari E. Congenital heart disease in patients with Turner's syndrome. Italian Study Group for Turner Syndrome (ISGTS). J Pediatr. 1998;133:688–92.
25. Lin AE, Garver KL. Monozygotic Turner syndrome twins correlation of phenotype severity and heart defect. Am J Med Genet. 1988;29:529–31.
26. Siggers DC, Polani PE. Congenital heart disease in male and female subjects with somatic features of Turner's syndrome and normal sex chromosomes (Ullrich's and related syndromes). Br Heart J. 1972;34:41–6.
27. Perloff JK. Physical examination of the heart and circulation. 3rd ed. Philadelphia: W.B. Saunders; 1998.
28. Campbell M, Suzman S. Coarctation of the aorta. Br Heart J. 1947;9:185–212.
29. Blumenthal S, Epps RP, Heavenrich R, et al. Report of the task force on blood pressure control in children. Pediatrics. 1977;59:I–II, 797–820.
30. Graham TP Jr, Burger J, Boucek RJ Jr, et al. Absence of left ventricular volume loading in infants with coarctation of the aorta and a large ventricular septal defect. J Am Coll Cardiol. 1989;14:1545–52.
31. Shinebourne EA, Tam AS, Elseed AM, Paneth M, Lennox SC, Cleland WP. Coarctation of the aorta in infancy and childhood. Br Heart J. 1976;38:375–80.
32. Hesslein PS, Gutgesell HP, Mcnamara DG. Prognosis of symptomatic coarctation of the aorta in infancy. Am J Cardiol. 1983;51:299–303.
33. Jentsch E, Liersch R, Bourgeois M. Prolapsed valve of the foramen ovale in newborns and infants with coarctation of the aorta. Pediatr Cardiol. 1988;9:29–32.
34. Bailie MD, Donoso VS, Gonzalez NC. Role of the renin-angiotensin system in hypertension after coarctation of the aorta. J Lab Clin Med. 1984;104:553–62.
35. Schneeweiss A, Sherf L, Lehrer E, Lieberman Y, Neufeld HN. Segmental study of the terminal coronary vessels in coarctation of the aorta: a natural model for study of the effect of coronary hypertension on human coronary circulation. Am J Cardiol. 1982;49:1996–2002.
36. Vlodaver Z, Neufeld HN. The coronary arteries in coarctation of the aorta. Circulation. 1968;37:449–54.
37. Goldberg MB, Scully AL, Solomon IL, Steinbach HL. Gonadal dysgenesis in phenotypic female subjects. A review of eighty-

seven cases, with cytogenetic studies in fifty-three. Am J Med. 1968;45:529–43.

38. Miro O, Jimenez S, Gonzalez J, De Caralt TM, Ordi J. Highly effective compensatory mechanisms in a 76-year-old man with a coarctation of the aorta. Cardiology. 1999;92:284–6.

39. Ward KE, Pryor RW, Matson JR, Razook JD, Thompson WM, Elkins RC. Delayed detection of coarctation in infancy: implications for timing of newborn follow-up. Pediatrics. 1990;86:972–6.

40. Schievink WI, Mokri B, Piepgras DG, Gittenberger-De Groot AC. Intracranial aneurysms and cervicocephalic arterial dissections as- sociated with congenital heart disease. Neurosurgery. 1996;39:685–9; discussion 689–690.

41. Edwards JE. Aneurysms of the thoracic aorta complicating coarctation. Circulation. 1973;48:195–201.

42. Shachter N, Perloff JK, Mulder DG. Aortic dissection in Noonan's syndrome (46 XY turner). Am J Cardiol. 1984;54:464–5.

43. Graham TP Jr, Atwood GF, Boerth RC, Boucek RJ Jr, Smith CW. Right and left heart size and function in infants with symptomatic coarctation. Circulation. 1977;56:641–7.

44. Baylis JH, Campbell M. The course and prognosis of coarctation of the aorta. Br Heart J. 1956;18:475–95.

45. Rudolph AM, Heymann MA, Spitznas U. Hemodynamic considerations in the development of narrowing of the aorta. Am J Cardiol. 1972;30:514–25.

46. Becker AE, Becker MJ, Edwards JE. Anomalies associated with coarctation of aorta: particular reference to infancy. Circulation. 1970;41:1067–75.

47. Liberthson RR, Pennington DG, Jacobs ML, Daggett WM. Coarctation of the aorta: review of 234 patients and clarification of management problems. Am J Cardiol. 1979;43:835–40.

48. Campbell M. Natural history of coarctation of the aorta. Br Heart J. 1970;32:633–40.

49. Reifenstein GH, Levine SA, Gross RE. Coarctation of the aorta; a review of 104 autopsied cases of the adult type, 2 years of age or older. Am Heart J. 1947;33:146–68.

50. Talner NS, Berman MA. Postnatal development of obstruction in coarctation of the aorta: role of the ductus arteriosus. Pediatrics. 1975;56:562–9.

51. Mcmahon CJ, Vick GW 3rd, Nihill MR. Right aortic arch and coarctation: delineation by three dimensional magnetic resonance angiogram. Heart. 2001;85:492.

52. Borow KM, Colan SD, Neumann A. Altered left ventricular mechanics in patients with valvular aortic stenosis and coarctation of the aorta: effects on systolic performance and late outcome. Circulation. 1985;72:515–22.

53. Gutgesell HP, Barton DM, Elgin KM. Coarctation of the aorta in the neonate: associated conditions, management, and early outcome. Am J Cardiol. 2001;88:457–9.

54. Leichtman DA, Schmickel RD, Gelehrter TD, Judd WJ, Woodbury MC, Meilinger KL. Familial Turner syndrome. Ann Intern Med. 1978;89:473–6.

55. Miettinen OS, Reiner ML, Nadas AS. Seasonal incidence of coarctation of the aorta. Br Heart J. 1970;32:103–7.

56. Hernandez FA, Miller RH, Schiebler GL. Rarity of coarctation of the aorta in the American Negro. J Pediatr. 1969;74:623–5.

57. Van Der Horst RL, Gotsman MS. Racial incidence of coarctation of aorta. Br Heart J. 1972;34:289–94.

58. Sehested J, Baandrup U, Mikkelsen E. Different reactivity and structure of the prestenotic and poststenotic aorta in human coarctation. Implications for baroreceptor function. Circulation. 1982;65:1060–5.

59. Brili S, Dernellis J, Aggeli C, et al. Aortic elastic properties in patients with repaired coarctation of aorta. Am J Cardiol. 1998;82:1140–3, A1110.

60. Alpert BS, Bain HH, Balfe JW, Kidd BS, Olley PM. Role of the renin-angiotensin-aldosterone system in hypertensive children with coarctation of the aorta. Am J Cardiol. 1979;43:828–34.

61. Warren DJ, Smith RS, Naik RB. Inappropriate renin secretion and abnormal cardiovascular reflexes in coarctation of the aorta. Br Heart J. 1981;45:733–6.

62. Perloff JK. Normal myocardial growth and the development and regression of increased ventricular mass. In: Perloff JK, Child JS, Aboulhosn J, editors. Congenital heart disease in adults. 3rd ed. Philadelphia: W.B. Saunders; 2009.

63. Bahabozorgui S, Nemir P Jr. Coarctation of the abdominal aorta. Am J Surg. 1966;111:224–9.

64. Bergamini TM, Bernard JD, Mavroudis C, Backer CL, Muster AJ, Richardson JD. Coarctation of the abdominal aorta. Ann Vasc Surg. 1995;9:352–6.

65. Roques X, Bourdeaud'hui A, Choussat A, et al. Coarctation of the abdominal aorta. Ann Vasc Surg. 1988;2:138–44.

66. Bahabozorgui S, Bernstein RG, Frater RW. Pseudocoarctation of aorta associated with aneurysm formation. Chest. 1971;60:616–7.

67. Wang W-B, Lin G-M. Pseudocoarctation and coarctation. Int J Cardiol. 2009;133:e62–4.

68. Schellhammer F, Von Den Driesch P, Gaitzsch A. Pseudocoarctation of the abdominal aorta. Vasa. 1997;26:308–10.

69. Joseph M, Leclerc Y, Hutchison SJ. Aortic pseudocoarctation causing refractory hypertension. N Engl J Med. 2002;346:784–78.

70. Chun K, Colombani PM, Dudgeon DL, Haller JA Jr. Diagnosis and management of congenital vascular rings: a 22-year experience. Ann Thorac Surg. 1992;53:597–602; discussion 602–593.

71. Brockmeier K, Demirakca S, Metzner R, Floemer F. Images in cardiovascular medicine. Double aortic arch. Circulation. 2000;102:E93–4.

72. Yamada M, Horigome H, Ishii S. Pseudocoarctation of the aorta coexistent with coarctation. Eur J Pediatr. 1996;155:993.

73. Bilgic A, Ozer S, Atalay S. Pseudocoarctation of the aorta. Jpn Heart J. 1990;31:875–9.

74. Mulder BJM, Van Der Wall EE. Optimal imaging protocol for evaluation of aortic coarctation; time for a reappraisal. Int J Cardiovasc Imaging. 2006;22:695–7.

75. Abbott ME. Coarctation of the aorta of adult type; statistical study and historical retrospect of 200 recorded cases with autopsy; of stenosis or obliteration of descending arch in subjects above age of two years. Am Heart J. 1928;3:574.

76. Folger GM Jr, Stein PD. Bicuspid aortic valve morphology when associated with coarctation of the aorta. Catheter Cardiovasc Diagn. 1984;10:17–25.

77. Fernandes SM, Sanders SP, Khairy P, et al. Morphology of bicuspid aortic valve in children and adolescents. J Am Coll Cardiol. 2004;44:1648–51.

78. Niwa K, Perloff JK, Bhuta SM, et al. Structural abnormalities of great arterial walls in congenital heart disease: light and electron microscopic analyses. Circulation. 2001;103:393–400.

79. Wallace RB, Nast EP. Postcoarctation mycotic intercostal arterial pseudoaneurysm. Am J Cardiol. 1987;59:1014–5.

80. Henderson RA, Ward C, Campbell C. Dissecting left subclavian artery aneurysm: an unusual presentation of coarctation of the aorta. Int J Cardiol. 1993;40:69–70.

81. Shamsa K, Perloff JK, Lee E, Wirthlin RS, Tsui I, Schwartz SD. Retinal vascular patterns after operative repair of aortic isthmic coarctation. Am J Cardiol. 2010;105:408–10.

82. Deeg KH, Singer H. Doppler sonographic diagnosis of subclavian steal in infants with coarctation of the aorta and interrupted aortic arch. Pediatr Radiol. 1989;19:163–6.

83. Yu C-H, Chen M-R. Clinical investigation of systemic-pulmonary collateral arteries. Pediatr Cardiol. 2008;29:334–8.

84. Johns KJ, Johns JA, Feman SS. Retinal vascular abnormalities in patients with coarctation of the aorta. Arch Ophthalmol. 1991;109:1266–8.

85. Freed MD, Keane JF, Van Praagh R, Castaneda AR, Bernhard WF, Nadas AS. Coarctation of the aorta with congenital mitral regurgitation. Circulation. 1974;49:1175–84.

86. Celano V, Pieroni DR, Morera JA, Roland JM, Gingell RL. Two-dimensional echocardiographic examination of mitral valve abnormalities associated with coarctation of the aorta. Circulation. 1984;69:924–32.

87. Rosenquist GC. Congenital mitral valve disease associated with coarctation of the aorta: a spectrum that includes parachute deformity of the mitral valve. Circulation. 1974;49:985–93.

88. Isner JM, Donaldson RF, Fulton D, Bhan I, Payne DD, Cleveland RJ. Cystic medial necrosis in coarctation of the aorta: a potential factor contributing to adverse consequences observed after percutaneous balloon angioplasty of coarctation sites. Circulation. 1987;75:689–95.

89. Baron MG. Radiologic notes in cardiology: obscuration of the aortic knob in coarctation of the aorta. Circulation. 1971;43:311–6.

90. Smallhorn JF, Anderson RH, Macartney FJ. Morphological characterisation of ventricular septal defects associated with coarctation of aorta by cross sectional echocardiography. Br Heart J. 1983;49:485–94.

Truncus Arteriosus

Vasiliki Patsiou, Alexandra Bekiaridou,
Andreas S. Papazoglou, and Dimitrios V. Moysidis

Abstract

This chapter aims to discuss a rare congenital heart defect called truncus arteriosus (TA). "TA is characterized by a ventricular septal defect (VSD), a single truncal valve, and a common ventricular outflow tract (OT)." Oxygenated and deoxygenated blood is mixed at the VSD level, supplying the systemic, pulmonary, and coronary circulation with deoxygenated blood and thereby giving birth to the cyanotic clinical presentation of neonatal heart failure. TA demands definitive surgical intervention. Otherwise, the prognosis is unfavorable. Nevertheless, patients need further revision operations throughout their later lives. Late surgical management is a new entity, which seems to be instrumental in cases where the diagnosis is missed.

Keywords

Truncus arteriosus · Congenital heart disease · Cyanotic Neonates · Fallot tetralogy · VSD · Prenatal screening Common tract · Interrupted arch · Pulmonary hypertension

Abbreviations

CE   Collet and Edwards
CHD   Congenital heart disease
OT   Outflow tract
PVR   Pulmonary vascular resistance
TA   Truncus arteriosus
VSD   Ventricular septal defect

Introduction

"Truncus arteriosus (TA) is a rare form of congenital heart disease (CHD)" occurring only in 1–3% of patients with CHD, with an annual incidence of 7 per 100,000 live births and without a racial or sex predisposition [1]. It was first reported in 1798 in a case autopsy by J. Wilson, with the anatomical morphology being described later in 1864 in a six-month-old infant by G. Buchanan [2]. It falls under the cyanotic congenital defects as it concerns a combination of heart abnormalities resulting in a low blood oxygen level in neonates.

Under normal conditions, the embryonic TA should give rise to the aorta and the pulmonary trunk throughout fetal development. Persistent TA develops when the septation of these two major arteries is inadequate or fails.

Surgical intervention is deemed required for the treatment of TA. Cases not addressed with surgical intervention are associated with extremely high mortality rates in infancy. Following surgical repair, long-term outcomes are satisfactory but residual, and potential complications burden the prognosis. Despite surgery, patients need continuous, long-term cardiology follow-up to prevent adverse clinical outcomes.

V. Patsiou (✉) · A. Bekiaridou · A. S. Papazoglou · D. V. Moysidis
Medicine School, Aristotle University of Thessaloniki,
Thessaloniki, Greece

© The Author(s), under exclusive license to Springer Nature Switzerland AG 2023
G. Tagarakis et al. (eds.), *Clinical and Surgical Aspects of Congenital Heart Diseases*,
https://doi.org/10.1007/978-3-031-23062-2_8

Pathophysiology

"The primitive heart develops from five dilations during the prenatal period: TA, conus cordis, primitive ventricle, primitive atria, and sinus venosus" [3]. However, due to inadequate or failed septation of the embryonic common arterial trunk during the fifth week of development, a persistent aortopulmonary trunk is created, consisting of a single OT, rather than two vascular channels, in conjunction with a common truncal valve (semilunar). This valve might have one to four cusps (usually three) [4]. The ductus arteriosus is a normal and essential fetal structure steering blood to the right ventricle, away from the high-resistance pulmonary circulation [5]. After birth, it closes spontaneously. In some cyanotic congenital defects, however, ductus arteriosus must remain patent to sustain systemic circulation.

Persistent TA can be linked to a variety of cardiac, aortic, and pulmonary structural anomalies [6, 7].

Numerous cardiac abnormalities may be correlated with TA, many of which variously impact the prognosis. Structural lesions of the truncal valve, including dysplastic and supernumerary leaflets, are usually reported and lead to valvular stenosis or regurgitation (moderate or severe) in up to 20% of the patients [8, 9]. Atrial septal defect, aberrant subclavian artery, left superior caval vein, and right aortic arch are also prevalent but with modest correlations. In addition to the above relatively common lesions identified in the spectrum of TA, further abnormalities have been less commonly documented, such as double aortic arch, complete atrioventricular septal defect, and several functional variations of univentricular heart.

Etiology

As in many other innate cardiac defects, the exact causes and the underlying mechanisms of TA malformation are still unknown. Important etiologic components in some cases of human TA seem to be the abnormalities encountered in the development of cells from the neural crest that occupy the outflow region of the normal developing heart. Genetically, it has been found that approximately 30–40% of patients with TA have microdeletions within the chromosome band 22q11.2 [10], which contains several related genes. Specifically, this chromosomal abnormality is likely to impair the cardiac neural crest cell migration and development [11], eventually resulting in structural abnormalities in TA. Although extensive research is being conducted to elucidate the correlation between TA and band 22q11, only the TBX1 gene appears to be involved in the pharyngeal arch and conotruncal development.

Other risk factors that may be associated with the development of TA are the following:

Research studies provide evidence for a relationship with poorly controlled diabetes mellitus in pregnant women [12, 13].

- Certain medications and various chemicals (e.g., retinoic acid, bis-diamine) are considered teratogenic and responsible for predisposition to TA in animal models. However, no verified evidence suggests that they contribute significantly to this anomaly in humans.
- Smoking and excessive alcohol consumption during pregnancy as well as the infection of a pregnant woman with German measles (rubella) seem to play a role in the onset of TA.
- DiGeorge syndrome, also known as velocardiofacial syndrome, is a rare disorder that comprises thymic and parathyroid gland abnormalities, conotruncal cardiac defects, and dysmorphic facies. In most cases, it is caused by deletions in the band 22q11, and it is classified as a clinical variant of the broad CATCH-22 syndrome [14]. The presence of DiGeorge syndrome has been ascertained in a 30–35% of patients with TA. These patients have the above-mentioned genetic mutation in their genotype.

Diagnosis

The severity of TA may vary, and thus the disease is characterized by variable clinical presentations. Prenatally, most cases are diagnosed between 20 and 25 weeks. Currently, most of the TA cases are diagnosed during the neonatal period. Indeed, only a small portion of patients is diagnosed through screening in utero with prenatal ultrasonography. Rarely, for some cases, the diagnosis may be validated later in infancy or even in adulthood, with a pejorative prognosis.

Prenatal Diagnosis

It is done by ultrasound studies during the pregnancy, and it can be suspicious but not confirmatory [15, 16].

Postnatal Diagnosis

Diagnosis also includes early postnatal screening and is based on clinical and radiological signs of a shunt. Pulmonary blood flow and PVR are the determinant factors for clinical presentation.

The clinical recognition of infants with TA begins with symptoms of acute cardiac heart failure: poor feeding, weak cry, insufficient weight, lethargy, tachypnea, costal–sternal retractions, grunting, nasal flaring, tachycardia, or hepatomegaly [17, 18]. In most patients, heart failure is rapidly worsening if left untreated. The newborn will appear moderately cyanotic, with clubbing, respiratory distress, and an oxygen saturation of <95%. Nevertheless, "cyanosis is not a constant and permanent feature. It can be minimal, intermittent, or even absent due to the large pulmonary flow, which can overcome the need for oxygen" [19]. This variety in patients' clinical presentation is often perplexed by the presence of concurrent abnormalities, such as valvular regurgitation (50% of patients) and clinical coarctation (10% of patients). Concurrent anomalies are linked to adverse prognosis and worse symptoms [15].

Investigations

Although chest radiography and electrocardiogram (ECG) share limited specificity, they can raise clinical suspicion about the presence of TA [16–20] (Fig. 1).

Transthoracic (TTE) and transesophageal echocardiography (TEE) with color flow and Doppler studies can establish a firm diagnosis, providing anatomical details. Antenatally, the mid-trimester or routine ultrasound scan includes the careful assessment of fetal anatomy to detect significant anatomical abnormalities, including the examination of the four chambers and ventricular OTs of the fetal heart. The identification of the mechanism, severity, and consequences of TA relies primarily on the assessment of pulmonary arterial pressures, atrial and ventricular volumes, the defect in the wall between the left and right ventricle, and the morphologic characteristics of a single artery, the common OT, overriding the ventricles and giving supply to both the systemic and pulmonary circulation

[19, 21]. Furthermore, at least one of the pulmonary arteries will rise from the ascending aorta or the transverse arch until the origin of the left subclavian artery, according to the classification of the TA (Fig. 2). Substantial pulmonary overcirculation may indicate left atrial enlargement. Furthermore, postnatal TTE can provide critical information for other concurrent anomalies, aiding the preoperative preparation and monitoring the perioperative management.

As echocardiography provides high sensitivity and specificity (Fig. 3), the need for cardiac catheterization is limited. Cardiac catheterization can clarify certain anatomic and hemodynamic aspects, such as the precise PVR, which is not clearly identified by echocardiography. However, MRI or CT angiography may supplant the need for cardiac catheterization by giving further details of associated anomalies before surgery [15].

Moreover, genetic testing is recommended to be included in the management routine for all patients born with TA due to the frequent association with 22q11 genetic mutations and DiGeorge syndrome [22].

Differential Diagnosis

Imaging modalities have increased the pre- and postnatal diagnostic success rates of TA up to greater than 90%. Nevertheless, there are limited cases where structures cannot be identified clearly on prenatal echocardiography. Single arterial trunk overriding a VSD is a common sonographic finding in both TA and tetralogy of Fallot (ToF). Indeed, TA may be diagnosed as ToF or pulmonary atresia with a VSD. Because TA is a complex conotruncal anomaly with multiple subtypes, diagnosis requires multiple imaging in three-dimensional and four-dimensional ultrasonography. Postnatally, auscultation in conjunction with the clinical presentation can clarify the diagnosis. In particular, a murmur

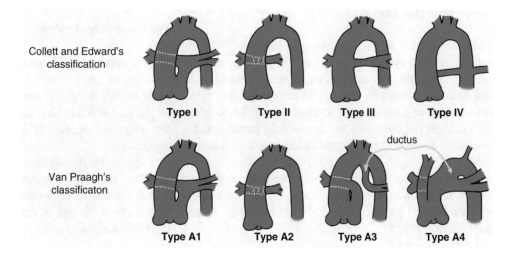

Fig. 1 Collett and Edwards's (top panel) and Van Praagh's (bottom panel) classification systems

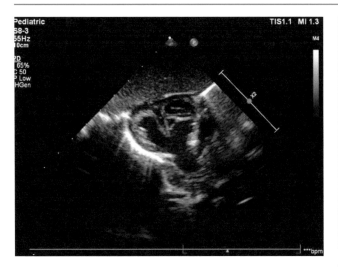

Fig. 2 Fetal echocardiography of truncus arteriosus (aorta and pulmonary artery), which bestrides a high ventricular septal defect. (Case courtesy of Dr. Anastasia Keivanidou, AHEPA University Hospital)

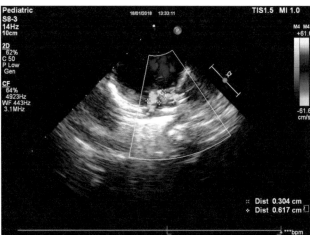

Fig. 3 Ultrasound of the aorta and main pulmonary artery sharing a TA. Mixture of blood is clearly seen. (Case courtesy of Dr. Anastasia Keivanidou, AHEPA University Hospital)

will be audible in TA but not in ToF, while cyanosis in TA will be milder.

Management

Palliative Treatment

The main goal is the patient's stabilization and the balance of the blood flow in the pulmonary and systemic circulation. First, heart failure is treated vigorously with diuretics, inotropic agents, and angiotensin-converting-enzyme (ACE) inhibitors to achieve proper fluid balance [23]. Supplemental oxygenation in clinical practice may worsen pulmonary overcirculation and should be avoided. Furthermore, metabolic derangements, electrolyte abnormalities, anemia, and hypoglycemia should be corrected to reduce complications.

Corrective Treatment

The heterogeneity of this clinical condition makes its surgical management even more complex. The presence of truncal valve regurgitation, concomitant interrupted aortic arch, and anomalous coronary anatomy constitutes a further burden. Definitive early surgical intervention of TA together with a single-stage repair of any concomitant cardiovascular anomalies throughout the neonatal period is well-established. "The VSD is closed so that the left ventricle blood flow is driven into the root of the common arterial trunk. A conduit with or without a valve is placed to reconstitute the continuity between the right ventricle and the confluence of pulmonary arteries" [23, 24].

Reports support that the TA can be repaired safely with low morbidity and mortality, not only in neonates, but also in infants, and older children. Late surgical therapy has also been applied to children from developing countries who often miss early diagnosis or early surgical treatment [25]. Nevertheless, as the degree of pulmonary vascular obstructive disease advances, the operative mortality and the probability of poor late results or late death are increased. Nowadays, the late management of TA has begun to gain ground, although it is a clinical challenge, and its indications have not been defined [26].

Lastly, although rarely used today, pulmonary artery banding is a surgical technique for the palliation (protection of pulmonary vascular bed) of TA to limit the pulmonary blood flow in case of a pulmonary over-circulation caused by large left-to-right shunts. This strategy led to only minor improvements in the clinical course of the disease, with substantial early and intermediate mortality rates [27].

Postoperative Period

Truncal valve regurgitation is a major, life-threatening complication of the TA. Further operations will be needed in patients with the progression of truncal valve insufficiency or with a quadricuspid truncal valve [28]. The presence of any diastolic murmur is indicative of valve or conduit regurgitation.

Endocarditis prophylaxis is recommended preoperatively and for the first postoperative for 6 months. Additionally, branch pulmonary artery stenosis and pulmonary hypertension are both considered common sequelae. In some cases, patients with postoperative pulmonary hypertension require medical support, with the administration of sildenafil and NO, without favoring survival. Other complications reported are tamponade, sternitis, mediastinitis, coronary ischemia, and secondary pericardial drainage.

Prognosis

Several factors might impact the prognosis of children receiving surgical treatment, which are classified as either modifiable or not [29]. Perioperative morbidity seems limited and concerns mainly patients with complex CHD, low cardiac output, cardiopulmonary bypass aftereffects, and transient arrhythmias. Patients in the early postoperative stage, especially those who undergo early repair, demonstrate minimal late mortality rates [30]. On the other hand, patients with complications such as significant truncal valve regurgitation or aortic arch interruption have less favorable results.

The clinical course of TA without surgical intervention is not thoroughly clarified. Until recently, the median age of death without surgery varied from 2 weeks to 3 months in most patients, with mortality approaching 100% by the age of one year. Patients with TA who survived into adulthood with unrepaired structural abnormalities have also been reported, but they constitute a decreasing minority. Progressive metabolic acidosis and cardiac dysfunction are the final results of this clinical sequelae. Systemic perfusion is insufficient as a consequence of blood mixture and failure to fulfill the body's metabolic demands.

Follow-Up

Since the late 1980s, when complete repair in the neonatal period came into widespread application as a treatment strategy, techniques of perioperative management have dramatically changed. Although existing data seem to be limited, contemporary studies demonstrate more positive outcomes in patients undergoing surgery. However, there is a minimal proportion of patients who present late mortality after early repair of TA. Most cases in which premature deaths occurred are likely to be related to reinterventions. Nevertheless, the truncal valve reintervention seems to be a low-risk operation in terms of mortality [31].

Most children require revision operations throughout their lives. Usually, the right ventricular OT is reconstructed with a nonviable conduit (i.e., duration of 3 years or less after implantation). When a conduit is placed during early infancy, its size becomes inadequate as the child grows. Thus, the conduit must be revised during childhood. Specifically, a

subsequent intervention is needed on the right ventricular OT. Admittedly, the results of these required reoperations and catheter-based reinterventions depend not only on the technique but also on the materials used. When the patient's tissue (homograft) is used as a part of this OT, there is the potential for growth of the conduit as the child grows, presenting prolonged durability.

A 28-year-follow up study in 83 patients showed that about 30% of patients remained without reoperation 10 years after TA repair. In 2010, more than 90% of patients were in good or very good clinical condition [32]. Moreover, another 20-year retrospective review in 165 patients demonstrated that 10- to 20-year survival and functional status were substantially good in infants who underwent complete repair of TA [33]. Conduit replacement or revision was considered almost necessary in those patients.

Multiple Choice Questions
1. Which of the following statements about truncus arteriosus is correct?
   A. Infants with TA usually are in distress in the first few days of life.
   B. Supplemental oxygen is always necessary.
   C. All conduits used for TA have a lack of growth potential through time.
   D. The prognosis does not depend on the age of surgical repair.
2. Which of the following genetic disorders increases a patient's risk of developing truncus arteriosus?
   A. Edward's syndrome (trisomy 18)
   B. Down syndrome
   C. DiGeorge syndrome
   D. Patau syndrome
3. What other congenital heart defect isis the other congenital heart defect most commonly present in truncus arteriosus?
   A. Atrial septal defect
   B. Pulmonary stenosis
   C. Tetralogy of Fallot
   D. Ventricular septal defect
4. The truncal valve most frequently has:
   A. One leaflet
   B. Two leaflets
   C. Three leaflets
   D. Four leaflets
   E. Five leaflets
5. Diagnosis is facilitated primarily by:
   A. MRI
   B. CT
   C. Cardiac catheterization
   D. Echocardiography

6. A 5-day-old full-term neonate with a cleft palate and dysmorphic facial features is undergoing repair of truncus arteriosus. After sternotomy, it is noted that the thymus is absent. Results of genetic testing are pending. Which electrolyte abnormality would you MOST likely expect on the patient's pre-op labs?
   A. Hypoglycemia
   B. Hypocalcemia
   C. Hypercalcemia
   D. Hyponatremia
7. Which of the following *does not* belong in the differential diagnosis of truncus arteriosus?
   A. Tetralogy of Fallot
   B. Pulmonary atresia with a ventricular septal defect
   C. Aortic dissection
   D. Sepsis
8. Which of the following *does not* belong in the palliative treatment of patients with truncus arteriosus?
   A. Inotropic agents
   B. Diuretics
   C. Prostaglandin
   D. Supplemental oxygen
9. Which of the following is a common finding in the electrocardiogram?
   A. ST-segment elevation
   B. Combined ventricular hypertrophy with higher QRS voltage
   C. Low electrocardiographic QRS voltage
   D. Q wave
10. The transthoracic echocardiography will show:
    A. A common outflow tract overriding the ventricles
    B. Only a ventricular septal defect
    C. Ventricular inversion
    D. An atrial septal defect

Answers
1. The answer is A.
   Most infants show symptoms in the first days of life and, if left untreated, do not survive beyond 6 months. Therefore, early surgical repair is crucial. As for the conditions, their technical specifications regarding growth are matter of current research.
2. The answer is C.
   About 33% of neonates with truncus arteriosus have a genetic disorder (stems from a deletion in the genome) called DiGeorge syndrome.
3. The answer is D.
   A ventricular septal defect (VSD) is commonly present in this CHD. The VSD will be near the truncus arteriosus, allowing blood to mix in the right and left ventricles and enter the truncus artery. It is very uncommon for one not to be present.
4. The answer is C.
   The common semilunar valve may have one to four cusps with tricuspid most frequently seen.
5. The answer is D.
   Transthoracic echocardiography is a feasible, integrated approach to raising suspicion for truncus arteriosus.
6. The patient has a phenotype consistent with 22q11.2 deletion syndrome. These patients may have hypoparathyroidism resulting in hypocalcemia, dysmorphic facial features, cleft palate, gastrointestinal and genitourinary abnormalities, developmental delay, and psychiatric disorders.
7. The answer is C.
   Aortic dissection is not a part of the differential diagnosis.
8. The answer is D.
   Supplemental oxygen might worsen pulmonary overcirculation.
9. The answer is B.
   Ventricular hypertrophy is a common finding in congenital heart diseases.
10. The answer is A.
    Echocardiography will show a common outflow tract overriding the ventricles and giving blood supply to the pulmonary and systemic circulation.

References

1. Bhansali S, Phoon C. Truncus arteriosus. In: Critical heart disease in infants and children. 2020. pp. 661–669.e2. [Online]. https://www.ncbi.nlm.nih.gov/books/NBK534774/. Accessed 6 July 2021.
2. XIII. A description of a very unusual formation of the human heart. Philos Trans R Soc Lond. 1798;88:346–356. https://doi.org/10.1098/rstl.1798.0014.
3. Moorman A, Webb S, Brown NA, Lamers W, Anderson RH. Development of the heart: (1) formation of the cardiac chambers and arterial trunks. Heart. 2003;89(7):806–14. https://doi.org/10.1136/HEART.89.7.806.
4. de la Cruz MV, Cayre R, Angelini P, Noriega-Ramos N, Sadowinski S. Coronary arteries in truncus arteriosus. Am J Cardiol. 1990;66(20):1482–6. https://doi.org/10.1016/0002-9149(90)90539-D.
5. Schneider DJ, Moore JW. Patent ductus arteriosus. Circulation. 2006;114(17):1873–82. https://doi.org/10.1161/CIRCULATIONAHA.105.592063.
6. Collett RW, Edwards JE. Persistent truncus arteriosus; a classification according to anatomic types. Surg Clin North Am. 1949;29(4):1245–70. https://doi.org/10.1016/S0039-6109(16)32803-1.

7. Van Praagh R. Truncus arteriosus: what is it really and how should it be classified? Eur J Cardiothorac Surg. 1987;1(2):65–70. https://doi.org/10.1016/1010-7940(87)90014-5.

8. Chowdhury D, Kodavatiganti R. Truncus arteriosus. In: Case studies in pediatric anesthesia. 2019. pp. 306–309. https://doi.org/10.1017/9781108668736.068.

9. Konstantinov IE, et al. Truncus arteriosus associated with interrupted aortic arch in 50 neonates: a Congenital Heart Surgeons Society study. Ann Thorac Surg. 2006;81(1):214–22. https://doi.org/10.1016/J.ATHORACSUR.2005.06.072.

10. McDonald-McGinn DM, Hain HS, Emanuel BS, Zackai EH. 22q11.2 deletion syndrome. 1993. pp. 621–626.e1. [Online]. https://pubmed.ncbi.nlm.nih.gov/20301696/. Accessed 6 July 2021.

11. Vitelli F, Morishima M, Taddei I, Lindsay EA, Baldini A. Tbx1 mutation causes multiple cardiovascular defects and disrupts neural crest and cranial nerve migratory pathways. Hum Mol Genet. 2002;11(8):915–22. https://doi.org/10.1093/HMG/11.8.915.

12. Ferencz C, Rubin JD, McCarter RJ, Clark EB. Maternal diabetes and cardiovascular malformations: predominance of double outlet right ventricle and truncus arteriosus. Teratology. 1990;41(3):319–26. https://doi.org/10.1002/TERA.1420410309.

13. Papazoglou AS, et al. Maternal diabetes mellitus and its impact on the risk of delivering a child with congenital heart disease: a systematic review and meta-analysis. J Matern Fetal Neonatal Med. 2022;35(25):7685–94. https://doi.org/10.1080/14767058.2021.1960968.

14. Wilson DI, Burn J, Scambler P, Goodship J. DiGeorge syndrome: part of CATCH 22. J Med Genet. 1993;30(10):852. https://doi.org/10.1136/JMG.30.10.852.

15. Jaggers J, Cole CR. Truncus arteriosus. In: Critical heart disease in infants and children. 2021. pp. 661–669.e2. https://doi.org/10.1016/B978-1-4557-0760-7.00055-3.

16. Swanson TM, Selamet Tierney ES, Tworetzky W, Pigula F, McElhinney DB. Truncus arteriosus: diagnostic accuracy, outcomes, and impact of prenatal diagnosis. Pediatr Cardiol. 2009;30(3):256–61. https://doi.org/10.1007/S00246-008-9328-7.

17. Truncus arteriosus—NORD (National Organization for Rare Disorders). https://rarediseases.org/rare-diseases/truncus-arteriosus/. Accessed 16 Feb 2022.

18. Congenital heart defects—facts about truncus arteriosus | CDC. https://www.cdc.gov/ncbddd/heartdefects/truncusarteriosus.html. Accessed 16 Feb 2022.

19. Gotsch F, et al. Prenatal diagnosis of truncus arteriosus using multiplanar display in 4D ultrasonography. J Matern Fetal Neonatal Med. 2010;23(4):297. https://doi.org/10.3109/14767050903108206.

20. Bibevski S, et al. Truncus arteriosus. In: Pediatric and congenital cardiology, cardiac surgery and intensive care. 2014. pp. 1983–2001. https://doi.org/10.1007/978-1-4471-4619-3_48.

21. Sharland G. Cardiology and undefined 2002. In: Echocardiographic features of common arterial trunk. Elsevier. [Online]. https://sci-hub.ru/https://www.sciencedirect.com/science/article/pii/S1058981302000061?casa_token=tCrcfJFw4BgAAAAA:7-5HzvccdlB9pDpwtNbuO0SxjJ41-tNZlMwiTwOu_zhVZmTRvd-3nm3CibgAlhPderx_CCy16w. Accessed 16 Feb 2022.

22. Pierpont ME, et al. Genetic basis for congenital heart defects: current knowledge: a scientific statement from the American Heart Association Congenital Cardiac Defects Committee, Council on Cardiovascular Disease in the Young: endorsed by the American Academy of Pediatrics. Circulation. 2007;115(23):3015–38. https://doi.org/10.1161/CIRCULATIONAHA.106.183056.

23. Persistent truncus arteriosus—pediatrics—Merck manuals professional edition. https://www.merckmanuals.com/en-pr/professional/pediatrics/congenital-cardiovascular-anomalies/persistent-truncus-arteriosus. Accessed 13 Feb 2022.

24. Raisky O, et al. Common arterial trunk repair: with conduit or without? Eur J Cardiothorac Surg. 2009;36(4):675–82. https://doi.org/10.1016/J.EJCTS.2009.03.062.

25. Gouton M, Lucet V, Bical O, Leca F. Late management of truncus arteriosus: 20 years of humanitarian experience. Cardiol Young. 2018;28(2):302–8. https://doi.org/10.1017/S1047951117002050.

26. Alamri RM, et al. Surgical repair for persistent truncus arteriosus in neonates and older children. J Cardiothorac Surg. 2020;15(1):1–7. https://doi.org/10.1186/S13019-020-01114-1/TABLES/5.

27. McFaul RC, Mair DD, Feldt RH, Ritter DG, McGoon DC. Truncus arteriosus and previous pulmonary arterial banding: clinical and hemodynamic assessment. Am J Cardiol. 1976;38(5):626–32. https://doi.org/10.1016/S0002-9149(76)80013-6.

28. Martínez-Quintana E, Portela-Torrón F. Truncus arteriosus and truncal valve regurgitation. Transl Pediatr. 2019;8(5):360–2. https://doi.org/10.21037/TP.2019.02.01.

29. Williams JM, de Leeuw M, Black MD, Freedom RM, Williams WG, McCrindle BW. Factors associated with outcomes of persistent truncus arteriosus. J Am Coll Cardiol. 1999;34(2):545–53. https://doi.org/10.1016/S0735-1097(99)00227-2.

30. Marcelletti C, McGoon DC, Danielson GK, Wallace RB, Mair DD. Early and late results of surgical repair of truncus arteriosus. Circulation. 1977;55(4):636–41. https://doi.org/10.1161/01.CIR.55.4.636.

31. Henaine R, et al. Fate of the truncal valve in truncus arteriosus. Ann Thorac Surg. 2008;85(1):172–8. https://doi.org/10.1016/J.ATHORACSUR.2007.07.039.

32. Tlaskal T, et al. Long-term results after correction of persistent truncus arteriosus in 83 patients. Eur J Cardiothorac Surg. 2010;37(6):1278–84. https://doi.org/10.1016/j.ejcts.2009.12.022.

33. Rajasinghe H. Long-term follow-up of truncus arteriosus repaired in infancy: a twenty-year experience. J Thorac Cardiovasc Surg. 1997;113(5):869–78. https://doi.org/10.1016/s0022-5223(97)70259-9.

Tricuspid Atresia

Nikolaos Otountzidis and Christos Tsagkaris

Abstract

Tricuspid atresia (TA) "is a rare cyanotic congenital heart defect, defined by total agenesis or absence of the tricuspid valve, resulting in an obstruction of the blood flow between the right atrium and ventricle." Therefore, a right-to-left shunt at the atrial level is obligatory for survival, resulting in the mixing of the systematic and pulmonary venous circulation. The impaired oxygen saturation and the underlying pathophysiological changes in the left ventricle lead to the clinical manifestations of the disease that include cyanosis and cardiac failure in the early life. The severity of the clinical presentation depends upon the flow in the pulmonary circulation. Apart from the postnatal diagnosis in neonates or young infants, most recent advances in fetal echocardiography permit the accurate prenatal diagnosis of the TA. Without the appropriate treatment, TA is associated with high mortality rates. Several surgical procedures such as the corrective Fontan operation have altered the clinical course of this congenital defect. This resulted in an improvement of patients' life expectancy and quality of life.

Keywords

Tricuspid atresia · Cyanosis · Fontan procedure Bidirectional Glenn · Cavopulmonary shunt · Palliation Univentricular heart · Heart defect · Pulmonary circulation · Tricuspid valve · Congenital defect

Introduction

"Tricuspid atresia (TA) is a severe congenital disease that belongs to the group of cyanotic congenital heart defects (CHD), characterized by total agenesis or absence of the tricuspid valve" [1]. As a result, there is no physical communication between the right atrium and the right ventricle. TA was firstly described by Kreysig in 1817 [1].

Epidemiology

TA is present in 0.1 per 1000 live births, while it represents approximately 1% of all congenital heart defects, making it the third most common cyanotic CHD [2]. TA may also be part of other congenital syndromes, such as chromosomal anomalies, VACTERL syndrome, and others [3].

Embryology and Genetic Background

The genetic background of the TA remains unclear. Embryologically, the atrioventricular valves are created after the formation of endocardial cushions (primitive valves, 31–35 embryonic day), via the transition of endothelial and mesenchymal cells with the coordination of many different signaling pathways (especially erbB, NOTCH, and Wnt) [4–6]. Cells from the endocardial cushions enter the extracellular matrix in order to differentiate the tissue into valve leaflets, while small remaining muscle bands form the papillary muscles and the chordae tendonae [5]. A glycosaminoglycan, called hyaluronan, seems to have an important role in the development of the valves, as the lack of hyaluronan has been proven to lead to defects in the endocardial cushion development in experimental models [7–9]. Moreover, other matrix components like fibronectin, fibulins, versican, and collagen participate in the formation of the heart valves [5]. A fault to these embryogenesis stages of the tricuspid valve

N. Otountzidis (✉)
Aristotle University of Thessaloniki, Thessaloniki, Greece

C. Tsagkaris
University of Crete, Heraklion, Greece

© The Author(s), under exclusive license to Springer Nature Switzerland AG 2023
G. Tagarakis et al. (eds.), *Clinical and Surgical Aspects of Congenital Heart Diseases*,
https://doi.org/10.1007/978-3-031-23062-2_9

may lead to TA. Recent studies indicate specific gene mutations, like those in *RASA1* and *NFATC1* genes, responsible for familial and inherited presentations of the TA, respectively [10, 11]. The recurrence risk of TA in a next pregnancy is estimated to be relatively low (1–2%) [12]. Maternal diabetes mellitus is also referred to as a risk factor for the presence of TA in infants [13, 14].

Pathogenesis

In a heart with TA, the following characteristics are present [15]:

- Fibrous thickening (most common) in the anatomical site of the tricuspid valve
- Lack of communication between the morphologically defined right atrium and ventricle
- Right ventricular hypoplasia with right atrial dilatation
- Interatrial communication via an atrial septal defect or a patent foramen ovale
- Normal morphology of the left ventricle and the mitral valve
- Ventricular septal defect (VSD, present in 90% of the cases [16])

The blockage on the site of the tricuspid valve leads to modifications in the blood flow. The blood from the superior and inferior vena cava returns normally to the right atrium; however, the flow to the right ventricle is not possible due to TA. Therefore, the presence of interatrial communication is necessary in order for the blood of the right atrium to flow in the left atrium and through the mitral valve into the left ventricle. Therefore, with normal great vessel anatomy, blood from the venous circulation mixes with the oxygenated blood returning to the pulmonary veins [15]. The pulmonary circulation is then supplied with the presence of a VSD, which allows the filling of the right ventricle (Fig. 1). However, when the VSD is absent or insufficient, or the outflow tract is severely obstructed, the presence of a patent ductus arteriosus (PDA) or collateral vessels between the two circulations are the alternate mean of pulmonary blood supply. With the presence of D-transposition of great arteries (Type II TA), the blood from the left ventricle flows into the pulmonary artery, while the systematic circulation is supplied by the right ventricle through the VSD [15, 16].

The above-mentioned alterations in the blood flow result in a univentricular system with an overworking left ventricle so that a normal cardiac output can be preserved. In patients with TA, significantly different dimensions of the left ventricle are found, compared to normal individuals, with larger ventricle diameter, width, spherical index, and volume measurements, with concurrent smaller chamber length to be present in TA [17]. These factors tend to return to normal after the surgical treatment of the defect [17].

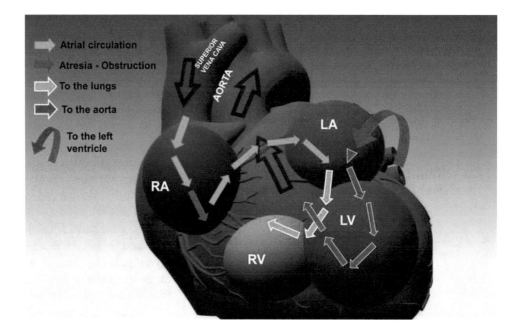

Fig. 1 Blood circulation in a heart with TA. *RA* right atrium, *RV* right ventricle, *LA* left atrium, *LV* left ventricle

Classification

TA can be classified according to the morphology of the atretic valve, the X-ray appearance of the pulmonary circulation, and the associated anatomical defects [18]. The morphology of the valve can be grouped into five types: (a) muscular (most common type, 76%), (b) membranous (12%), (c) valvular (6%), (d) Ebstein's (6%), and (e) atrioventricular canal type (rare) [19]. Based on the X-ray findings on the pulmonary vascular marking, three different groups have been described: (a) decreased markings, (b) normal or increased markings, and (c) initially normal or increased alternating to decreased markings [20]. Although these classification systems have historical value, their clinical importance is minor.

The most widely used and unified classification system is based on the TA associate abnormalities, and it was proposed by Rao [18]:

1. Type I: Normally related great arteries
2. Type II: D-transposition of the great arteries (TGA)
3. Type III: Other than type II malpositions of the great arteries
4. Type IV: Persistent truncus arteriosus

Each type can be further subdivided into three types according to the pulmonary arteries' status:

- Subtype a: Pulmonary atresia
- Subtype b: Pulmonary stenosis or pulmonary hypoplasia
- Subtype c: Normal anatomy of the pulmonary arteries

Clinical Presentation

Up to 80% of infants with TA will develop symptoms in the first month of their life [15]. The main factor determining the clinical presentation and the severity of the disease is the pulmonary blood flow. Based on the above, two different categories can be described: patients with obstruction in the pulmonary flow (usually due to the VSD) and patients with unrestricted flow.

When the pulmonary circulation is obstructed, the patients present with cyanosis early, in the first days of life. The timing of the cyanosis is proportional to the severity of the obstruction, while other signs of low oxygenation can also be present such as tachypnoea and respiratory acidosis. Moreover, in infants with severe obstruction or even pulmonary atresia, the cyanosis presents right after the closure of the ductus arteriosus. During clinical examination, central cyanosis, tachypnoea, and clubbing (in older infants or children, chronic conditions) may be present with a normal heart rate. A holosystolic murmur at the left lower sternal border

and/or a continuous murmur can be heard, indicating a VSD or a PDA, respectively. Due to pulmonary obstruction, in some cases, a systolic murmur may be present in the upper left sternal border [15].

When the pulmonary blood flow remains unobstructed, the infants usually present with the clinical picture of heart failure. The symptoms appear later than in the first group, typically without cyanosis, and they are characteristic of the underlying heart failure, including fatigue, dyspnea, low food intake, and growth restriction. Most of these patients also have TGA (Type II TA). Clinical examination reveals signs of congestive heart failure, including tachypnoea, elevated heart rhythm, and hepatomegaly [15].

Diagnosis

The diagnosis of TA, as in many congenital heart defects, can be set either before or after birth. With the rapidly growing advancements in antenatal ultrasound screening and the specialization of sonographers, nowadays, most cases of TA are diagnosed intra-utero, at least in countries with well-organized prenatal screening programs.

Prenatal Diagnosis

TA is diagnosed prenatally in 0.2–0.9 cases per 10,000 births, while the proportion of the diagnoses before birth varies between 12 and 100% in different countries [21]. The initial diagnosis of TA is set at a median gestational age of 22 weeks [3]. Lack of patency of the tricuspid valve and the presence of a VSD should be sought in the ultrasound [12]. Except TA, other associate defects such as great vessel transposition and pulmonary stenosis can be depicted, giving further information for postnatal management. However, the prenatal diagnosis of the TA does not seem to have significantly improved the survival rates of the patients [22].

Postnatal Diagnosis

Infants or children with TA that were not diagnosed during the fetal period may present with the signs and symptoms attributed in the section "Clinical Presentation". The oxygen saturation measurement using pulse oximetry constitutes an easily accessible tool with high specificity and sensitivity for the detection of CHD [23].

The electrocardiogram (ECG) in TA presents with left axis deviation in the frontal plane, which can be partly explained by the left ventricle hypertrophy and the hypoplastic right ventricle [24]. Other signs of left ventricle hypertrophy are also common. Moreover, due to the consequent dilatation of the right (and in some cases the left) atrium, high amplitude P waves are also noted. The lead V6 may indicate the pulmonary flow status, as in patients with the restricted flow, the ECG depicts swallow Q and short R waves, while in patients with unrestricted flow, the Q waves are deep and the R waves tall [24].

Referring to imaging studies, chest X-ray in TA is indicative of pulmonary blood flow. When the blood flow is restricted, the radiograph generally demonstrates normal heart dimensions. The pulmonary vasculature is poorly depicted, while in patients with small pulmonary artery a concavity may be seen on its normal radiological site. With normal or increased pulmonary flow, the heart is portrayed as enlarged, with good visualization of the pulmonary vessels. In both cases, a prominent right heart border is the delineation of the dilatated right atrium [25].

Echocardiography is the gold standard technique for the diagnosis of the TA. The atretic valve can be exactly determined. In the anatomical site of the tricuspid valve, a dense hyperechoic band can be seen, representing the most common "muscular type" of TA, with concurrent attachment of the anterior valve leaflet to the left of the interatrial septum [15, 26]. Other typical findings include the right and left atrial dilatation, the characteristic hypoplastic right ventricle, and the left ventricle hypertrophy. Doppler imaging can be used to further analyze the pressure difference in the atrial and ventral septum defects and, more significantly, to identify and estimate the right ventricle outflow obstruction. The possible TGA may be recognized through the visualization of the great vessels' characteristics close to the heart (bifurcation of the pulmonary artery and aortic arch, respectively) [15].

While the use of interventional procedures for diagnosis is nowadays restricted, they remain useful for the estimation of hemodynamic data and the planning of the relevant surgical procedures. Cardiac magnetic resonance imaging (MRI) is nowadays a considerable alternative, indicating similar results with routine catheterization [27].

Management and Treatment

The initial management of patients presenting with TA includes a thermically suitable environment, especially for neonates, with usually moderate administration of O_2 (up to 40%) and concurrent correction of the biochemical values [25]. Neonates with severe pulmonary obstruction or critical VSD that are PDA dependent and present severe cyanosis after birth will be benefited from the administration of prostaglandin (PGE1) [28]. Prostaglandin will maintain the patency of the ductus arteriosus in order to provide adequate flow in the pulmonary circulation, improving oxygen saturation. In older patients with signs and symptoms of cardiac

failure, anticongestive therapy with diuretics, digoxin, and afterload-reducing agents should be considered [15]. Although angiotensin-converting enzyme inhibitors (ACEi) are commonly used, randomized evidence suggests that their use does not improve patients' clinical outcomes [29].

After initial stabilization and detailed examination, the first surgical step in the treatment of patients with severe obstruction is the modified Blalock–Thomas–Taussig shunt (BTTS), performed in patients under 3 months old [15, 30]. The original procedure was first described in 1945 for patients with pulmonary stenosis in tetralogy of Fallot, but rapidly expanded in other CHD, like TA [30, 31]. The original BTTS surgery includes a direct anastomosis of the right or the left subclavian artery to the ipsilateral pulmonary artery, while in the modified BTTS, a synthetic graft (Gore-Tex or Dacron) is positioned between the subclavian artery or the brachiocephalic trunk and a pulmonary artery branch [32]. This provides adequate blood flow in the pulmonary circulation with improvement in systematic oxygen saturation. Recent evidence, however, suggests that a PDA stent is a more effective and safer alternative than the BTTS for the initial shunt [33].

In cases with the normal or increased pulmonary flow, pulmonary artery banding can result in a reduction of the blood volume. This is of great significance in patients with TGA concerning high pulmonary pressure [25]. However, in patients with normal great vessel anatomy, it is more common for the VSD to close spontaneously; thus, this procedure will eventually lead to restricted pulmonary flow [34]. Therefore, conservative treatment is the first step in the management of these patients. Nowadays, an absorbable (polydioxanone) band can be used in order to temporally restrict the flow till the closure of the VSD, reducing the number of reoperations [35, 36].

Other interventions that should be addressed include the atrial septostomy in cases with the restricted interatrial flow, reconstruction of narrow pulmonary arteries, and balloon dilatation procedures (stenotic pulmonary valve, aortic concartion, etc.) [37–39]. In particular, in patients with type II TA (TGA), VSD enlargement procedures and the Damus–Kaye–Stansel operation (anastomosis between the aorta and the pulmonary trunk) can be performed in order to overcome the systemic ventricular outflow obstruction [15, 40]. Before the final operation, the pulmonary vasculature and pressure should be analyzed in detail, and any aortopulmonary collateral vessels should be occluded [25].

The final corrective surgery for the TA is the Fontan operation. This procedure allows the bypassing of the atretic valve via a cavopulmonary connection. It is usually performed in two stages.

The first stage includes a superior cavopulmonary anastomosis, such as the bidirectional Glenn or the hemi-Fontan operation. During bidirectional Glenn, the superior vena cava is directly anastomosed to the right pulmonary artery [41]. The term "bidirectional" is used to highlight the blood flow in both lungs. This anatomical modification allows the blood from the upper body to return solely in pulmonary circulation. This leads to better oxygen saturation in cyanotic patients and lower blood load in the functional left ventricle [42]. The procedure can be performed between 2 and 6 months of age [43, 44]. The hemi-Fontan operation remains on the same principle. The difference relies on the fact that the superior vena cava retains its connection with the right atrium when anastomosed to the right pulmonary artery, while the junction between the vein and the atrium is surgically obstructed via a homograft [45]. This may lead to a more suitable anatomy for the upcoming Fontan operation, though it generally constitutes a more complex procedure [45].

All the above-mentioned surgical procedures should respect the anatomical structures for the final corrective Fontan operation. The procedure is generally performed in children older than 2 years of age with a weight of 15 kg or more [25]. The Fontan operation was first described in 1971 for the surgical correction of TA [46]. By this procedure, the systemic and the pulmonary circulation are completely separated. The original technique included: (a) anastomosis between the superior vena cava and the distal end of the right pulmonary artery (Glenn's procedure), (b) anastomosis between the right atrium and the proximal end of the right pulmonary artery with the intersection of an aortic valve homograft, (c) closure of the atrial septal defect, (d) intersection of a pulmonary valve homograft between the inferior vena cava and the right atrium, and (e) ligation of the pulmonary trunk [46]. Thus, there is a total separation between the saturated and the desaturated circulation, as the blood from the right atrium flows directly to the pulmonary arteries, resulting in a normal circulation in terms of physiology. This complex operation has undergone many modifications since its initial description and nowadays two different techniques are mainly used: the extracardiac conduit technique and the intracardiac lateral tunnel technique.

The extracardiac is the most commonly used technique and results in the total return of the venous blood to the pulmonary arteries without the interference of the heart. The superior vena cava is anastomosed directly to the right pulmonary artery (Glenn's procedure), while the inferior vena cava is connected to the pulmonary artery through a conduit [47]. Therefore, this Fontan modification is the operation of choice if a bidirectional Glenn shunt precedes. The intracardiac lateral tunnel technique is differentiated by the formation of a composite interatrial channel, which leads the blood from the inferior to the superior vena cava and then to the right pulmonary vein, as mentioned before. The main outcome of both procedures is the passive return of the systemic venous volume to the pulmonary circulation. According to a recent meta-analysis, the extracardiac procedure provides better long-term survival and a lower rate of postoperative arrythmias, when compared to the intracardiac approach [48]. Moreover, fenestration (an anastomosis between the Fontan circulation and the pulmonary venous atrium) during the Fontan operation was shown to improve the short-term outcomes and constitutes common practice for most cardiac surgeons [49].

After a successful Fontan operation, further pharmacological treatment is also required. This includes thromboprophylaxis through antiplatelet or anticoagulant agents and possibly pulmonary pressure-reducing agents [50]. However, other common treatments, like inotropes and afterload-reducing agents, have shown no effect on the reduced outflow of the Fontan circulation [51].

Outcome and Follow-Up

Without the appropriate surgical treatment, TA results in up to 90% mortality rates during the first year of life [20]. After the Fontan operation, the survival of the patients with TA rises at 93% in the first year and at 82% after 10 years, while in the overall TA population, the survival lies at 81% and 64% in 1 and 15 years, respectively [52]. More recent data report an overall 8-year survival of 84% [53]. The highest mortality rates are generally mentioned between the initial neonatal palliation (e.g., BTTS) and the first stage of the Fontan operation (superior cavopulmonary shunt) [52, 54].

The Fontan procedure, however, is not without complications. Pleural effusions, arrythmias, thromboembolic events, and protein-losing enteropathy remain among the most frequent [16, 55]. Other conditions, such as renal dysfunction, liver fibrosis, and neuropsychological disorders, have also been reported [50]. The surgical procedure itself, the passive venous circulation with the consequent elevated venous pressure, and low cardiac output result in the manifestation of these complications. Moreover, in women with Fontan circulation, the miscarriage rates climb up to 50% [54]. Heart transplantation remains the final solution for the patient with failing Fontan [16].

Regarding the peculiarity of the Fontan operation, an outpatient visit for clinically well Fontan patients every 6–12 months is highly recommended according to the American Heart Association [50]. Most recent guidelines on adult patients with TA and Fontan circulation suggest an annual evaluation, or even more frequently if they present a New York Heart Association (NYHA) stage of III or IV [56]. Finally, up to 60% of the patients that have undergone a Fontan operation will require another intervention in the next 20 years [57]. Given the high mortality presented between the first palliation procedure and the cavopulmonary shunt operation, a recent paper studied the effectiveness of a home monitoring program on these death rates [58]. The result was that this well-organized program (that includes, for example, daily oxygen saturation measurements) leads to a decrease in the death rates by up to 30% [58]. This indicates that a standardized follow-up pattern is of great significance in order to minimize the adverse events of the TA.

Conclusion

TA represents a rare yet severe CHD with high mortality rates. The current surgical options extend the patients' longevity and quality of life; however, serious adverse events are yet to be diminished. Novel advancements in pharmacological protocols and surgical techniques are expected to alter the prognosis of these patients, minimizing the complications of the disease. In this context, the follow-up will be transitioned to adulthood, indicating the need for an experienced adult congenital disease approach.

Multiple Choice Questions
1. One of the following defects is necessary for the survival in the TA:
   A. Interatrial communication
   B. Pulmonary atresia
   C. Transposition of great vessels
   D. Aortic coarctation
2. Which of the following is true about the diagnosis of TA?
   A. The diagnosis can be set solely via the clinical examination.
   B. Interventional procedures are necessary for diagnosis.
   C. The ECG is the gold standard for diagnosis.
   D. Echocardiography is the gold standard for diagnosis.

Answers
1. Correct answer: A.

   As there is no communication between the right atrium and the right ventricle due to the atretic tricuspid valve, interatrial communication is necessary for the blood to flow into the left chambers and, from there, to the systematic and pulmonary (via the VSD) circulation. The other choices represent possible associated cardiac defects.
2. Correct answer: D.

   Echocardiography remains the gold standard for the prenatal and the postnatal diagnosis of the TA, as the atretic valve can be directly determined. Although the ECG can depict some characteristic findings for the TA, these can be present in various cardiac diseases. The clin-

ical examination can set the suspicion for a congenital heart defect. Interventional procedures are not necessary for the initial diagnosis; however, they can be useful for surgical planning.

References

1. Rashkind WJ. Tricuspid atresia: a historical review. Pediatr Cardiol. 1982;2:85–8. https://doi.org/10.1007/BF02265624.
2. Liu Y, Chen S, Zühlke L, Black GC, Choy MK, Li N, et al. Global birth prevalence of congenital heart defects 1970-2017: updated systematic review and meta-analysis of 260 studies. Int J Epidemiol. 2019;48:455–63. https://doi.org/10.1093/ije/dyz009.
3. Berg C, Lachmann R, Kaiser C, Kozlowski P, Stressig R, Schneider M, et al. Prenatal diagnosis of tricuspid atresia: intrauterine course and outcome. Ultrasound Obstet Gynecol. 2010;35:183–90. https://doi.org/10.1002/uog.7499.
4. Armstrong EJ, Bischoff J. Heart valve development: endothelial cell signaling and differentiation. Circ Res. 2004;95:459–70. https://doi.org/10.1161/01.RES.0000141146.95728.da.
5. Schroeder JA, Jackson LF, Lee DC, Camenisch TD. Form and function of developing heart valves: coordination by extracellular matrix and growth factor signaling. J Mol Med. 2003;81:392–403. https://doi.org/10.1007/s00109-003-0456-5.
6. Beis D, Bartman T, Jin SW, Scott IC, D'Amico LA, Ober EA, et al. Genetic and cellular analyses of zebrafish atrioventricular cushion and valve development. Development. 2005;132:4193–204. https://doi.org/10.1242/dev.01970.
7. Camenisch TD, Spicer AP, Brehm-Gibson T, Biesterfeldt J, Augustine ML, Calabro A Jr, et al. Disruption of hyaluronan synthase-2 abrogates normal cardiac morphogenesis and hyaluronan-mediated transformation of epithelium to mesenchyme. J Clin Invest. 2000;106:349–60. https://doi.org/10.1172/JCI10272.
8. Baldwin HS, Lloyd TR, Solursh M. Hyaluronate degradation affects ventricular function of the early postlooped embryonic rat heart in situ. Circ Res. 1994;74:244–52. https://doi.org/10.1161/01.res.74.2.244.
9. Mjaatvedt CH, Yamamura H, Capehart AA, Turner D, Markwald RR. The Cspg2 gene, disrupted in the hdf mutant, is required for right cardiac chamber and endocardial cushion formation. Dev Biol. 1998;202:56–66. https://doi.org/10.1006/dbio.1998.9001.
10. Nozari A, Aghaei-Moghadam E, Zeinaloo A, Alavi A, Ghasemi Firouzabdi S, Minaee S, et al. A pathogenic homozygous mutation in the Pleckstrin homology domain of RASA1 is responsible for familial tricuspid atresia in an Iranian consanguineous family. Cell J. 2019;21:70–7. https://doi.org/10.22074/cellj.2019.5734.
11. Abdul-Sater Z, Yehya A, Beresian J, Salem E, Kamar A, Baydoun S, et al. Two heterozygous mutations in NFATC1 in a patient with tricuspid atresia. PLoS One. 2012;7:e49532. https://doi.org/10.1371/journal.pone.0049532.
12. Petropoulos AC, Valiyeva Q, Xudiyeva A, Behbudov V, Ismaylova M, Kalangos A. Prenatal diagnosis and management of tricuspid valve atresia: a case report and review of literature. J Neonatol Clin Pediatr. 2018;5:21.
13. Wren C, Birrell G, Hawthorne G. Cardiovascular malformations in infants of diabetic mothers. Heart. 2003;89:1217–20. https://doi.org/10.1136/heart.89.10.1217.
14. Papazoglou AS, Moysidis DV, Panagopoulos P, Kaklamanos EG, Tsagkaris C, Vouloagkas I, et al. Maternal diabetes mellitus and its impact on the risk of delivering a child with congenital heart

disease: a systematic review and meta-analysis. J Matern Fetal Neonatal Med. 2022;35(25):7685–94. https://doi.org/10.1080/14767058.2021.1960968.

15. Rao PS. Tricuspid atresia. Curr Treat Options Cardiovasc Med. 2000;2:507–20. https://doi.org/10.1007/s11936-000-0046-6.

16. Murthy R, Nigro J, Karamlou T. Tricuspid atresia. In: Ungerleider RM, Meliones JN, McMillan KN, editors. Critical heart disease in infants and children. 3rd ed. Elsevier; 2019. p. 765–77.

17. Chen LJ, Zhang YQ, Tong ZR, Sun AM. Evaluation of the anatomic and hemodynamic abnormalities in tricuspid atresia before and after surgery using computational fluid dynamics. Medicine (Baltimore). 2018;97:e9510. https://doi.org/10.1097/MD.0000000000009510.

18. Rao PS. A unified classification for tricuspid atresia. Am Heart J. 1980;99:799–804. https://doi.org/10.1016/0002-8703(80)90632-8.

19. Weinberg PM. Anatomy of tricuspid atresia and its relevance to current forms of surgical therapy. Ann Thorac Surg. 1980;29:306–11. https://doi.org/10.1016/s0003-4975(10)61476-2.

20. Dick M, Fyler DC, Nadas AS. Tricuspid atresia: clinical course in 101 patients. Am J Cardiol. 1975;36:327–37. https://doi.org/10.1016/0002-9149(75)90484-1.

21. Bakker MK, Bergman JEH, Krikov S, Amar E, Cocchi G, Cragan J, et al. Prenatal diagnosis and prevalence of critical congenital heart defects: an international retrospective cohort study. BMJ Open. 2019;9:e028139. https://doi.org/10.1136/bmjopen-2018-028139.

22. Wald RM, Tham EB, McCrindle BW, Goff DA, McAuliffe FM, Golding F, et al. Outcome after prenatal diagnosis of tricuspid atresia: a multicenter experience. Am Heart J. 2007;153:772–8. https://doi.org/10.1016/j.ahj.2007.02.030.

23. Plana MN, Zamora J, Suresh G, Fernandez-Pineda L, Thangaratinam S, Ewer AK. Pulse oximetry screening for critical congenital heart defects. Cochrane Database Syst Rev. 2018;3:CD011912. https://doi.org/10.1002/14651858.CD011912.pub2.

24. Davachi F, Lucas RV Jr, Moller JH. The electrocardiogram and vectorcardiogram in tricuspid atresia. Correlation with pathologic anatomy. Am J Cardiol. 1970;25:18–27. https://doi.org/10.1016/0002-9149(70)90810-6.

25. Rao PS. Diagnosis and management of cyanotic congenital heart disease: part I. Indian J Pediatr. 2009;76:57–70. https://doi.org/10.1007/s12098-009-0030-4.

26. Orie JD, Anderson C, Ettedgui JA, Zuberbuhler JR, Anderson RH. Echocardiographic-morphologic correlations in tricuspid atresia. J Am Coll Cardiol. 1995;26:750–8. https://doi.org/10.1016/0735-1097(95)00250-8.

27. Brown DW, Gauvreau K, Powell AJ, Lang P, del Nido PJ, Odegard KC, et. Cardiac magnetic resonance versus routine cardiac catheterization before bidirectional Glenn anastomosis: long-term follow-up of a prospective randomized trial. J Thorac Cardiovasc Surg. 2013;146:1172–8. https://doi.org/10.1016/j.jtcvs.2012.12.079.

28. Akkinapally S, Hundalani SG, Kulkarni M, Fernandes CJ, Cabrera AG, Shivanna B, et al. Prostaglandin E1 for maintaining ductal patency in neonates with duct-dependent cardiac lesions. Cochrane Database Syst Rev. 2018;2:CD011417. https://doi.org/10.1002/14651858.CD011417.pub2.

29. Hsu DT, Zak V, Mahony L, Sleeper LA, Atz AM, Levine JC, et al. Enalapril in infants with single ventricle: results of a multicenter randomized trial. Circulation. 2010;122:333–40. https://doi.org/10.1161/CIRCULATIONAHA.109.927988.

30. Trusler GA, Williams WG. Long-term results of shunt procedures for tricuspid atresia. Ann Thorac Surg. 1980;29:312–6. https://doi.org/10.1016/s0003-4975(10)61477-4.

31. Blalock A, Taussig HB. Landmark article May 19, 1945: the surgical treatment of malformations of the heart in which there is pulmonary stenosis or pulmonary atresia. By Alfred Blalock and Helen B. Taussig. JAMA. 1984;251:2123–38. https://doi.org/10.1001/jama.251.16.2123.

32. Williams JA, Bansal AK, Kim BJ, Nwakanma LU, Patel ND, Seth AK, et al. Two thousand Blalock-Taussig shunts: a six-decade experience. Ann Thorac Surg. 2007;84:2070–5. https://doi.org/10.1016/j.athoracsur.2007.06.067.

33. Boucek DM, Qureshi AM, Goldstein BH, Petit CJ, Glatz AC. Blalock-Taussig shunt versus patent ductus arteriosus stent as first palliation for ductal-dependent pulmonary circulation lesions: a review of the literature. Congenit Heart Dis. 2019;14:105–9. https://doi.org/10.1111/chd.12707.

34. Rao PS. Natural history of the ventricular septal defect in tricuspid atresia and its surgical implications. Br Heart J. 1977;39:276–88. https://doi.org/10.1136/hrt.39.3.276.

35. Bonnet D, Sidi D, Vouhé DR. Absorbable pulmonary artery banding in tricuspid atresia. Ann Thorac Surg. 2001;71:360–1. https://doi.org/10.1016/S0003-4975(00)02153-6.

36. Daley M, Brizard CP, Konstantinov IE, Brink J, Jones D, d'Udekem Y. Absorbable pulmonary artery banding: a strategy for reducing reoperations. Eur J Cardiothorac Surg. 2017;5:735–9. https://doi.org/10.1093/ejcts/ezw409.

37. Rao PS, Thapar MK, Galal O, Wilson AD. Follow-up results of balloon angioplasty of native coarctation in neonates and infants. Am Heart J. 1990;120:1310–4. https://doi.org/10.1016/0002-8703(90)90241-o.

38. Fuchigami T, Nishioka M, Akashige T, Higa S, Nagata N. Off-pump atrial septectomy for infants with restrictive atrial septal defect. Ann Thorac Surg. 2017;103:e111–3. https://doi.org/10.1016/j.athoracsur.2016.07.060.

39. Torigoe T, Sato S, Kanazawa H. Percutaneous transluminal pulmonary valvuloplasty in a child with tricuspid atresia, ventricular septal defect, and severe pulmonary valve stenosis: usefulness of the femoral artery approach. Catheter Cardiovasc Interv. 2014;83:774–7. https://doi.org/10.1002/ccd.25193.

40. Yang CK, Jang WS, Choi ES, Cho S, Choi K, Nam J, et al. The clinical outcomes of damus-kaye-stansel procedure according to surgical technique. Korean J Thorac Cardiovasc Surg. 2014;47:344–9. https://doi.org/10.5090/kjtcs.2014.47.4.344.

41. Pridjian AK, Mendelsohn AM, Lupinetti FM, Beekman RH 3rd, Dick M 2nd, Serwer G, et al. Usefulness of the bidirectional Glenn procedure as staged reconstruction for the functional single ventricle. Am J Cardiol. 1993;71:959–62. https://doi.org/10.1016/0002-9149(93)90914-x.

42. Allgood NL, Alejos J, Drinkwater DC, Laks H, Williams RG. Effectiveness of the bidirectional Glenn shunt procedure for volume unloading in the single ventricle patient. Am J Cardiol. 1994;74:834–6. https://doi.org/10.1016/0002-9149(94)90450-2.

43. Salik I, Mehta B, Ambati S. Bidirectional Glenn procedure or Hemi-Fontan. [Updated 2020 Oct 16]. In: StatPearls [Internet]. Treasure Island: StatPearls Publishing. 2021. https://www.ncbi.nlm.nih.gov/books/NBK563299/. Accessed 31 Aug 2021.

44. Bradley SM, Mosca RS, Hennein HA, Crowley DC, Kulik TJ, Bove EL. Bidirectional superior cavopulmonary connection in young infants. Circulation. 1996;94:II5–II11.

45. Douglas WI, Goldberg CS, Mosca RS, Law IH, Bove EL. Hemi-Fontan procedure for hypoplastic left heart syndrome: outcome and suitability for Fontan. Ann Thorac Surg. 1999;68:1361–7. https://doi.org/10.1016/s0003-4975(99)00915-7.

46. Fontan F, Baudet E. Surgical repair of tricuspid atresia. Thorax. 1971;26:240–8. https://doi.org/10.1136/thx.26.3.240.

47. Marcelletti C, Corno A, Giannico S, Marino B. Inferior vena cava-pulmonary artery extracardiac conduit. A new form of right heart bypass. J Thorac Cardiovasc Surg. 1990;100:228–32.

48. Ben Ali W, Bouhout I, Khairy P, Bouchard D, Poirier N. Extracardiac versus lateral tunnel Fontan: a meta-analysis of long-term results. Ann Thorac Surg. 2019;107:837–43. https://doi.org/10.1016/j.athoracsur.2018.08.041.

49. Lemler MS, Scott WA, Leonard SR, Stromberg D, Ramaciotti C. Fenestration improves clinical outcome of the fontan procedure: a prospective, randomized study. Circulation. 2002;105:207–12. https://doi.org/10.1161/hc0202.102237.

50. Rychik J, Atz AM, Celermajer DS, Deal BJ, Gatzoulis MA, Gewillig MH, et al. Evaluation and management of the child and adult with Fontan circulation: a scientific statement from the American Heart Association. Circulation. 2019. https://doi.org/10.1161/CIR.0000000000000696.

51. Gewillig M, Brown SC. The Fontan circulation after 45 years: update in physiology. Heart. 2016;102:1081–6. https://doi.org/10.1136/heartjnl-2015-307467.

52. Sittiwangkul R, Azakie A, Van Arsdell GS, Williams WG, McCrindle BW. Outcomes of tricuspid atresia in the Fontan era. Ann Thorac Surg. 2004;77:889–94. https://doi.org/10.1016/j.athoracsur.2003.09.027.

53. Alsoufi B, Schlosser B, Mori M, McCracken C, Slesnick T, Kogon B, et al. Influence of morphology and initial surgical strategy on survival of infants with tricuspid atresia. Ann Thorac Surg. 2015;100:1403–9. https://doi.org/10.1016/j.athoracsur.2015.05.037.

54. Kulkarni A, Patel N, Singh TP, Mossialos E, Mehra MR. Risk factors for death or heart transplantation in single-ventricle physiology (tricuspid atresia, pulmonary atresia, and heterotaxy): a systematic review and meta-analysis. J Heart Lung Transplant. 2019;38:739–47. https://doi.org/10.1016/j.healun.2019.04.001.

55. Kverneland LS, Kramer P, Ovroutski S. Five decades of the Fontan operation: a systematic review of international reports on outcomes after univentricular palliation. Congenit Heart Dis. 2018;13:181–93. https://doi.org/10.1111/chd.12570.

56. Stout KK, Daniels CJ, Aboulhosn JA, Bozkurt B, Broberg CS, Colman JM, et al. 2018 AHA/ACC guideline for the management of adults with congenital heart disease: executive summary: a report of the American College of Cardiology/American Heart Association task force on clinical practice guidelines. Circulation. 2019;139:e637–97. https://doi.org/10.1161/CIR.0000000000000602.

57. Downing TE, Allen KY, Goldberg DJ, Rogers LS, Ravishankar C, Rychik J, et al. Surgical and catheter-based reinterventions are common in long-term survivors of the Fontan operation. Circ Cardiovasc Interv. 2017;10:e004924. https://doi.org/10.1161/CIRCINTERVENTIONS.116.004924.

58. Gardner MM, Mercer-Rosa L, Faerber J, DiLorenzo MP, Bates KE, Stagg A, et al. Association of a home monitoring program with interstage and stage 2 outcomes. J Am Heart Assoc. 2019;8:e010783. https://doi.org/10.1161/JAHA.118.010783.

Teratology of Fallot (TOF)

Abbas Mohammad

Abstract

TOF is one of the most common congenital heart diseases. It is characterized by the presence of four structural defects including (a) RVO obstruction, (b) large VSD, (c) overriding of aorta on VSD, and (d) right ventricular hypertrophy. The etiology of TOF is not fully understood but there are many aspects suspected to contribute in the developing of TOF. These aspects include genetic aspect, embryological aspect, anatomical aspect, and hemodynamic aspect. The severity of clinical features of TOF mainly depends on the severity of RVO obstruction. The clinical features vary with age. In newborn, the patient may be normal or have cyanosis according to the severity of RVO obstruction and patency of ductus arteriosus. In infants, the commonest features are poor feeding and failure to thrive. In older children, the patient may develop severe cyanosis in presence of exacerbating factors including exercise, stress, metabolic (acidosis and dehydration), drugs (beta receptor against), and ductus arteriosus closure. This condition is called "hypercyanotic spell" which is characterized by squatting posture to compensate for the cyanosis. This condition is treated by simple procedure (such as knee-chest posture), beta-agonist, and alpha-adrenergic agonist (phenylephrine). The TOF is diagnosed by (a) clinical features including history and physical examination, (b) laboratory tests including full blood count, coagulation profile, arterial blood gases, and blood culture, (c) ECG, and (d) imaging including CXR, echocardiography, and MRI. There are many differential diagnoses for TOF which may have cyanosis and should be distinguished from TOF. These differential diagnoses include cardiac, respiratory, chest wall, vascular, hematological, and neurological diseases. TOF management depends on many factors including age of the patient, severity of RVO obstruction and clinical features, and presence of complications. The medical treatment for a patient with TOF is unclear to be beneficial and some patients may benefit from afterload—reducing drugs like sildenafil and nitric oxide specifically in those with severe pulmonary insufficiency and pulmonary hypertension. The option of choice for a patient with TOF is surgical treatment but also its not curative. The surgical treatment includes the correction of surgical defects and either replacement or repair of the pulmonary valve. The bioprosthetic valve is preferable to the mechanical valve. The surgery does not eliminate the risk of arrhythmia so some patients may need AICD or radiofrequency ablation. The surgery has many complications which are divided into (a) short-term complications including cardiac tamponade, rebleeding, continuous raising of RV pressure, right ventricular failure, atrial arrhythmia, wound infection, heart block, and residual VSD and (b) long-term complications including continuous RVO obstruction, pulmonary valve sufficiency, both ventricular and atrial arrhythmia, right ventricular failure, and endocarditis. Patient with TOF needs primary and secondary prevention from endocarditis by using prophylactic antibiotics in some invasive procedures. In the long term, the patient may need reoperation or re-replacement of pulmonary valve. The TOF has many complications which are divided into (a) short-term complications including paradoxical emboli and hypercyanotic spell (b) long-term complications including arrhythmias, pulmonary valve regurgitation, CHF, and sudden death.

Keywords

Teratology of Fallot · Hypercyanosis · Heart block
Heart failure · Acrocyanosis · Pulmonary valve
Overriding aorta · Right-sided aorta · Hypercyanotic
spell · Phenylephrine

A. Mohammad (✉)
Thi Qar University, College of Medicine, Al-Nasiriyah, Iraq

© The Author(s), under exclusive license to Springer Nature Switzerland AG 2023
G. Tagarakis et al. (eds.), *Clinical and Surgical Aspects of Congenital Heart Diseases*,
https://doi.org/10.1007/978-3-031-23062-2_10

Introduction

Before discussing TOF, we discuss the heart anatomy and physiology related to TOF. The heart looks like a house. It has four rooms (chambers). In between, there are doors (valves) to the inside and outside which allow unidirectional blood flow. These heart rooms are separated by walls of different thickness (septi). The blood passes from outside to inside then travels between heart rooms through the valves and then outside to whole body. The blood comes back from the whole body as the deoxygenated blood by the superior vena cava and inferior vena into the right atrium and then into the right ventricle through the tricuspid valve. After that, its passes into the pulmonary artery through the pulmonary valve. The travel to the lung undergoes gas exchange process which occurs between pulmonary capillaries and alveoli to recurring of oxygen and removal of CO_2 then comes back to the left atrium by pulmonary veins. Then pass into left ventricle through the mitral valve. From the left ventricle it passes into aorta through aortic valve, then travel to the whole body as oxygenated blood. The heart rooms are connected parallelly. Many congenital defects may convert this connection from parallel to series connection. One of the most common of these defects is TOF. It is considered the most common cyanotic congenital heart disease. It is characterized by four structural defects including RVO obstruction, VSD, RVH, and overriding aorta. These defects differ in severity from patient to patient and the severity of defects (especially RVO obstruction) reflect the severity of the disease. Also, the TOF may be associated with other cardiac malformations such as right-sided aorta, ASD, anomalous coronary artery, PDA, bilateral superior vena cava, and additional VSD [1, 2].

Epidemiology

TOF is the most common congenital heart disease. It represents about 7–10% of all congenital heart disease and represents about 230–630 per million births. During adulthood, the percentage of TOF is about 0.1 in 350 to 0.1 in 450 people. In patients younger than 15 years, it represents about 33.3% of all congenital heart disease. The cause of TOF is unknown and most cases of TOF have no family history of TOF (sporadic cases). It most commonly occurs in males than females. When the parents are affected the chance of a sibling being affected is about 1–5%. Sometimes the TOF is associated with other extracardiac congenital defects such as bone anomalies (craniofacial and skeletal defects), hypospadias, cleft lip, and palate. Some genetic studies show that there is some genetic base for TOF including deletion mutation of 22q11 and submicroscopic genetic alternations [3].

Today, there is a large patient group in adulthood who have done cardiac surgery early in life, but the number is not exactly known because they have poor compliance for follow-up but approximately two-third of children who have repaired TOF early in childhood can reach adulthood. A study was done on 168 patients of 16 years old and older who had repaired TOF. The study shows their survival rate is about 94%. The 30 years survival rate for childhood TOF is about 75%. In adulthood, the male and female are approximately equally affected clinically, but this result is not exactly priced due to shortage of data on adults [4].

Pathophysiology

Around the 20th day of gestation, the heart starts to form by fusion of both endocardial tubes to form one tubular structure which is called the cardiac tube. The latter then looped and folded to form the atrium which has a cranial and dorsal pole, followed by moving down of primitive ventricles to the right and ventrally. The dominant heart room during embryonic and fetal life is the right ventricle which mainly contributes to supply of the placenta, lung, and lower part of the body. It receives about 65% of venus blood return during this period. The right ventricle is composed of three parts including:

1. Trapiculated apical myocardium
2. Inlet which consists of a tricuspid valve with papillary muscle and chordae tendineae
3. Conus or infundibulum

Embryonic Aspect of TOF

During embryonic life, the main contributor to TOF is unknown but thought that there is cephalic and anterior divination of the infundibular septum causing misaligned and overriding aorta that causes outflow obstruction of the right ventricle.

Anatomical Aspects of TOF

There are four structural defects in patients with TOF.

1. Right ventricular outflow obstruction: the severity of right ventricular outflow obstruction determines the severity of signs and symptoms. There is a different site for obstruction included in Table 1 with their percentages [5].

   When there is right ventricular obstruction, there is back pressure on the right ventricle causing right ventricular hypertrophy. The wall thickness of the right ventricle

Table 1 The sites of RVO obstruction and their percentages

Site	Percentage %
Infundibulum	50%
Pulmonary valve	20–25%
Infundibulum with pulmonary valve	20–25%
Supravalvular region and pulmonary artery	Rare

becomes equal to those of the left ventricle. Also, there is hypertrophy of crista supraventricular. The infundibulum of the right ventricle becomes a distinct channel that is located anterior to the VSD. This region will be smaller. Also, there is an increase in trabeculation leading to RVO obstruction. The RVO obstruction may result due to a structural defect of the pulmonary valve, which may be unicuspid or bicuspid while the pulmonary trunk will be more narrow and thinner than normal. Sometimes, there is atretic pulmonary valve so the condition is called pulmonary atresia with VSD which was previously called pseudo-truncus arteriosus [6].

2. Overriding aorta: In about two-third of cases, the aortic root overrides the right ventricle. The overriding is different from one patient to another (15–95% of the aortic orifice). The most characteristic feature of the TOF is biventricular aortic origin with large VSD. In about 25% of cases, there is right-sided aorta. There is dilatation of ascending aorta and inversely proportional to the size of the main pulmonary artery.

3. VSD: It is large and has different sites including perimembranous, subaortic, or infracristal type. Also, in some cases, there is multiple restrictive VSD, atrioventricular canal, or supracristal VSD. The characteristic feature of VSD is the presence of continuous fibrous tissue in the posteroinferior rim of structural defect between aortic and mitral valves. In about 80% of cases, the size of VSD is equal to the size of an artic orifice. The pressure in both ventricles is equal.

4. Right ventricular hypertrophy: occur due to back pressure on the right ventricle due to RVO obstruction. If there is no dilatation of the right ventricleit is hypertrophy, and on precordial palpation it is non-pulsatile (silent) [7].

Hemodynamic Aspect of TOF

1. Fetal circulation: The fetal circulation is not affected by the presence of TOF and there is no interference with umbilico-placental blood circulation. So, there is a good blood supply to the fetus and there is normal fetal growth.

2. Neonatal circulation: after birth, when the neonate takes the first breath and the lungs become ventilated, the pulmonary vascular resistance decrease rapidly and the blood flow to the lung increase. Delivery of the placenta will increase systemic vascular resistance. When there is TOF with RVO obstruction, there is a little blood flow to the lung unless there is ductus arteriosus still patent which

can maintain the pulmonary blood flow from the aorta and increase oxygen saturation which stimulates the ductus arteriosus to constrict. For unknown causes, the ductus arteriosus remains patent in patients with TOF for a period longer than in normal neonates [8].

If the ductus arteriosus is closed early and there is severe RVO obstruction, the pulmonary blood flow will decrease severely and cause low oxygen saturation of systemic blood (35–40% oxygen saturation) and there is severe cyanosis. When ductus arteriosus is not closed early and remain patent for a longer period, the collateral circulation develops and this new vessel maintains pulmonary blood flow even after the closure of the ductus arteriosus so there is no cyanosis (acyanotic phase). In this condition, there is a small chance for the development of congestive heart failure. The clinical features severity depends on the degree of RVO obstruction (systemic vascular resistance to pulmonary vascular resistance). The clinical course of TOF is divided into four phases according to hemodynamic stability:

In summary:

- The right-to-left shunt decreased by increased systemic vascular resistance. So, the pulmonary blood flow increases and also increases oxygen saturation.
- The ratio of systemic to pulmonary blood flow determines the severity of the disease.
- The presence of cyanosis depends on pulmonary blood flow which depend on the degree of RVO obstruction, the presence aortic and brachial collateral circulation, and the patency of ductus arteriosus. When there is mild RVO obstruction or there is good collateral circulation or PDA, the cyanosis disappears but some patients develop CHF and pulmonary HTN. In general, CHF is uncommon because the biventricular pressure is equal through the large VSD (Table 2).

Table 2 The phases of TOF according to hemodynamic stability

Phase	Description
Precyanotic phase	There is small pulmonary vascular resistance and mild RVO obstruction. The pulmonary blood flow is approximately adequate
Early cyanotic phase	There is exertional cyanosis because there is a balance between pulmonary and systemic circulation
Cyanotic phase	There is an increase in RVO obstruction and decreased pulmonary blood flow with the development of right-to-left shunt through the large VSD
Severe cyanotic phase	There is atresia of the pulmonary artery or severe RVO obstruction, so there is no pulmonary blood flow. Also, deoxygenated blood from right ventricle is pumped to the body through the aorta. During this phase, the pulmonary blood flow can be maintained only by PDA. If the PDA is closed, the flow is maintained by collateral circulation from the aorta and its branches

Genetic Aspect of TOF

TOF may be associated with many genetic diseases/syndromes including the following examples:

1. San-Luis valley and kabuki syndrome
2. Alagille syndrome
3. Syndrome or velocardiofacial syndrome
4. Cat's eye syndrome

The deletion mutation of 22q11.2 is present in about 8–23% of TOF cases. The common region size deleted from DNA is more than 2 megabases and about more than 25 genes. Deletion of the half of amount of one or more of these genes may result in the development of phenotype. Those patients with those genetic mutations have more chance to develop psychological disorders such as schizophrenia or mental retardation in the later life. TOF is present in about 10–15% of Alagille syndrome (is inherited as autosomal dominant. Characterized by cardiac defect, bile duct defect, ocular defect, and characteristic face). This syndrome arises due to a defect in gene known as the Jagged1 gene which codes for a specific protein on the cell membrane that act as a ligand for the transmembrane receptor. Also, there is a gene related to the disease which is called Nkx2. 5 which is associated with ASD and TOF [3].

Embryological Aspect of TOF

Until now, the embryological defect that results in the development of TOF is not fully understood. Some studies suggest that TOF defects result from a single embryological defect which is the development of proportionally unequal ventricles. The left has a large aorta and the right has a small pulmonary trunk with stenosis due to deviation of the outlet septum or conus more anteriorly. This deviation also results in the development of VSD and infundibular RVO narrowing giving rise to pulmonary stenosis. The degree of overriding aorta and sub-valvular stenosis is determined by the severity of antero-cephalic deviation. Another embryological factor for TOF is maldevelopment of the right ventricular conus which result in infundibular RVO narrowing and inadequate development of the main pulmonary artery. This hypothesis called "van Praagh hypothesis" is popular but has some limitations. It is a wide detailed hypothesis but in summary, the truncus arteriosus is unequally separated by a spiral septum that results in antero-cephalic deviation of septal conus which results in the development of structural defects of TOF. The TOF is sometimes called the "Monology of Fallot" because all structural defects result from a single embryological defect [4, 9].

Associated Anomalies

The TOF is commonly associated with cardiac and extracardiac anomalies and it may be a part of genetic syndromes. These anomalies are divided into vascular anomalies and structural cardiac anomalies:

- *Vascular Anomalies*
  1. Congenital coronary artery anomalies: The congenital coronary artery defect include either abnormal course or abnormal distribution or both. For example, single coronary ostium, single circumflex artery originated from RCA, left anterior descending artery originated from RCA, fistula between pulmonary artery and coronary arteries, anastomosis between right atrium or bronchial arteries and coronary arteries, the right ventricle crossed by large anterior ventricular arteries or large conus artery. Congenital coronary artery anomalies remain the most common congenital defects associated with TOF
  2. Left subclavian artery aberrancy
  3. Persistent left SVC
  4. Left pulmonary artery hypoplasia or sometimes absence of pulmonary artery
  5. Right aortic arch
  6. Anomalous systemic venous return.
- *Structural cardiac anomalies*
  1. Absence of pulmonary valve
  2. Ostium secundum ASD
  3. Primum ASD
  4. Complete AV canal.

Clinical Features

- *Pediatric age group*:
  The most common clinical feature of TO in infants is failure to thrive and poor feeding. When the ductus arteriosus is closed without the development of collateral circulation and when there is severe pulmonary stenosis, the patient develops cyanosis. But when there is mild pulmonary stenosis and adequate pulmonary blood flow, the patient does not develop cyanosis and remain without symptoms until a decrease in pulmonary blood flow. Some neonates have no cyanosis at birth but with time the patient will have attacks of cyanosis on feeding or crying. This condition is called "hypoxic tet spells" or "hypercyanotic spells" which is dangerous and unpredictable and can occur even in patients without cyanosis. The mechanism of tet spell is the rapid development of RVO obstruction due to right ventricular infundibular spasm which can be decreased by specific techniques, especially in older

children. The common technique used by children is squatting. Also, it has diagnostic value. It is highly specific for children with TOF. The squatting can compensate for the tet spell by decreasing the venous blood return from lower limbs which is relatively low oxygenated and allow venous blood return only from abdomen, upper limbs, head, and neck which is relatively highly oxygenated. Also, to increase systemic vascular resistance, increase left ventricular pressure and decrease the left to right shunt. With increasing age, exertional dyspnea increase. Sometimes, in children, the collateral arteries ruptured and result in hemoptysis. Rarely, the patient remains asymptomatic in adult life. In general, cyanosis increase with age, but there are some factors that may increase in infants including:

- Exercise
- Stress
- Metabolic (acidosis and dehydration)
- Drugs (beta receptor against)
- Ductus arteriosus closure.

The right-to-left shunt causes cyanosis due to a high percentage of deoxygenated blood in systemic circulation which in turn result in polycythemia. The direction of the shunt depends on the degree of pulmonary stenosis. When the stenosis is not severe, the pressure inside both ventricles is equal and the shunt across VSD is bidirectional. When the stenosis is very mild and the pressure inside the right ventricle is lower than the left ventricle, the direction of shunt is left to right which causes normal systemic oxygen saturation. This condition is called "pink TOF." Recurrent hypoxia and TIA may result in mental retardation. The other symptom is headache that is considered a constant symptom. The headache is due to CNS complications including brain abscess and venous sinus thrombosis. A brain abscess is one of the important causes of death in patients with TOF if not recognized. It more commonly occurs in those of 2-years old age. Some patients develop anemia instead polycythemia which can cause cerebral thrombosis. Hemoptysis also may occur due to rupture of bronchial collateral circulation or pulmonary thrombosis due to low blood flow and polycythemia. The aortic engorgement may compress the trachea causing wheezing and stridor. Also, the CNS problem may result in loss of normal nasal Resonance due to velopharyngeal dysfunction [10].

- *Adult age group*:
    In adult, the clinical features of adult with TOF depend on the severity of structural defects. The fact that should be understood taken in care that the repairing surgery for TOF is palliative surgery not curative surgery because the surgery repairs defects not repair the cause. So, in long term, the RV Anatomical and pulmonary vessels changes are ongoing and is not prevented by surgery. So, all patients who have repaired TOF will come back with clinical symptoms due to right ventricular failure. But the majority of those patients remain asymptomatic for at least two decades after repairing surgery, then after symptom-free period the patient develops asymptomatic pulmonary valve insufficiency. This insufficiency increases with time to become symptomatic insufficiency. At this time the most clinical presentation for those patients are palpitations and exercise intolerance [11].

Physical Examination

General inspection: With time the TOF increase in severity. In adulthood, the patient develops palpitation and exertional dyspnea. Also, there is a clinical feature of right ventricular dysfunction including raised JVP, evidence of systemic venous congestion including ascites, hepatomegaly, and peripheral edema. On JVP examination, there is A wave that occurs when there is severe pulmonary stenosis that causes RVH which resists emptying of the right atrium causing late diastolic atrial contraction [12, 13].

Auscultation: On Auscultation, there is low-pitched diastolic murmur which is very difficult to be heard in most patients because it has a short period this murmur occurs due to pulmonary valve insufficiency. This can be missed even in severe insufficiency. The other finding on auscultation is ejection click that occurs due to aortic dilatation. This aortic dilatation may cause aortic valve insufficiency in some patients which result in the development of mid-diastolic murmur in the aortic area. The other type of murmur also may be found due to VSD is pansystolic murmur and RVO obstruction (ejection systolic murmur). The pulmonary valve insufficiency is easily missed in a patient with TOF and with time leads to the development of right ventricular failure. So most of those patients in adulthood require correction of pulmonary valve function either by replacement or just repair [14].

Hypercyanotic Spells

It is characteristic phenomenon for patients with TOF. The incidence of this phenomenon increase to peak between 6 and 24 months of age. It rarely occurs after 2 years of age. The aggravating factors to this condition include crying, feeding, and defecation but sometimes occur spontaneously without aggravating factors, especially in patients who have severe cyanosis. There is a poor correlation between hypercyanotic spell and degree of cyanosis. It is a more common short period after steep awaking. It is characterized by paroxysmal dyspnea, limpness, deep cyanosis, CNS symptoms (CVA, convulsion), or death. Mechanism of spell is rapid RVO obstruction due to infundibular spasms which increase the pressure inside the right ventricle more than the left ventricle and as a result the right-to-left shunt increases across VSD and pumping of the blood from the right ventricle into the aorta also increased. As the result, the deoxygenated blood is pumped to the whole body and increases cyanosis. This hypothesis is called "Paul hypothesis" which is the most accepted hypothesis until now. While the mechanism of aggravating factors (crying, feeding, and defecation especially after waking) is that the respiratory center in the brain becomes sensitive to a sudden change in cardiac output after a long period of sleeping. After awaking, there is a sudden increase in activity. So sudden increase in heart rate, venous return, and cardiac output in presence of RVO obstruction as a result of the pressure inside the right ventricle increase more than the left ventricle and increase right-to-left shunt. Also, there is an infundibular spasm which enforces the condition. The deoxygenated blood is pumped to whole body causing high arterial Pco_2 and low arterial PO_2 also decrease in arterial ph. At the same time, tissue hypoxia causes metabolic acidosis and a further decrease in arterial ph. At this time, the sensitive respiratory centre after prolonged sleeping will be over stimulated by chemical change (change in PH) causing further increase in cardiac output, heart rate, and hyperpnea. This cycle will further be repeated causing a further increase in severity each time. Also, arrhythmia like rapid AF and paroxysmal SVT may develop causing further deterioration by increasing heart rate and cardiac output. This cycle continues until clinical cyanotic spell is established which is interrupted by the simple procedures or progresses to death. The most common one of this procedure is squatting which is a characteristic procedure for a patient with TOF. It is adapted by older child after simple exercise to relieve dyspnea. It is commonly seen between 2 and 10 years of age when a child gets walking. Also, there are equivalent procedures including underneath leg down with sitting, standing with crossed leg, knee-chest posture, and lying down posture. Squatting and its equivalent are used to reverse the dyspnea. The squatting can compensate for the tet spell by decreasing the venous blood return from lower limbs which is relatively low oxygenated and allow venous blood return only from the abdomen, upper limbs, head, and neck which is relatively highly oxygenated. Also, to increase systemic vascular resistance, increase left ventricular pressure and decrease the left to right shunt across VSD.

Diagnosis

The diagnosis of TOF depends on history, physical examination, laboratory investigations, ECG, cardiac catheterization, and imaging studies:

- Laboratory investigations: laboratory tests used to evaluate TOF including:
  1. *Full blood count*: in most patients the CBC show mild anemia, but when there is no cyanosis, CBC shows polycythemia in rare conditions
  2. *Coagulation profile*: in some patients with bleeding and cyanosis, the coagulation profile shows abnormal findings.
  3. *Arterial blood gases*: ABG is used to evaluate the condition of Po2, acid-base balance, and lactate level. In patients undergoing surgery for repairing TOF, the most prognostic factor for mortality are base and lactate levels
  4. *Blood culture*: used to exclude sepsis or endocarditis in a patient with fever because a patient with TOF is vulnerable to endocarditis due to presence of structural defects.
- ECG: due to the presence of pressure load in right ventricle, the ECG shows right axis deviation, RBBB, and RVH. The significant degree for RVH is when the QRS duration is 180 ms or more because it may cause sudde death due to arrhythmia. Also, the other productive finding for the develoment of sudden death due to arrhythmia is the rate of widening of QRS duration. When the rate of QRS widening is more than 3.5 ms/year, it becomes associated with a high risk of sudden death. Also, not only abnormal increase QRS is significant but the rapid change in QRS duration is significant even with normal QRS duration. Another predictive risk for sudden death is heart rate variation. in some patients with TOF, the patient has atrial arrhythmia on ECG as AF and atrial tachycardia [15].
- Cardiac catheterization: the catheterization is not the study of choice for patient with TOF but may use to evaluate the pressure load in the pulmonary artery and RV. Also used to evaluate the pulmonary vessel condition, size, and location of VSD. Also, it is necessary when there is suspicion of pulmonary hypertension and anomalous coronary artery when there is concern about pulmonary arterial disease and when the heart anatomy is difficult to be evaluated by Echocardiography.

- Imaging:
  1. *Chest X-ray*: in some patients with TOF, the chest X-ray is normal but in other patients there is cardiomegaly due to RVH. The pathognomic radiological finding of TOF on chest x-ray is boot—shaped heart. This important radiological feature results due to small size pulmonary artery with an upright elevation of the cardiac apex due to RVH. Also, there is an oligemic lung field due to decreased pulmonary blood flow. In adult, this radiological feature is not always seen.
  2. *Echocardiography*: in adults echocardiography is used to assess structural defects. Color-flow echocardiography is more important than traditional echocardiography because it can evaluate the following:
     - If there is residual VSD, ASD, and PDA
     - Overall heart function
     - Cardiac valves status
     - Severity and grade of RVO obstruction.
  3. *Magnetic Resonance Imaging*: MRI is the gold standard imaging modality to assess the size and function of RV. Also used to assess the volume of pulmonary regurgitation, so it is the first imaging of choice in patients suspected to have pulmonary valve defect. Also, it is used to evaluate the size of the aorta, severity of RVO obstruction, state of pulmonary vessels, RVH, VSD, intrathoracic pressure, blood flow, and

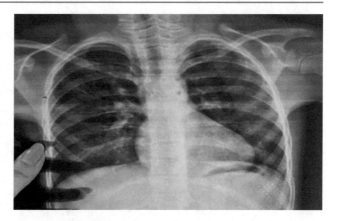

Fig. 1 X-ray of a patient with TOF

gradients. The MRI differs from other modalities by its ability to detect stenosis in branches of the pulmonary artery which can increase the severity of pulmonary valve regurgitation and development of collateral circulation between the aorta and pulmonary circulation which is common when there is pulmonary atresia. Some centers use MRI for screening of pediatrics with TOF even in asymptomatic patients to provide baseline information that can be used for monitoring of patient every 3–7 years to detect any change [16, 17] (Fig. 1).

Differential Diagnosis

See Table 3.

Table 3 Differential diagnosis of TOF (conditions associated with cyanosis)

Clinical features									
Differential diagnosis		Symptoms			Signs				
Class	Conditions	Chest pain	Dyspnea	Fever	Central cyanosis	Peripheral cyanosis	Peripheral edema	Finger clubbing	By auscultation
Cardiac conditions									
Congenital heart disease	TOF	May be present	May be present	No	Yes	No	No	May be present	Harsh systolic murmur
	Isolated pulmonary valve stenosis	Yes	Yes	No	Yes	No	No	May be present	Ejection systolic murmur
	PDA	May be present	May be present	No	Yes	No	No	May be present	Continuous machinery murmur
	TPG	May be present	Yes	No	Yes	No	No	May be present	Both systolic and diastolic murmurs
	Truncus arteriosus	May be present	May be present	No	Yes	No	No	May be present	Ejection systolic murmur
	AV canal defect	May be present	Yes	No	Yes	May be present	No	May be present	Ejection systolic murmur
	Ebstein anomaly	May be present	May be present	No	Yes	No	No	No	Loaded S1 heart sound
	Total anomalous pulmonary venous return	May be present	Yes	No	Yes	No	No	May be present	Systolic murmur in the pulmonary area
Acquired heart disease	MI	Yes	Yes	May be present	Yes	No	No	No	There are S3, S4 heart sounds
	Valvular heart defects	No	Yes	No	No	Yes	No	Yes	Murmurs according to pathology
	Heart failure	Yes	Yes	May be present	No	Yes	No	Yes	S3 with coarse basal crackle
	Cardiogenic shock	No	Yes	No	Yes	May be present	No	Yes	Muffled heart sounds
	Cardiomyopathy	Yes	Yes	No	Yes	No	No	Yes	There are S3, S4 heart sounds
	Cardiac tumor	May be present	Yes	No	Yes	No	May be present	May be present	Early diastolic murmur
Vascular									
Arterial disease	Thromboembolism	Yes	No	No	No	Yes	No	May be present	Normal
	Raynaud's phenomenon	No	No	No	No	Yes	No	Yes	Normal
	Acrocyanosis	No	No	No	No	Yes	No	May be present	Normal
Venous disease	Venous congestion	No	No	No	No	Yes	Yes	Yes	Normal
	SVC syndrome	May be present	No	No	No	Yes	Yes	May be present	Normal
Pulmonary conditions									

Table 3 (continued)

Clinical features								
Differential diagnosis		Symptoms			Signs			
Class	Conditions	Chest pain	Dyspnea	Fever	Central cyanosis	Peripheral cyanosis	Peripheral edema	Finger clubbing	By auscultation
Airway diseases	Foreign body	May be present	Yes	No	No	Yes	No	No	Wheeze with decreased breathing sounds
	Chronic bronchitis	May be present	Yes	May be present	Yes	No	No	Yes	Wheeze and crackle
	Bacteria Trecheatitis	Yes	Yes	Yes	No	Yes	No	No	Stridor (mostly inspiratory
	Epiglotitis	No	Yes	Yes	No	Yes	No	No	Presence of Stridor
	Severe croup	No	Yes	May be present	No	Yes	No	No	Presence of Stridor
	Atelectasis	Yes	Yes	May be present	Yes	No	No	No	Wheeze with diminished breathing sounds (localized)
	Obstructive sleep apnea	No	Yes	No	Yes	No	No	No	Normal auscultation
Parenchymal lung disease	Asthma	May be present	Yes	No	Yes	No	No	May be present	
	COPD	Yes	Yes	May be present	No	Yes	May be present	May be present	Inspiratory crackle, wheeze, and decrease breathing sounds
	Pneumonia	Yes	Yes	Yes	Yes	No	No	May be present	Crackle and wheeze with pleural friction
	Alveolitis	Yes	Yes	May be present	Yes	May be present	No	May be present	Crackle and wheeze
	TB	Yes	Yes	Yes	Yes	No	No	May be present	Expiratory wheeze with decreased breathing sounds in severe asthma
	ARDS	Yes	Yes	May be present	Yes	No	No	May be present	Inspiratory crackle, wheeze, and decrease breathing sounds
	Lung cancer	May be present	Yes	No	Yes	No	No	May be present	Wheeze, Stridor with the absence of breathing sounds
	Pulmonary fibrosis	Yes	Yes	No	Yes	No	No	Yes	Bilateral fine crackle
	Cystic fibrosis	May be present	Yes	May be present	No	Yes	No	Yes	Crackle and wheeze
	Pneumoconiosis	May be present	Yes	No	Yes	No	No	May be present	Expiratory wheeze
Pulmonary vascular diseases	Pulmonary embolism (massive)	Yes	Yes	May be present	Yes	No	May be present	No	Loaded P2 heart sound, crackle, and diminished breathing sounds
	Pulmonary HTN	May be present	Yes	No	No	No	No	Yes	Pulmonary arterial bruit
	Pulmonary AV malformation	Yes	Yes	No	No	Yes	No	May be present	Murmurs of tricuspid and pulmonary regurgitations
Chest wall diseases	Pneumothorax	Yes	Yes	No	No	Yes	No	No	Diminished breathing sounds
	Flail chest	Yes	Yes	No	No	Yes	No	No	Normal auscultation

(continued)

Table 3 (continued)

Clinical features									
Differential diagnosis		Symptoms			Signs				
Class	Conditions	Chest pain	Dyspnea	Fever	Central cyanosis	Peripheral cyanosis	Peripheral edema	Finger clubbing	By auscultation
Hematological disorders									
Hematological disorders	Polycythemia	May be present	Yes	May be present	Yes	Yes	No	Yes	Normal
	Methemoglobinemia	Yes	Yes	May be present	Yes	No	No	No	Wheezing
Neurological disorders									
Neurological disorders	Coma	No	No	No	Yes	No	Yes	No	Wheezing
	Seizure	No	Yes	May be present	Yes	No	No	No	Normal
	Head trauma	No	Yes	No	Yes	No	No	No	Normal
	Breathing-holding attacks	May be present	Yes	No	Yes	No	No	No	Wheezing

Management

All patients with TOF need preoperative and follow-up care. This follow-up includes monitoring of body weight, progressive cyanosis, and the parents should be educated to distinguish the hypercyanotic spell early with early treatment [18, 19].

Treatment of Hypercyanotic Spells

The hypercyanotic spell is one of the threatening conditions in a patient with TOF and it is one of the important cardiological emergency topics. The early treatment of spell is important because late diagnosis and treatment may result in brain death due to ischemia. The management of spell starts with simple maneuvers. The most commonly used maneuver is squatting (discussed previously) and knee-chest posture. The patient should remain calm and giving off oxygen and avoidance of stimulation. If severe cyanosis is persisting, acidosis will develop. If these simple maneuvers failed to reverse cyanosis, the next step is using medical treatments including:

- Stabilization of patient by using supportive measures including intravenous fluid, oxygen, treatment of acidosis, and using morphine
- Increasing of pulmonary blood flow by using beta-blockers to relieve infundibular spasm adequate RV filling
- Increasing of systemic vascular resistance to increase pulmonary blood flow by using alpha-adrenergic agonist (phenylephrine) which is the last medical option.

In a newborn when there is profound cyanosis, alprostadil (prostaglandin) is beneficial to maintain PDA to allow passage of blood from aorta into pulmonary artery and increased pulmonary blood flow. In those newborns, the surgery is indicated during neonatal period. If medical therapy is failed to reverse severe cyanosis, urgent Blalock–Taussig shunt is indicated (making of a synthetic shunt between systemic and pulmonary circulation by using the tube to increase pulmonary blood flow). Another surgical option is extract-corporeal membrane oxygenation. Preoperative using of beta-blocker is beneficial while arranging for surgery [20] (Table 4).

Medical Treatment of TOF

In a patient with pulmonary insufficiency, the medical treatment including afterload reducing drugs is not beneficial and does not prevent the condition progression. Some patients especially those with severe pulmonary hypertension are put on sildenafil which may have some benefits, but it is unclear if it is beneficial for long term or not due to a lack of studies and it is unknown to prevent long-term progression of the condition. The other drug that is used for pulmonary insufficiency is nitric oxide which is suggested to be effective for pulmonary hypertension and pulmonary insufficiency [21, 22].

Surgical Treatment of TOF

The ideal surgery for repairing of TOF is primary repairing in infants by using of cardiopulmonary bypass. Surgery should include VSD closing and RVO obstruction relieving by resection of the stenosis of infundibulum. Before using pulmonary bypass, a shunt should be placed between systemic and pulmonary circulation.

Table 4 The lines of management of hypercyanotic spell

Line no.	Options	Description
First line	Simple Maneuvers	• Squatting • Knee chest posture
	Supportive care	• Intravascular volume replacement by fluid or blood when needed • IV morphine to keep the child calm when needed • Correction of acidosis by using sodium bicarbonate when needed • Oxygen supplement to a degree that does not stimulate the child.

Second line	Beta blockers	• Propranolol
		  Dose:
		   – Parental rout: 0.15–0.25 mg/kg given as initial bolus dose. Can be repeated in 15 min
		   – Oral route: 2–8 mg/kg/day given in 6 h divided dose
		• Esmolol
		  Dose: initial IV bolus dose of 100–500 µg/kg followed by infusion dose of 50–500 µg/kg

	Supportive care	As mentioned in first line
Third line	Phenylephrine	Dose: initial IV bolus dose of 5–10 µg/kg followed by infusion dose of 0.1–0.5 µg/kg
	Supportive care	As mentioned in first line
Newborn with severe cyanosis and low pulmonary blood flow	Alprostadil	Given IV in a dose of 0.02–0.1 µg/kg
	Supportive care	As mentioned in first line

Note: one of the adverse side effects of Alprostadil is apnea and conversion to mechanical ventilation. so, the apnea should be monitored

Surgery of TOF in Adults

In an adult risk-benefit ratio of surgery should be taken into care because some patients have irreversible RV failure which does not benefit from any surgery other than transplantation [23].

Time of Surgery

The time of surgery in an adult with TOF is controversial. In past, surgery was done when there is a long QRS duration (more than 180 ms on ECG) some surgeons prefer the surgery when the patient has symptoms. Other surgeons say that when the patient has RV insufficiency, replacement of the pulmonary valve is the only recommended procedure. Others still say that the earlier surgery is more beneficial depending on the finding of echocardiography not on the clinical picture of the patient. The arguments about the time of surgery in an adult are conflicting but the universal argument for all surgeons is that the waiting of patient to become symptomatic before doing surgery is an unbeneficial option because there is irreversible damage to the right ventricle. Also, pulmonary valve replacement should be done before the development of RV sufficiency. The surgery is not needed when there is normal RV function, no or mild dilatation of the RV, and the patient is asymptomatic [24].

Procedure of Surgery

The surgery is done by cardioplegia and using cardiopulmonary bypass. The first structural defect repaired is VSD closure after cardiac arrest. The VSD is closed by a patch followed by infundibular dilatation and then repairing of the pulmonary valve. For pulmonary valve insufficiency, transmural patch is not used for the adult patient due to the risk of pulmonary valve insufficiency late in life. So, the pulmonary valve is either repaired or replaced without using of transmural patch. The best choice for pulmonary valve insufficiency is the replacement of valve. This option can improve the function of RV and reduce its size in long term. But the risk of arrhythmia is the same and not affected by options of pulmonary insufficiency correction [25, 26].

Choosing the Type of Valve (Bioprosthetic or Mechanical Valve)

The best type of valve used for pulmonary valve replacement is a bioprosthetic valve not a mechanical valve due to three reason

1. Increased risk of thrombosis associated with mechanical valve which needs anticoagulant lifelong that put the patient at risk of bleeding
2. Lower blood flow in the right ventricle and pulmonary circulation
3. In female, using mechanical valve with anticoagulant (warfarin) is a strong limitation to getting pregnant due to the difficulty using of warfarin during pregnancy (it is teratogenic). There are two types of bioprosthetic valves which are homograft (human tissue) and animal tissue (Porcine heart valve or pericardium of bovine). The main problem associated with bioprosthetic valve is that has no longer survival. On average about 47. 5% (40–55% as a range) will survive only one-decade post-replacement and then damaged. So bioprosthetic valve is not suitable for young patients because there is a high chance for repeating surgery and re-replacement with a new valve once or more in the future that increases the chance of surgery complication.

Using of AICD (Automatic Implantable Cardioverter-Defibrillator)

As mentioned above, the surgery does not eliminate the risk of arrhythmia. So, in some patients who persist to expert ventricular arrhythmia that put the patient at risk of sudden, AICD is indicated. AICD was implanted under local anesthesia.

Radiofrequency Ablation

In a patient with TOF who has a trial or ventricular arrhythmia, the other option for treatment of this arrhythmia is ablation which is a recent technique.

Postoperative Monitoring

The patients who get open cardiac surgery should be sent to ICU with restricting monitoring of hemodynamic measures. In a study on postoperative opening cardiac surgery patients found that the short-term results depend on the inotropic amount and pressure support during admission to ICU. The patients who need more support have a more worse result. Any postoperative patient of open-heart surgery should stay intubated and on mechanical ventilation until stabilization of respiratory and cardiac status. The intravascular volume and peripheral tissue perfusion should be maintained along with an adequate cardiac output by using of atrial pacemaker on need. Daily body weight should be checked to assess the volume condition. A permanent pacemaker is indicated when the heart rate is not back to normal value within 5 days in a patient on a temporary pacemaker due to heart block.

Outcomes of Surgery

There are various results of surgery among patients with TOF. The mortality rate is about 6–10%. The 5 years survival rate is more than 90% and 10 years survival rate is more than 86% after the replacement of the pulmonary valve. The studies show excellent short-term outcomes while there are poor long-term outcomes. Some patients will need re-replacement of the pulmonary valve especially bioprosthetic valve and may need the insertion of pacemaker, while other patients may continue to have elevated RV pressure. Some studies that follow postoperative patients show that the replacement of the pulmonary valve reverses or reduces the progression of pulmonary valve insufficiency. These complications including tricuspid insufficiency and RV failure. While the risk of arrhythmia is not affected by surgery, some studies show that there is a reduced risk of arrhythmia in the short postoperative period but in long-term, there are no differences in risk. So, the risk of arrhythmia generally is not affected by surgery [27, 28].

Complications of Surgery

The complications of TOF repairing surgery are divided into short-term and long-term complications.

Short-term Complications
1. Cardiac tamponade
2. Rebleeding
3. Continuous raising of RV pressure
4. Right ventricular failure
5. Atrial arrhythmia
6. Wound infection
7. Heart block
8. Residual VSD

Long-term Complications
1. Continuous RVO obstruction
2. Pulmonary valve sufficiency
3. Both ventricular and atrial arrhythmia
4. Right ventricular failure
5. Endocarditis: which persists lifelong risk, but it is lower than those in unrepaired TOF.

Arrhythmia is considered the most common cause of death after surgery especially ventricular arrhythmia, which is the most common type. Ventricular arrhythmia-related sudden death is reported in about 0.5% of patients with TOF within 10 years postoperatively. While in patients with early surgery, the risk of arrhythmia is about 1% [29].

Prophylaxis for Infective Endocarditis

It is commenced before surgery and continues 6 months postoperatively. Lifelong use of prophylaxis during invasive procedures (such as surgical dental procedures, respiratory system procedures, and infected skin) is indicated in patients with postoperative residual defects at the site or near bioprosthetic valve. [30] (Table 5).

For cardiac surgery 'the aim of the prophylaxis is against staphylococcus spp., so the prophylaxis of choice is cephalosporin (cephalexin). But in general, choosing of antibiotic depends on the susceptibility result for each hospital. For other invasive (such as surgical dental procedures and invasive respiratory system procedures infected skin) the aim of prophylaxis is against enterococci, so the prophylactic of choice is penicillin (ampicillin or amoxicillin). It is indicated before mentioned invisible in all followings:

Table 5 The drugs of choice and their doses

Option	Dose
Cephalexin	Single oral dose of 50 mg/kg given 1 h before invasive procedures. Maximum dose is 2000 mg/dose
Amoxicillin	Single oral dose of 50 mg/kg given 1 h before invasive procedures. Maximum dose is 2000 mg/dose
Ampicillin	Single IV or IM dose of 50 mg/kg is given half an hour before invasive procedures. Maximum dose is 2000 mg/dose

1. Any patient with uncorrected CHD or those with palliative shunt
2. Any patient with corrected CHD but there is a residual structural defect at the site or near bioprosthetic valve.

Secondary prevention

Any patient with TOF should receive seasonal vaccination against respiratory syncytial virus. Also, taking antibiotic for infected endocarditis is indicated before invasive procedures such as surgical dental procedures or invasive procedures for any patient with uncorrected TOF or corrected TOF with residual defects at the site or near the device. Female with TOF should have counseling before getting pregnant because there is 10-folds increase in the risk of TOF in off siblings if there is a first-degree relative who has TOF. For a pregnant female, who has a previous child with CHD or she has CHD, fetal echocardiography is indicated during pregnancy. Female with corrected TOF should undergo a complete cardiological assessment before pregnancy [31, 32].

Patient Education

The patients should be informed that the surgery is not a curative option and other surgery may be needed in the future. Female with TOF should be informed about the risk of her children having TOF or other CHD so counseling is indicated before getting pregnant and cardiac assessment by echocardiography is indicated during the pregnancy.

Reoperation

The percentage of patients who underwent surgical correction of TOF during childhood and need reoperation in the future is about5%. The most important indications for short-term reoperation

1. Residual RVO obstruction with pressure more than 60 mmHg
2. Residual VSD with a shunt of to 2:1

The residual VSD Significance depends on its size. When it is small, there is no clinical significance but when it is large in size, there is a clinical significance because it caused volume overload which is intolerable to the patient. In a patient who undergo reoperation, there is a dramatic improvement and low-risk operation. Sometimes, there is a progression of pulmonary valve sufficiency and development of RV insufficiency. The pulmonary valve may be re-repaired or re-replaced in about 5% of patients with TOF

who underwent surgery during childhood. But in general, there is increasing long-term survival rates due to excellent surgery outcomes at the present time. Most of those patients presented with the clinical features of pulmonary valve regurgitation which is treated by replacement with bioprosthetic valve which is better than mechanical valve to avoid high risk of thrombosis [33].

- Indications of pulmonary valve re-replacement in corrected TOF
  1. *Asymptomatic patient: if there are two or more of the following criteria:*
     (a) Index of right ventricular end-systolic volume is more than 80%
     (b) Index of right ventricular end-diastolic volume is 155% or more
     (c) Ejection fraction of the right ventricle is less than 47%
     (d) Ejection fraction of the left ventricle is less than 55%
     (e) Large RVO tract aneurysm
     (f) Wide QRS complex more than 162nd right-sided heart volume overload sustained arrhythmia
     (g) Significant hemodynamic abnormalities including:
        – RVO obstruction with right ventricular systolic pressure is 0.7 systemic or more
        – Severe pulmonary artery stenosis (pulmonary blood less than 30% in affected branch) not corrected by transcatheter interventions
        – Tricuspid regurgitation in a moderate degree of more severe
        – Pulmonary to systemic shunt through residual VSD or ASD is 1:5 or more
        – Severe aortic valve insufficiency.
  2. *Symptomatic patients*: if there are symptoms (such as the feature of CHF, arrhythmia-induced syncope, and exercise intolerance not related to extracardiac condition) with one or more of the criteria mentioned above.

Prognosis

During recent years, the postoperative survival rate for a patient with TOF is increasing and decreasing early mortality. According to data from American and European cardiothoracic surgery registries, the perioperative mortality rate is lower than 3%. Some factors can affect the perioperative mortality rate including:

1. Oxygen saturation
2. Gradient pressure through pulmonary valve
3. Pulmonary arteries size
4. Pulmonary valve function

The perioperative mortality rate is high among patients with the following factors:

1. Repairing with a transannular patch which is considered only in severe TOF when the pulmonary annulus Z score is between −2 and −3
2. Prematurity
3. Associated coronary anomalies
4. Small size of body
5. Genetic anomalies

A follow-up for a medium period shows no significant change in mortality rate while the long-term rate is about 68.5%. The most important factors in long-term outcomes are the severity of pulmonary valve insufficiency and residual RVO obstruction. In recent years, the adulthood surviving for a patient with TOF is increased than those patients need a special care lifelong and with increased rate of adulthood survival, the rate of reoperation is also increased. During following of patients with repaired TOF, the registries found that about 44% of patients need reoperation by surgery or catheter intervention beyond the age of 35 years. Other study found that about 19–29% of patients with repaired TOF reoperated beyond the age of 30 years. A study found that the risk of reoperation and 10-years survival rate is lower among patients with the transarterial repair which is about 80% that need no reoperation. Another study found that about 75% need no reoperation within 25 years postoperatively. The single case-control analysis compared with outcomes of transarterial and transventricular repair. It found that the pulmonary valve replacement amount for patients with transarterial repair is lower than those with transventricular repair. But use of transannular patch increases the risk of reoperation [34–36].

Follow-Up

Any patient undergoing surgical repairing of TOF should be assessed by a cardiologist. The recommendation of CCA/AHA is that any adult with corrected TOF should undergo a scheduled assessment by adult CHD specialized cardiologist. The frequency of assessment can increase according to clinical pictures and the result of assessment. The other important advice is that echocardiography and MRI should be performed only by expert physician. The other guideline from the European society of cardiology is the same recommendations as CCA /AHA including the following of adult with corrected TOF by an expertise cardiologist. Female with corrected TOF should get counseling before pregnancy and during pregnancy. For a patient with corrected TOF, every 1–5 years should undergo RV function assessment and check pulmonary valve state for valve insufficiency or

stenosis by echocardiography. This schedule of assessment is variable from patient to other. Yearly assessment is indicated if there is a valve problem (stenosis or insufficiency), RV dilatation progression, or symptomatic patient. The other modalities for assessment of RV function are MRI and CT scan. The MRI provides accurate assessment by producing a 3D picture of RV volume, so now it is used for time detection of replacement of pulmonary valve. In some patients, multiple imaging modalities are used due to their significant clinical picture and the result of the previous assessment. [37, 38].

Complications of TOF

- Short-term complications

1. Paradoxical emboli: patient with unrepaired TOF has communication between the venous circulation and arterial circulation, so there is a risk of paradoxical emboli because venous embolism can pass through the large VSD and enter the left ventricle or directly into the aorta then impacted in the arterial circulation causing ischemia of the supplied organ. Also, there is an increase in the risk of intravenous catheter-related air embolism because air bubbles pass through the catheter into the venous system can pass through the VSD causing arterial air embolism. So intravenous catheters should be used with caution in patients with unrepaired TOF. There is no need for anticoagulant prophylaxis in a patient with unrepaired TOF but when there is a risk of venous thrombosis it should be identified and managed
2. Hypercyanotic spell: discussed previously.

- Long-term complications
  1. Ventricular arrhythmia: there is a medium risk of ventricular arrhythmia in a patient with unrepaired TOF. The risk of development of ventricular arrhythmia is one of the limiting factors for long-term outcomes. A retrospective study was done in the period of 1960–1993 for patients who have unrepaired TOF. The result of the study was as follows
     - No ventricular arrhythmia in 28% of patients
     - Minor ventricular arrhythmia in 51% of patients
     - Non-sustained VT in 10.5% of patients
     - Sustained VT in 9% of patients

     The most important risk factor for ventricular arrhythmia is the widening of QRS complex. So, monitoring of QRS width is important for the detection of the risk of arrhythmia. If there is a widening of QRS, further assessment with other electrophysiological studies is necessary. A recommendation by some of the expertise clinicians for periodic monitoring with

Holter as an arrhythmia screening test. Other clinicians use exercise test as a screening test [39–41].

2. Atrial arrhythmia: there is a medium risk of atrial arrhythmia which is one of the common long-term complication of corrected TOF which start to increase in the previous decade. A retrospective analysis was done on an adult who underwent surgical repair of TOF during childhood. It shows that about one-third of included patients have atrial arrhythmia in the form of SVT, AF, atrial flutter, and sinus node block.

3. Pulmonary valve regurgitation with right-sided heart failure: the risk is high. A one to study done on 100 adult patients who underwent surgical correction of TOF in childhood and by using MRI imaging show that poor left ventricle and right ventricle functions are independent risk factor for a poor clinical condition. Congestive [42].

4. Congestive heart failure: the long-term risk of development of CHF in patients with TOF is low. The symptoms may be present in a patient with minimal RVO obstruction and most commonly treated with furosemide, but the diuresis-induced hypercyanotic spell should be considered. In patients with repaired TOF, the CHF is not a common long-term complication. One study done on 100 adult patients with repaired TOF during childhood found the following results (percentages or stages of CHF):
   – Patients with NYHA class I about 48%
   – Patients with NYHA class II about 40%
   – Patients with NYHA class III about 12%

5. Sudden death: there is a low risk of sudden death in patients with repaired TOF. The sudden death occurs due to ventricular arrhythmia (VF and VT) which is the most common cardiac-related death in a patient with corrected TOF. There is a belief that sudden cardiac death is associated with the progression of right heart failure. There is an increase in the risk of sudden death per year from 0.06 to 0.2% 10 years postoperatively. Prospective study done in the US during the period of 1958–1996 shows that about 11 of each 445 patients with corrected TOF died suddenly. Another study on an adult patient who underwent surgical repairing of TOF during childhood found that 100% of patients who died suddenly have moderate to severe pulmonary valve insufficiency [43–48].

Multiple Choice Questions

1. The severity of clinical features of TOF mainly depends on the severity of which of the following:
   A. VSD
   B. Overriding of aorta
   C. Degree of RVO obstruction
   D. Patient age

2. By physical examination of the patient with TOF, all of the following murmurs may be heard except:
   A. Low-pitched diastolic murmur of pulmonary valve insufficiency
   B. Pansystolic murmur of RVO obstruction
   C. Ejection systolic murmur of VSD
   D. Mid diastolic murmur of aortic valve insufficiency

3. All of the following are associated anomalies for TOF except:
   A. Congenital coronary artery anomalies
   B. ASD
   C. Right-sided aortic arch
   D. Right subclavian artery aberrancy

4. All of the following are aggregating factors for hypercyanotic spell except:
   A. Isoproterenol
   B. DKA
   C. Diarrhea
   D. Indomethacin

5. A 4-year-old boy with uncorrected TOF presented with severe cyanosis and dyspnea while playing football. The oxygen saturation was 80%. What is the first step in the treatment of this patient?
   A. Propranolol
   B. Phenylephrine
   C. Knee–chest posture
   D. Alprostadil

6. In Tetralogy of Fallot, the tetralogy comprises all EXCEPT
   A. Pulmonary stenosis.
   B. Left ventricular hypertrophy.
   C. Overriding of the ventricular septal defect by the aorta.
   D. Left ventricular hypertrophy.

7. Palliative Blalock–Taussig shunt is done:
   A. Between pulmonary vein and aorta
   B. Between pulmonary artery and aorta
   C. Between subclavian artery to subclavian vein
   D. Between pulmonary artery and subclavian artery

8. The most common site of RVO obstruction in a patient with TOF is:
   A. Pulmonary valve
   B. Infundibulum
   C. Supravalvular region
   D. All of the above regions

9. Patient have increase in RVO obstruction and decrease pulmonary blood flow with the development of the right-to-left shunt through the large VSD. According to hemodynamic phases of TOF, this phase is
   A. Precyanotic phase
   B. Cyanotic phase
   C. Severe cyanotic phase
   D. None of above

10. All of the following are long-term complications of TOF except:
    A. Arrhythmia
    B. Congestive heart failure
    C. Hypercyanotic spell
    D. Pulmonary valve regurgitation

Answers

1. C.

   The severity of clinical features of TOF mainly depends on the degree of RVO obstruction which determines the pulmonary blood flow volume and degree of arterial blood oxygenation

2. A.

   The low-pitched diastolic murmur of pulmonary valve insufficiency is very difficult to be heard even in severe insufficiency and commonly missed by auscultation

3. D.

   The TOF may be associated with left subclavian artery aberrancy not right

4. D.

   Indomethacin is prostaglandin which prevent the closure of PDA and maintains the pulmonary blood flow in case of severe RVO obstruction. Isoproterenol is a beta agonist.

5. C.

   The first step in the treatment of a patient with TOF is knee–chest posture to increase systemic vascular resistance.

6. B.

   The patient with TOF has right ventricular hypertrophy due to back pressure resulting from RVO obstruction.

7. D.

   Palliative Blalock–Taussig shunting was done between pulmonary artery and subclavian artery to improve the pulmonary blood flow. But it is not a curative choice and the patient need correcting surgery later.

8. B.

   The most common site of RVO obstruction in a patient with TOF is infundibulum which represents about 50% of cases.

9. B.

   These criteria are related to the cyanotic phase.

10. C.

    Hypercyanotic spell is a short-term complication.

References

1. Bailliard F, Anderson RH. Tetralogy of fallot. Orphanet J Rare Dis. 2009;4:1–2.
2. Sheikh AM, Kazmi U, Syed NH. Variations of pulmonary arteries and other associated defects in tetralogy of fallot. Springerplus. 2014;3:467.
3. Refaat MM, Ballout J, Mansour M. Ablation of atrial fibrillation in patients with congenital heart disease. Arrhythm Electrophysiol Rev. 2017;6(4):191–4.
4. Maury P, Sacher F, Rollin A, et al. Ventricular arrhythmias and sudden death in tetralogy of Fallot. Arch Cardiovasc Dis. 2017;110(5):354–62.
5. Rauch R, Hofbeck M, Zweier C, et al. Comprehensive genotype-phenotype analysis in 230 patients with tetralogy of Fallot. J Med Genet. 2010;47(5):321–31.
6. Dabizzi RP, et al. Associated coronary and cardiac anomalies in the tetralogy of Fallot. An angiographic study. Eur Heart J. 1990;11(8):692–704.
7. Bhardwaj V, Kapoor PM, Irpachi K, Ladha S, Chowdhury UK. Basic arterial blood gas biomarkers as a predictor of mortality in tetralogy of Fallot patients. Ann Card Anaesth. 2017;20(1):67–71.
8. Bokma JP, de Wilde KC, Vliegen HW, et al. Value of cardiovascular magnetic resonance imaging in noninvasive risk stratification in tetralogy of Fallot. JAMA Cardiol. 2017;2(6):678–83.
9. Gabriele B, Maurizio B, Marco B. Does pharmacological therapy still play a role in preventing sudden death in surgically treated tetralogy of Fallot? Mini Rev Med Chem. 2018;18(6):490–4.
10. Scalone G, Gomez-Monterrosas O, Fiszer R, Szkutnik M, Galeczka M, Bialkowski J. Combined strategy of Waterston shunt percutaneous occlusion and medical treatment with sildenafil for management of pulmonary hypertension in an adult patient with corrected tetralogy of Fallot. Postepy Kardiol Interwencyjnej. 2017;13(3):277–8.
11. McRae ME, Coleman B, Atz TW, Kelechi TJ. Patient outcomes after transcatheter and surgical pulmonary valve replacement for pulmonary regurgitation in patients with repaired tetralogy of Fallot: a quasi-meta-analysis. Eur J Cardiovasc Nurs. 2017;16(6):539–53.
12. Bhagra CJ, Hickey EJ, Van De Bruaene A, Roche SL, Horlick EM, Wald RM. Pulmonary valve procedures late after repair of tetralogy of Fallot: current perspectives and contemporary approaches to management. Can J Cardiol. 2017;33(9):1138–49.
13. Yuan SM, Shinfeld A, Raanani E. The Blalock-Taussig shunt. J Card Surg. 2009;24(2):101–8.
14. Saxena A, Ramakrishnan S, Tandon R, et al; Working Group on Management of Congenital Heart Diseases in India. Consensus on timing of intervention for common congenital heart diseases. Indian Pediatr. 2008;45(2):117–126.
15. Lindsey CW, Parks WJ, Kogon BE, Sallee D 3rd, Mahle WT. Pulmonary valve replacement after tetralogy of Fallot repair in preadolescent patients. Ann Thorac Surg. 2010;89(1):147–51.
16. Boening A, Scheewe J, Paulsen J, et al. Tetralogy of Fallot: influence of surgical technique on survival and reoperation rate. Thorac Cardiovasc Surg. 2001;49(9):355–60. https://doi.org/10.1055/s-2001-19013.
17. Frigiola A, Hughes M, Turner M, Taylor A, Marek J, Giardini A, Hsia TY, Bull K. Physiological and phenotypic characteristics of late survivors of tetralogy of Fallot repair who are free from pulmonary valve replacement. Circulation. 2013;128:1861–8.
18. Knauth AL, Gauvreau K, Powell AJ, Landzberg MJ, Walsh EP, Lock JE, del Nido PJ, Geva T. Ventricular size and function assessed by cardiac MRI predict major adverse clinical outcomes late after tetralogy of Fallot repair. Heart. 2008;94:211.
19. Geva T, Sandweiss BM, Gauvreau K, Lock JE, Powell AJ. Factors associated with impaired clinical status in long-term survivors of tetralogy of Fallot repair evaluated by magnetic resonance imaging. J Am Coll Cardiol. 2004;43:1068.
20. Davlouros PA, Karatza AA, Gatzoulis MA, Shore DF. Timing and type of surgery for severe pulmonary regurgitation after repair of tetralogy of Fallot. Int J Cardiol. 2004;97 Suppl 1:91.

21. Qureshi A, Behzadi A. Foreign-body aspiration in an adult. Can J Surg. 2008;51(3):E69–70. PMC 2496600.

22. Liston SL, Gehrz RC, Siegel LG, Tilelli J. Bacterial tracheitis. Am J Dis Child. 1983;137(8):764–7.

23. Spicuzza L, Caruso D, Di Maria G. Obstructive sleep apnoea syndrome and its management. Ther Adv Chronic Dis. 2015;6(5):273–85. https://doi.org/10.1177/2040622315590318. PMC 4549693. PMID 26336596.

24. Kim V, Criner GJ. Chronic bronchitis and chronic obstructive pulmonary disease. Am J Respir Crit Care Med. 2013;187(3):228–37.

25. Peroni DG, Boner AL. Atelectasis: mechanisms, diagnosis and management. Paediatr Respir Rev. 2000;1(3):274–8.

26. Lee JS, Im JG, Ahn JM, Kim YM, Han MC. Fibrosing alveolitis: prognostic implication of ground-glass attenuation at high-resolution CT. Radiology. 1992;184(2):451–4.

27. Simonetti AF, Viasus D, Garcia-Vidal C, Carratalà J. Management of community-acquired pneumonia in older adults. Ther Adv Infect Dis. 2014;2(1):3–16.

28. Bělohlávek J, Dytrych V, Linhart A. Pulmonary embolism, part I: epidemiology, risk factors and risk stratification, pathophysiology, clinical presentation, diagnosis and nonthrombotic pulmonary embolism. Exp Clin Cardiol. 2013;18(2):129–38.

29. Khurshid I, Downie GH. Pulmonary arteriovenous malformation. Postgrad Med J. 2002;78(918):191–7.

30. Luh SP. Review: diagnosis and treatment of primary spontaneous pneumothorax. J Zhejiang Univ Sci B. 2010;11(10):735–44.

31. Macris MP, Ott DA, Cooley DA. Complete atrioventricular canal defect: surgical considerations. Tex Heart Inst J. 1992;19(3):239–43.

32. Safi LM, Liberthson RR, Bhatt A. Current management of Ebstein's anomaly in the adult. Curr Treat Options Cardiovasc Med. 2016;18(9):56.

33. Bailliard F, Anderson RH. Tetralogy of Fallot. Orphanet J Rare Dis. 2009;4:2.

34. Yoo BW, Park HK. Pulmonary stenosis and pulmonary regurgitation: both ends of the spectrum in residual hemodynamic impairment after tetralogy of Fallot repair. Korean J Pediatr. 2013;56(6):235–41.

35. Stein P. Total anomalous pulmonary venous connection. AORN J. 2007;85(3):509–20; quiz 521–4.

36. Martins P, Castela E. Transposition of the great arteries. Orphanet J Rare Dis. 2008;3:27.

37. Van Praagh R. Truncus arteriosus: what is it really and how should it be classified? Eur J Cardiothorac Surg. 1987;1(2):65–70.

38. Maganti K, Rigolin VH, Sarano ME, Bonow RO. Valvular heart disease: diagnosis and management. Mayo Clin Proc. 2010;85(5):483–500.

39. Kannan M, Vijayanand G. Mitral stenosis and pregnancy: current concepts in anaesthetic practice. Indian J Anaesth. 2010;54(5):439–44.

40. Das S, Maiti A. Acrocyanosis: an overview. Indian J Dermatol. 2013;58(6):417–20.

41. Lyaker MR, Tulman DB, Dimitrova GT, Pin RH, Papadimos TJ. Arterial embolism. Int J Crit Illn Inj Sci. 2013;3(1):77–87.

42. Block JA, Sequeira W. Raynaud's phenomenon. Lancet. 2001;357(9273):2042–8.

43. Cohen R, Mena D, Carbajal-Mendoza R, Matos N, Karki N. Superior vena cava syndrome: a medical emergency? Int J Angiol. 2008;17(1):43–6.

44. Fan CM. Venous pathophysiology. Semin Intervent Radiol. 2005;22(3):157–61.

45. Ashurst J, Wasson M. Methemoglobinemia: a systematic review of the pathophysiology, detection, and treatment. Del Med J. 2011;83(7):203–8.

46. Spivak JL. The optimal management of polycythaemia vera. Br J Haematol. 2002;116(2):243–54.

47. Goldman RD. Breath-holding spells in infants. Can Fam Physician. 2015;61(2):149–50.

48. Hotchkiss RS, Moldawer LL, Opal SM, Reinhart K, Turnbull IR, Vincent JL. Sepsis and septic shock. Nat Rev Dis Primers. 2016;2:16045.

Total Anomalous Pulmonary Venous Return

Morad Al Mostafa

Abstract

Congenital heart diseases range from diseases that can have minor symptoms and do not require treatment to diseases that pose a threat to life and need urgent surgical intervention. They are the most common among congenital diseases, which have a health, psychological, and financial burden on the infected children and their family. This chapter discusses one of these congenital heart diseases, total anomalous pulmonary venous return, which is a cardiac abnormality in which pulmonary veins are not connected right.

We have studied the latest scientific research, articles, and studies related to total anomalous pulmonary venous return, the etiology, and the types of this defect, which includes supracardiac, cardiac, infracardiac, and mixed TAPVR.

The chapter also discusses the diagnosis, signs and symptoms, pathophysiology, and the effect of this defect on the normal blood flow and normal function of the heart.

Due to recent developments and the accumulation of experiences in the field of treating congenital heart diseases, it has become possible to treat total anomalous pulmonary venous return. The concept of surgery is to create a communication between pulmonary veins and the left atrium and to close any abnormal connections. The surgical approach, risks , benefits, and complications of surgical correction are discussed in this chapter.

Keywords

Total anomalous pulmonary venous return · Pulmonary veins · Heart chambers · TAPVR · Cyanosis Supracardiac · Infracardiac · Obstructed TAPVR Hypertrophy · Atria · Venous confluence · Catheterization

Introduction

Congenital cardiac abnormality, where there are defects in the structure of the heart, is the most prevalent birth defect, accounting for approximately 33% of all birth defects worldwide [1].

Congenital heart disease is a term used to describe cardiac abnormalities that develop before birth. During pregnancy, such anomalies can happen in the baby. The defect can be in the heart walls, heart valves, or the blood vessels.

Every year, 1.4 million children worldwide are born with congenital cardiac disease. A tiny hole in the heart might alter the way blood flows through it or cause life-threatening complications. Although there are serious defects, they can be treated through surgery, and there are defects that exist without causing problems or symptoms.

Etiology

There is no obvious reason behind it. The reason in most children diagnosed with total anomalous pulmonary venous return is unknown [2] (Fig. 1).

Congenital heart defect has a major effect on children's lives, and it is a main cause of prenatal morbidity and mortality, despite medical and surgical improvements. This effect varies based on the disease's nature and intensity. But in general, this disease is a financial and psychological burden on children and families.

The pulmonary veins transfer oxygen-rich blood from the lungs to the left atrium, where it is pumped via aorta from the

M. Al Mostafa (✉)
Jordan University of Science and Technology, Ar-Ramtha, Jordan

Fig. 1 Etiology

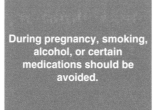

left ventricles to the body. In the absence of congenital car- diac defect, the right ventricle ejects oxygen-poor blood to the lungs via the pulmonary artery. There are two pulmonary veins returning blood from each lung, for a total of four pul- monary veins. Normally, they all attach to the left atrium of the heart.

TAPVR (total anomalous pulmonary venous return) or TAPVC (total anomalous pulmonary venous connection) is a cardiac abnormality in which pulmonary veins are not con- nected right. The four pulmonary veins connect to the heart by an anomalous route instead of the left atrium as they should, and this means that oxygen-rich blood goes to the wrong chamber.

In the right atrium, the oxygen-poor blood will mix with oxygen-rich blood returning via the pulmonary veins. This will prevent oxygen-rich blood from going to the rest of body. Other heart defects often occur with TAPVR and help infants have enough oxygen in their blood until they can have surgery.

In order for the child to live, there must be a road connect- ing the right and left part of the heart, allowing oxygen-rich blood to reach the left ventricle and then be pumped into the body through the aorta. Babies with TAPVR usually have an atrial septal defect (a hole between the left and right atrium) or patent foramen ovale, which enables oxygenated blood to reach the left heart.

As a result, the left ventricles contain a low amount of oxygen in the blood, which will be pumped to the body, and this leads to problems and symptoms related to the disease.

The rest of the blood is pumped from the right ventricle through the pulmonary artery into the lungs. Oxygen-rich blood will go an ineffective way back to the lungs instead of the path the body needs to get enough oxygen-rich blood. TAPVR cannot be tolerated for a long time [3].

Partial anomalous pulmonary venous return (PAPVR) is a defect that is not critical and severe as TAPVR, because not all the pulmonary veins have an anomalous route. One or more pulmonary veins attach to the left atrium as they should.

Total anomalous pulmonary venous return is classified into four types:

Darlings Classification

Supracardiac Total Anomalous Pulmonary Venous Return

Supracardiac TAPVC is the most common type accounting for approximately 45% of cases. In supracardiac TAPVC, the right and left pulmonary veins join a common pulmonary confluence that drains superiorly via a vertical vein (derived from a primitive anterior cardinal vein) into the left brachio- cephalic vein, the right superior vena cava, or less commonly the right azygos vein and then to the right atrium [4].

Supracardiac TAPVC is further classified into two subtypes:

1. *Connection to the Right SVC or Right Azygous Vein*
2. *Connection to the Left Innominate Vein (LIV)*

The hemodynamic state and clinical features depend on the presence or absence of obstructive lesions in the anomalous pulmonary venous channel and the size of the interatrial defect.

Supracardiac TAPVC causes right-sided hypertrophy because of volume overload and various degrees of pulmonary hypertension. If there is a restriction of the interatrial connection, pulmonary overcirculation will increases and systemic output will decrease.

Anatomic site of obstruction:

- Interatrial septum:
- Patients with large interatrial openings survive longer than those with restricted ones.
- Intrinsic narrowing of the anomalous vessels' wall
- Extrinsic pressure on the anomalous vessels when the vertical vein to the innominate vein passes between the left main bronchus and the left main pulmonary artery.

When the pulmonary veins are not obstructed, the patients may be asymptomatic at birth, but half of them will have heart failure within the first month. By the age of 6 months, the majority of patients will have heart failure. Untreated children have an 85% death rate in their first year of life.

Cardiac Total Anomalous Pulmonary Venous Return

Common pulmonary venous sinus drains either directly into the right atrium or into the coronary sinus [4].

Infracardiac Total Anomalous Pulmonary Venous Return

The pulmonary venous confluence drains by a descending vertical vein inferiorly anterior to the esophagus to the hepatic vein or portal veins (most common), IVC, and then to the right atrium.

This variant of TAPVR can induce pulmonary venous obstruction because the descending vertical vein drains into the portal venous system. Obstruction can be caused by a variety of factors, including intrinsic narrowing of the connecting vessel, the interposition of the hepatic sinusoids between the pulmonary veins and the heart, and constriction of ductus venosus. To allow pulmonary venous return to reach the left heart, an atrial septal defect is required [4].

The infracardiac type of total abnormal pulmonary venous return is the type mostly associated with obstructed pulmonary veins.

Mixed-Type TAPVC

It occurs when there is more than one level of anomalous venous connections, and it is the least common among other types, accounting for less than 10% of cases.

Signs and Symptoms

TAPVR (total anomalous pulmonary venous return) causes cyanosis, feeding difficulties, and tachypnea in newborns. This occurs because there is a combination of oxygenated and deoxygenated blood in the left heart that is pumped by aorta to the body [5].

Physiological manifestations depend on the distribution of the mixed venous blood between systemic and pulmonary circulation.

The state of the interatrial septum is important if the atrial septal defect is small and the amount of blood reaching the left ventricles and supplying the body will be reduced.

The pulmonary and systemic vascular resistance is approximately equal at birth. Because the pulmonary vascular resistance is decreased in the first weeks of life, there is a larger amount of mixed venous blood flow via the pulmonary circuit.

When there is TAPVC with pulmonary venous obstruction, patients will complain of dyspnea, tachycardia, and cyanosis within hours of birth. The elevated pressure will be transmitted to the pulmonary capillary bed and result in pulmonary hypertension and pulmonary edema. Once symptoms begin, there will be rapid progression to cardiorespiratory failure, necessitating emergent surgical surgery to correct this defect.

Total anomalous pulmonary venous return symptoms include:

- A bluish color of the skin, lips, and nails (cyanosis)
- Breathing difficulties
- Heart murmur
- Poor feeding or poor growth

Diagnosis

The total anomalous pulmonary venous return may be suspected in the first few months when the child presents with cyanosis and heart murmur. In infracardiac TAPVC with obstruction, there might be severe respiratory distress and acidosis.

- Chest X-RAY findings:
  TAPVC without pulmonary venous obstruction:
  - Evidence of pulmonary hypertension and pulmonary edema.
  - Right atrium and right ventricle are enlarged.
  - Pulmonary artery segment is prominent.
  - Left atrium and left ventricle are not enlarged.

- The supracardiac has a snowman appearance (figure of 8 heart or cottage loaf heart), where the head of the snowman is formed by brachiocephalic vein on top, the dilated vertical vein on the left, and the superior vena cava on the right. The right atrium represents the body of the snowman.

TAPVC with pulmonary venous obstruction:
- Ground glass appearance
- ECG findings:
  - Tall, peaked P waves
  - Right axis deviation
  - Right ventricular hypertrophy
  - Incomplete right bundle branch block
- Pulse oximetry:
- The reading will be low (in the mid to high 80s).
- Right ventricular hypertrophy is common in TAPVC with pulmonary obstruction, while right atrial enlargement is uncommon.
- The gold standard diagnostic test of total anomalous pulmonary venous return is the echocardiogram. The test's objectives are to confirm the diagnosis, to reveal any aberrant connections between the pulmonary veins, whether supracardiac, cardiac, or infracardiac, and to evaluate whether the pulmonary venous flow is obstructed.
- Cardiac catheterization is occasionally needed to make the diagnosis. In TAPVC without pulmonary venous obstruction, the venous site of anomalous connection can be identified. A balloon dilation can be used to enlarge the restrictive ASD for improved blood shunting between the left and right atria.
- Cardiac MRI

There are screening tests to look for birth abnormalities and other disorders during pregnancy. Some ultrasound findings may point to the possibility that a baby has TAPVR. If this is the case, a fetal echocardiography might be requested to confirm the diagnosis. Because there is not much blood going to the lungs in the uterine life, the pulmonary veins are difficult to spot on prenatal screening tests. This defect is easier to identify after delivery [6].

Treatment for Total Anomalous Pulmonary Venous Return

Total anomalous pulmonary venous connection includes supracardiac, cardiac, infracardiac, and mixed types. TAPVC's surgical correction results have improved over time, and surgical mortality has decreased as a result of the accumulation of experience in the surgical field and extensive postoperative care.

In all cases, total anomalous pulmonary venous return necessitates open heart surgery. To preserve the patient's life, early detection of the illness and urgent surgical surgery are required. Surgical treatment is timed differently based on the type of total abnormal pulmonary venous return and the state of the child. When surgery is undertaken on severely sick neonates, especially those with obstructed pulmonary venous return, the death rate is higher. Surgeons may wait up to 2 months to do surgery if the child is not dangerously ill. Although the surgery is not urgent in these children, there is usually no advantage in delaying it more than 1 or 2 months.

Corrective surgery is the definitive treatment. Obstructed total anomalous pulmonary venous return is a surgical emergency, while nonobstructed total anomalous pulmonary venous return is corrected by an elective surgery a few days after the diagnosis.

TAPVR repairing is done by open-heart surgery. In supracardiac and infra-cardiac TAPVR, an anastomosis between the pulmonary venous confluence and the left atrium is created and the vertical vein is divided and ligated. The goal of surgery is to create a communication between pulmonary veins and left atrium and to close any aberrant connections. Later in life, if the pulmonary veins become obstructed, further surgery or catheterization is needed [7].

Infants who have surgically corrected abnormalities may have long-term complications. A kid or adult with TAPVR should be followed up on a frequent basis to track the course of his or her health condition and avoid problems.

What are the risks of TAPVR surgery for a child?

- Bleeding
- Infection
- Stroke
- Arrhythmia
- Heart block
- Anesthetic complications
- Death

The outcome of surgical correction for complete anomalous pulmonary venous return is typically favorable, and these children are anticipated to grow normally as a result of regular circulation. Intensive postoperative medical care is required for severely sick babies who survive surgery. They are frequently placed on a ventilator for a lengthy period of time to allow their lungs to recover [8].

Follow-Up Care for TAPVR

Children with TAPVR who underwent surgical correction must continue to have a regular follow-up with a cardiologist.

Multiple Choice Questions

1. All of the followings are ECG findings of TAPVR except:
   A. Right axis deviation
   B. Pulmonale
   C. Right ventricular hypertrophy
   D. Findings of left atrial enlargement
2. Snowman appearance is found in:
   A. Supracardiac TAPVR
   B. Infracardiac TAPVR
   C. Cardiac TAPVR
   D. Mixed-type TAPVR
3. The gold standard diagnostic test of total anomalous pulmonary venous return is:
   A. Chest X-RAY
   B. Cardiac catheterization
   C. Echocardiogram
   D. Cardiac MRI
4. One of the followings is false regarding TAPVR:
   A. The outcome of surgical correction for complete anomalous pulmonary venous return is favorable.
   B. Infants who had surgically corrected abnormalities may have long-term complications.
   C. The goal of surgery is to create communication between pulmonary veins and the left atrium.
   D. In surgery on severely sick neonates with obstructed pulmonary venous return, the death rate is low.
5. The most type of TAPVR that is associated with obstructed pulmonary veins is:
   A. Supracardiac TAPVR
   B. Infracardiac TAPVR
   C. Cardiac TAPVR
   D. Mixed-type TAPVR
6. Regarding the etiology of TAPVR, it is attributed mostly to:
   A. The reason in most children is unknown.
   B. Maternal viral infection in pregnancy
   C. Smoking during pregnancy
   D. Defects in the genes and chromosomes of the child
7. The pulmonary venous confluence in infracardiac total anomalous pulmonary venous return drains in most cases to:
   A. Hepatic vein
   B. Portal veins
   C. Inferior vena cava
   D. None of the above
8. In the nonobstructed TAPVR, the majority of patients have heart failure at age:
   A. At birth
   B. 2 years
   C. 6 months
   D. First month
9. Pulmonary venous obstruction in infracardiac total anomalous pulmonary venous return can be caused by one of the following mechanisms:
   A. Intrinsic narrowing of the connecting vessel
   B. Constriction of ductus venosus
   C. Interposition of the hepatic sinusoids between the pulmonary veins and the heart
   D. All of the above
10. One of the following statements is true:
    A. When the atrial septal defect is large, the amount of blood reaching the left ventricles is reduced.
    B. Less amount of blood flow via the pulmonary circuit when pulmonary vascular resistance is decreased.
    C. A child with total anomalous pulmonary venous return will present with cyanosis and breathing difficulties.
    D. The infracardiac TAPVR has a snowman appearance.

Answers

1. D
2. A
3. C
4. D
5. B
6. A
7. B
8. C
9. D
10. C

References

1. Domadia S, et al. Neonatal outcomes in total anomalous pulmonary venous return: the role of prenatal diagnosis and pulmonary venous obstruction. Pediatr Cardiol. 2018;39(7):1346–54.
2. Shi X, et al. Next-generation sequencing identifies novel genes with rare variants in total anomalous pulmonary venous connection. EBioMedicine. 2018;38:217–27.
3. White BR, et al. Repair of total anomalous pulmonary venous connection: risk factors for postoperative obstruction. Ann Thorac Surg. 2019;108(1):122–9.

4. Shi G, et al. Total anomalous pulmonary venous connection: the current management strategies in a pediatric cohort of 768 patients. Circulation. 2017;135(1):48–58.
5. Yoshimura N, et al. Surgery for total anomalous pulmonary venous connection: primary sutureless repair vs. conventional repair. Gen Thorac Cardiovasc Surg. 2017;65(5):245–51.
6. Spigel ZA, et al. Total anomalous pulmonary venous connection: influence of heterotaxy and venous obstruction on outcomes. J Thorac Cardiovasc Surg. 2022;163(2):387–395.e3.
7. White BR, et al. Venous flow variation predicts preoperative pulmonary venous obstruction in children with Total anomalous pulmonary venous connection. J Am Soc Echocardiogr. 2021;34(7): 775–85.
8. Jaramillo FA, et al. Infracardiac type total anomalous pulmonary venous return with obstruction and dilatation of portal vein. Radiol Case Rep. 2017;12(2):229–32.

Multiple Malformations

Qasim Mehmood and Irfan Ullah

Abstract

The existence of two or more related or unrelated malformations in the patient is called multiple malformations, and they include the pentalogy of Cantrell, Shone syndrome, and Scimitar syndrome. Cantrell pentalogy is a rare anomaly characterized by sternal or pericardial defect, diaphragmatic defect, omphalocele, ectopia cordis, and various congenital cardiac abnormalities. Other cardiac malformations are Shone syndrome and Scimitar syndrome characterized by defects in the heart, major blood vessels, and lungs. Surgical intervention can be done to treat all of these defects.

Keywords

Multiple malformations · Congenital heart defects
Cantrell pentalogy · Omphalocele · Ectopia cordis
Shone syndrome · Aortic coarctation · Hypoplastic
ventricle · Scimitar syndrome · Turkish sword
Pulmonary hypertension

Introduction

When two or more unrelated structural anomalies of the heart coexist in a patient, they are referred to as multiple malformations. In other words, the existence of two or more malformations in the same baby and at the same time is called multiple malformations [1]. Pentalogy of Cantrell, Shone syndrome, and Scimitar syndrome are the classical anomalies that can be addressed under multiple malformations of the heart.

Cantrell Pentalogy

Cantrell pentalogy is a rare hereditary anomaly categorized by a constellation of five clinical features, which include sternal or pericardial defect, anterior diaphragmatic defect, omphalocele, ectopia cordis, and various congenital intracardiac abnormalities, including left ventricular diverticulum, ASD, VSD, and tetralogy of Fallot [2–5]. Clinical presentation varies in the degree of severity and can cause potentially lethal complications in the majority of cases. Most cases do not show the full presentation of PC and are called incomplete pentalogy of Cantrell. Complete pentalogy of Cantrell is only referred to those cases having all the five defects [6]. The term "Cantrell pentalogy," also called Cantrell deformity, was first introduced by Cantrell and co-workers in 1958 [3, 4] (Fig. 1).

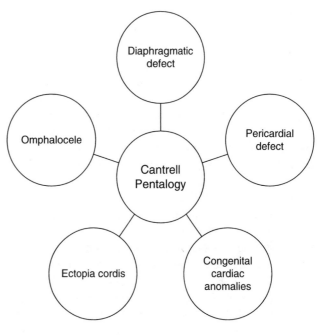

Fig. 1 Salient features of Cantrell pentalogy

Q. Mehmood (✉)
King Edward Medical University, Lahore, Pakistan

I. Ullah
Kabir Medical College, Gandhara University, Peshawar, Pakistan

Classification

The pentalogy of Cantrell can be classified as class 1, 2, and 3. A patient having all five defects present is categorized as class 1. The one having four of the five defects is categorized as class 2. The patient in which there is an incomplete expression of defects is categorized as class 3 [3, 4].

Etiology and Incidence

The pentalogy of Cantrell is very rare, and the exact prevalence is not known [6]. But an incidence of around 6 in 1 million live births has been reported in some studies [5]. The exact etiology is not known, but family history has been described in some cases suggesting the involvement of genetic factors [2]. Cantrell pentalogy has a slight male predilection with an MTF ratio of 2.7:1 [4].

Pathogenesis

The collection of malformations detected in Cantrell pentalogy is believed to result from the abnormal migration of the sternal anlage and myotomes [5] and defective formation of the intraembryonic mesoderm at about 14–18 days of gestation [6]. Abnormal migration of paired primordial structures results in the development of sternal and abdominal wall defects, while pericardial, intracardiac, and diaphragmatic anomalies are due to maldevelopment of septum transversum [4].

Diagnosis

Early diagnosis of Cantrell pentalogy is essential, and techniques include fetal ultrasound, echocardiography, and MRI. Cantrell pentalogy can be diagnosed by ultrasonography within the first 10 weeks of gestation [4]. Transverse abdominal ultrasound shows an omphalocele containing the heart prenatally, which is the hallmark of Cantrell pentalogy, and sagittal ultrasound shows both the liver and heart outside the chest of the fetus [7]. 3D ultrasound is an adjunctive to 2D ultrasound to visualize fetal abnormalities in various orthogonal planes [4]. To assess the degree of involvement of the heart in PC, echocardiography can be performed [6]. It has been recommended that MRI can also provide an optimal evaluation of fetuses with Cantrell pentalogy [4]. The degree of certain abnormalities such as the abdominal wall and pericardial defects can be assessed using MRI [6]. Chromosomal analysis of the fetus is also recommended to detect associated trisomies and Turner syndrome [4]. The differential diagnosis of Cantrell pentalogy includes ectopia cordis, omphalocele, limb body wall complex, and amniotic bands, so they should be kept in mind [2].

Clinical Characteristics

The clinical features of Cantrell pentalogy vary from patient to patient and can range from mild defects to serious, life-threatening complications. Ectopia cordis with omphalocele is the most severe presentation of Cantrell pentalogy expressed at birth. Omphalocele may be large or small, and in some cases, it is totally absent. Other forms of abdominal wall defects include diastasis of abdominal wall muscles and gastroschisis. Sternal abnormalities may range from the absence of the xiphoid process of the sternum to an abnormally short sternum or sternal cleft to absence of the sternum. Pericardial defects can also be seen in PC, especially in the diaphragmatic part of the pericardium. Affected babies may also have a congenital diaphragmatic hernia. Intracardiac abnormalities in Cantrell pentalogy include ventricular septal defect, atrial septal defect, dextrocardia, and tetralogy of Fallot. Other complex congenital heart defects can also be detected in Cantrell pentalogy, but their type and severity vary from person to person [6].

Associated Anomalies

Abnormalities associated with Cantrell pentalogy may be intracardiac or extra-cardiac. Intracardiac abnormalities include Ebstein's anomaly, septal defects, single atrium, or tetralogy of Fallot [4]. Extra-cardiac anomalies in this syndrome include craniofacial malformations such as cleft lip, cleft palate, or supernumerary nares; CNS abnormalities like craniorachischisis, encephalocele, hydrocephalus, cystic hygroma, or neural tube defects; and skeletal defects such as vertebral column anomalies, limb abnormalities—often an absence of radius or tibia, and clubfoot [3–5]. Abdominal abnormalities include polysplenia, malformation of the kidneys, and gallbladder agenesis [4, 6]. Other serious defects associated with the pentalogy of Cantrell include underdevelopment of the lungs, breathing difficulties, and abnormal function of the heart [6]. The co-existence of PC with other syndromes such as Edward syndrome, trisomy 13, and trisomy 18 has also been reported in some studies [3, 5]. Affected infants are also at a higher risk of developing widespread abdominal infections [6].

Treatment

The specific treatment strategy of Cantrell pentalogy depends on the nature of ectopia cordis, the size and type of the abdominal wall defect, and the associated cardiac and extra-cardiac abnormalities [4]. Most cases of PC, however, show a very poor prognosis. The aims and goals of surgical management of PC include repairing cardiac abnormalities, protecting the heart from compression, and making an adequate space in the chest cavity for the return of the heart [5].

After the prenatal diagnosis of PC, correction of the omphalocele, sternal defects, pericardial anomalies, and diaphragmatic defects should be done immediately after birth [4]. Surgical repair of the epigastrium or lower sternum may be required after an appropriate growth of lungs in the chest cavity, usually by 2–3 years [6]. Surgical repair is very difficult in the case of abdominal or thoracic hypoplasia. So, a multidisciplinary team of healthcare workers should be there to determine the best time of delivery. Following amniocentesis, showing abnormal karyotype, pregnancy can also be terminated [4].

Shone Syndrome

Shone syndrome, also known as Shone's anomaly [8], was first introduced by a Canadian pediatric cardiologist Dr. John Shone [9, 10]. He identified four lesions as specific clinical features of Shone syndrome, including coarctation of the aorta, subaortic narrowing, supra-valvular mitral valve ring, and parachute mitral valve [9–11]. But now, Shone syndrome is characterized by eight typical lesions [9]. A person must have at least three of these lesions to be diagnosed as Shone syndrome, and incomplete forms are common [12]. The clinical severity and prognosis depend on the complexity of each lesion and the degree of block across the left ventricular inflow and outflow tracts [10] (Fig. 2).

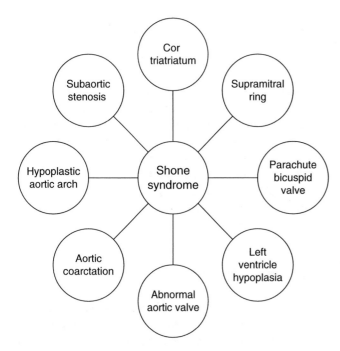

Fig. 2 Salient features of Shone syndrome

Etiology and Prevalence

Shone syndrome, a disease of unknown etiology, usually develops very early in the fetus. It is believed to affect both sexes, all races, and ethnic groups [8]. The exact prevalence is not known but is estimated to be less than 0.7%. There is often left ventricular hypoplasia leading to LV inflow and outflow tract obstruction [10].

Diagnosis

Shone syndrome can be diagnosed prenatally using fetal echocardiographs. Left ventricular dimensions and luminal diameters of the mitral and aortic valves are diagnostically very important. The abnormal echocardiographic findings seen in patients with Shone's anomaly include small sizes of the left ventricle and root of aorta, decreased luminal diameter of the mitral valve, and narrowed or stenosed aortic valve. All these abnormal dimensions are compared with normal cardiac measurements for accurate diagnosis [13].

Clinical Features

Generalized symptoms of congestive cardiac failure include difficulty in breathing, tachycardia, weakness, fatigue, edema in legs, and frequent pneumonia [8]. The first pathological finding in Shone syndrome is mitral valve obstruction, which leads to left ventricular hypoplasia, LV outflow tract obstruction, and coarctation of the aorta [12]. Specific clinical lesions characteristic of Shone anomaly are as follows:

Cor Triatriatum
Cor triatriatum results in the formation of a membrane in the left atrium, which divides it into two. Pulmonary edema or pulmonary hypertension may develop due to the backup of blood in the lungs. Management of cor triatriatum is often surgical, and the recurrence rate is low [9].

Supramitral Ring
The supramitral ring can lead to narrowing and obstruction of mitral valve [9]. The embryologic basis of this defect is not clear, but it is believed to result from an incomplete partition of endocardial cushion tissue [12]. The membrane is thick, fibrous, and looks like orange peel that can easily be peeled off the annulus. The clinical presentation may be variable, ranging from mild forms to severe obstruction. Surgical treatment of the supramitral ring is highly successful [9].

Parachute Bicuspid Valve

Papillary muscles provide attachment to chordae tendineae around the bicuspid valve and control their opening and closing [9]. When there is a single papillary muscle for chordal attachment in the left ventricle, the condition is called parachute mitral valve as the pattern of attachment of it to the mitral valve looks like a parachute [14]. This is often asymptomatic but can lead to either stenosis or regurgitation of the mitral valve in some cases [9].

Aortic Coarctation

Constriction of the aorta at different levels is called aortic coarctation [14]. An important clinical feature, present at the level of aortic media, is the partial disappearance of elastic tissue [12]. The clinical presentation of it is highly variable, ranging from milder forms in adults to more severe forms in infants. High blood pressure is a typical diagnostic finding and is difficult to control. Immediate surgical repair is needed in the case of infants and is the treatment of choice. Balloon angioplasty and stent replacement can be done in adult patients, and success rates of these procedures are quite high [9].

Hypoplastic Aortic Arch

A small aortic arch in Shone syndrome can lead to chronic high blood pressure as the left ventricle is pumping blood against higher resistance [9].

Subaortic Stenosis

It is also a common defect in patients with Shone syndrome [9]. A membranous or muscular thickening is formed under the aortic valve, which leads to LV outflow tract obstruction [14]. Clinical manifestations of subaortic stenosis may appear earlier, and surgical repair is the treatment of choice [9].

Bicuspid Aortic Valve

When the normal tricuspid aortic valve has only two cusps or leaflets, the condition is called bicuspid aortic valve. Not only two cusps are present, but their movement is also restricted. The narrow opening of the aortic valve leads to obstruction of blood flow through this valve. Valve repair or replacement can be done to treat this condition [9].

Hypoplastic Left Ventricle

Various lesions in Shone's anomaly can cause the left ventricles to become hypoplastic. These ventricles are usually stiff and are frequently missed on examination. One of the biggest morbidities in Shone's anomaly is left ventricular stiffness, which leads to decreased pumping activity of the ventricles. Pulmonary edema, pulmonary hypertension, and arrhythmias are quite common in these cases. Hypoplastic left ventricles are difficult to treat surgically, so they are managed using drugs like diuretics and ACE inhibitors [9].

Scimitar Syndrome

Scimitar syndrome, also named Halasz syndrome, congenital veno-lobar syndrome, vena cava broncho-vascular syndrome, mirror-image lung syndrome, or hypo-genetic lung syndrome, is a rare congenital heart deformity [15]. In Scimitar syndrome, pulmonary veins drain the right lung to IVC. Furthermore, there is right lung hypoplasia, pulmonary hypertension, and other cardiac anomalies [16]. Scimitar syndrome was described by Neill and his team [17] referring to the tubular opacity seen on chest radiography, which resembles a saber with a curved blade or a curved Turkish sword called a scimitar [16].

Epidemiology

Scimitar syndrome is very rare, with an estimated incidence of 3–6% [18]. The condition is more common in females, with an estimated MTF ratio of 1:2 [15].

Classification

Scimitar syndrome can be classically divided into infants and adult forms. Frequently the disease has a benign clinical course. The patient may be asymptomatic in infancy but can eventually develop heart failure, recurrent respiratory infections, or dyspnea on exertion [19, 20].

Etiology

The exact etiological basis of Scimitar syndrome is not known but is believed to result from an embryological defect in the development of the right lung bud [15]. This leads to right lung hypoplasia and failure of growth of the endodermal tissue, which forms pulmonary venous plexus. The endodermal tissue from the right lung fails to fuse with the mesodermal pulmonary vein outpouchings, which lead to the formation of a scimitar vein to drain the venous supply from the right lung [18].

Clinical Presentation

Scimitar syndrome has varied clinical presentations ranging from an asymptomatic state to severe pulmonary hypertension or heart failure. Signs and symptoms of this rare syndrome depend on the age of the patients at which they present. Infants present with poor growth, cyanosis, pulmonary arterial hypertension, and other complex cardiac abnormalities [21]. Adult patients usually have a benign course and may present with recurrent pulmonary infections and dyspnea on exertion. Hemoptysis may also be a rare presenting symptom in some patients [21]. On physical examination, there is a characteristic right-ward shift of the heart sounds and cardiac impulse often associated with a systolic murmur [15].

Diagnosis

The diagnosis of scimitar syndrome can be done by chest X-radiography, angiography, transthoracic or trans-esophageal echocardiography, or CT scan. Chest X-ray reveals a small, hypoplastic lung with blurred right heart borders. The anomalous vein draining the right lung can be seen as a shape of a Turkish sword, hence the name scimitar syndrome [17]. Besides chest X-ray, angiography, CT scan, and echocardiography can also be done for diagnosis [21]. Fetal echocardiography may be helpful in the prenatal diagnosis of scimitar syndrome by visualizing the anomalous pulmonary venous pathway [15]. Another diagnostic technique to visualize the abnormal vascular anatomy of this complex congenital anomaly is magnetic resonance imaging (MRI) [21].

Differential Diagnosis

Differential diagnoses of scimitar syndrome include pulmonary sequestration, right middle lobe atelectasis, congenital hypoplasia of the right lung, unilateral absence or aplasia of pulmonary artery [17], bronchopulmonary mass with systemic arterial blood supply [15], and Macleod's syndrome [21].

Treatment

Management of scimitar syndrome often involves a multidisciplinary approach. Medical intervention should be started immediately if the infants present with the signs of cardiac failure [15]. Surgical correction is considered in the case of significant pulmonary hypertension and heart failure. Careful lobectomy can also be performed if the anomalous vein drains only one lobe of the lung [20]. The main objective of surgical repair is to avoid the deleterious consequences of chronic heart overload [16].

Complications

Surgical correction of scimitar syndrome may lead to various complications like pulmonary hypertension and the Eisenmenger phenomenon [17].

Multiple Choice Questions

1. One of the five characteristic features of Cantrell Pentalogy is:
   A. Club foot
   B. Cleft lip
   C. Ectopia cordis
   D. Hyperpigmentation of skin
2. Scimitar means:
   A. Turkish wood
   B. Turkish sword
   C. Arabic dagger
   D. European knife

Answers

1. Option C: Ectopia cordis.
   Cantrell pentalogy is a rare anomaly characterized by five salient features: sternal or pericardial defect, deficiency of anterior diaphragm, omphalocele, ectopia cordis, and various congenital cardiac defects.
2. Option B: Turkish sword
   The word "scimitar" means "Turkish sword" referring to the tubular opacity seen on chest radiography, characteristic of Scimitar syndrome.

References

1. Ooki S. Multiple congenital anomalies after assisted reproductive tech-nology in Japan (between 2004 and 2009). Int Scholar Res Notices. 2013;2013:1–8. https://doi.org/10.5402/2013/452085.
2. Pentalogy of Cantrell|Genetic and Rare Disease Information Center (GARD). Nih.gov.2014 [cited 2021 Sep 5]. https://rarediseases.info.nih.gov/diseases/7359/pentalogy-of-cantrell.
3. Naburi H, Assenga E, Patel S, Massawe A, Manji K. Class II pentalogy of Cantrell. BMC Res Notes. 2015;8(1):1–6.
4. Chandran S, Ari D. Pentalogy of Cantrell: an extremely rare congenital anomaly. J Clin Neonatol. 2013;2(2):95.
5. Weerakkody Y. Pentalogy of Cantrell|radiology reference article|Radiopaedia.org [Internet]. Radiopaedia.org. 2014 [cited 2021 Sep 5]. https://radiopaedia.org/articles/pentalogy-of-cantrell-3.
6. Pentalogy of Cantrell—NORD (National Organization for Rare Disorders) [Internet]. NORD (National Organization for Rare Disorders). NORD; 2019 [cited 2021 Sep 5]. https://rarediseases.org/rare-diseases/pentalogy-of-cantrell/.
7. Diseases of the pediatric abdominal wall, peritoneum, and mesentery. Pentalogy of Cantrell. Textbook of gastrointestinal radiology, 3rd ed. 2008. p. 2371–2381. https://doi.org/10.1016/B978-1-4160-2332-6.50132-9.
8. Shone's Syndrome|Nicklaus Children's Hospital [Internet]. Nick-lauschildrens.org. 2021 [cited 2021 Sep 5]. https://www.nicklaus-childrens.org/conditions/shone-s-syndrome.
9. Shone Syndrome [Internet]. ACHA. 2021 [cited 2021 Sep 5]. https://www.achaheart.org/your-heart/educational-qas/types-of-heart-defects/shone-syndrome/.
10. Aslam S, Khairy P, Shohoudi A, Mercier LA, Dore A, Marcotte F, Miró J, Avila-Alonso P, Ibrahim R, Asgar A, Poirier N. Shone complex: an under-recognized congenital heart disease with substantial morbidity in adulthood. Can J Cardiol. 2017;33(2):253–9.

11. Pediatric case study of Shone's complex, a congenital heart condition [Internet]. Clevelandclinic.org. Consult QD; 2019 [cited 2021 Sep 5]. https://consultqd.clevelandclinic.org/pediatric-case-study-of-shones-complex-a-congenital-heart-condition/amp/.

12. Popescu BA, Jurcut R, Serban M, Parascan L, Ginghina C. Shone's syndrome diagnosed with echocardiography and confirmed at pathology. Eur J Echocardiogr. 2008;9(6):865–7.

13. Zucker N, Levitas A, Zalzstein E. Prenatal diagnosis of Shone's syndrome: parental counseling and clinical outcome. Ultrasound Obstet Gynecol. 2004;24(6):629–32.

14. Williams H. Shone's complex|Pediatric echocardiography [Internet]. Pedecho.org. 2015 [cited 2021 Sep 5]. https://pedecho.org/library/chd/shones-complex.

15. Scimitar syndrome [Internet]. StatPearls. StatPearls Publishing; 2021 [cited 2021 Sep 5]. https://www.statpearls.com/ArticleLibrary/viewarticle/28774.

16. Assoignon MP, Christiaens P, Laleman W. Correction of the scimitar syndrome, a rare cardiac venous anomaly, leading to Budd–Chiari syndrome: a case report. J Med Case Rep. 2014;8(1):1–4.

17. Iqbal S, Gaillard F. Scimitar syndrome (lungs)|radiology reference article|Radiopaedia.org [Internet]. Radiopaedia.org. 2011 [cited 2021 Sep 5]. https://radiopaedia.org/articles/scimitar-syndrome-lungs.

18. Salciccioli K. Scimitar syndrome|Pediatric echocardiography [Internet]. Pedecho.org. 2016 [cited 2021 Sep 5]. https://pedecho.org/library/chd/scimitar-syndrome.

19. Ramirez-Marrero MA, de Mora-Martin M. Scimitar syndrome in an asymptomatic adult: fortuitous diagnosis by imaging technique. Case Rep Vasc Med. 2012;2012:138541.

20. Vida VL, Padalino MA, Boccuzzo G, Tarja E, Berggren H, Carrel T, Çiçek S, Crupi G, Di Carlo D, Di Donato R, Fragata J. Scimitar syndrome: a European congenital heart surgeons association (ECHSA) multicentric study. Circulation. 2010;122(12):1159–66.

21. Gupta ML, Bagarhatta R, Sinha J. Scimitar syndrome: a rare disease with unusual presentation. Lung India. 2009;26(1):26.

Ectopia Cordis

Ibrahim Dheyaa Al-Hasani, Hayder Saad Salih,
Ali Mohammed Hatem, and Yousif Ahmed Hussein

Abstract

Ectopia cordis is a rare cardiac deformity resulting from the atypical early development of the primitive heart outside the embryonic disc. Hence, there is the abnormal placement of the heart outside the thoracic cavity due to a defect in the chest wall and abdominal wall associated with cardiac malformation, a defect in the parietal pericardium, diaphragm, and sternum. The etiology is not well understood and studies suggest that the disorder is related to chromosomal abnormalities, e.g., trisomy 18, Turner syndrome, and 17 q+. Diagnosis is done by physical examination on childbirth, the condition can also be diagnosed antenatally by ultrasound and most accurately through magnetic resonance accompanied by echocardiography in the prenatal period (MR/MDCT). Although the condition has a poor prognosis especially if associated with other congenital anomalies, the definitive treatment is done by surgery to reduce the heart into, correct thoracic and abdominal wall deformities, and later correct intracardiac defects.

Keywords

Ectopia cordis · Ventral wall defects · Pentalogy of Cantrell sternal · Abnormal cardiac position · Serum HCG · Cleft lip · Naked heart · Amniotic band syndrome Omphalocele · Cutler and Wilens

Introduction

"Ectopia cordis is a rare congenital anomaly caused by failure of maturation of the midline of the mesodermal part of the anterior chest wall and abdomen, rendering the heart in abnormal position outside the thoracic cavity, as well as sternal malformations, parietal pericardium diaphragm malformations, and internal cardiac defects" [1]. The abnormality is called true ectopia cordis when there are internal defects internally in addition to the abnormal position of the heart [2]. It's a sporadic heart lesion that was linked to chromosomal abnormalities, according to studies. It has a prevalence of 5.5–7.9 per million newborns. It is categorized into five groups based on its location: cervical, cervicothoracic, thoracic, thoracoabdominal, and abdominal. "There are two classifications suggested for ectopia cordis which are partial or total according to the location of the heart away from the thoracic cavity, and depending on the amount of cardiac size revealed outside the cavity" [3]. The heart may beat through the skin in partial ectopia cordis as it is placed just beneath the skin outside the chest wall. However, the heart is seen completely outside the chest not concealed by any skin layer in complete ectopia cordis [3–7]. Although the newborn cardiac surgery has been passed strides, ectopia cordis surgery is still a hurdle with a poor prognosis [8–10].

Associated Anomalies

The disease often coexists with other organ malformations that develop abnormally as in abdominal wall defects. Defects associated with ectopia cordis include:

1. Intracardiac defects [11]
   - Ventricular septal defect—100% of cases.
   - Atrial septal defect—53% of cases
   - Tetralogy of Fallot—20% of cases
   - Left ventricular diverticulum—20% of cases [11].
2. Non-cardiac defects
   - The disorder is associated with an increase in the incidence of Encephalocele, hydrocephalus as well as cleft lip and/or palate deformities, and craniorachischisis [8, 12, 13].

I. D. Al-Hasani (✉) · H. S. Salih · A. M. Hatem · Y. A. Hussein
College of Medicine, University of Baghdad, Baghdad, Iraq

© The Author(s), under exclusive license to Springer Nature Switzerland AG 2023
G. Tagarakis et al. (eds.), *Clinical and Surgical Aspects of Congenital Heart Diseases*,
https://doi.org/10.1007/978-3-031-23062-2_13

- Limb defects such as clubfoot can possibly be associated with ectopia cordis, as well as the absence of tibia or radius, and hypodactyly [14, 15].
- Defects in the formation of abdominal organs such as gallbladder agenesis and polysplenia [16].

Etiology

The normal embryonic development of the heart and the thoracic cavity commences as the mesoderm migrates to form the ventral body wall at day 8 of embryonic life. The heart is situated then in the cephalic side of the embryo as it lies finally between the ventral folding and lateral flexing by day 16 to 18 of embryonic life [17]. The midline fusion and formation of both thoracic and abdominal cavity is reached by the ninth week of gestation which will give the steps of cardiac and thoracic development its final steps [8, 10–18].

Mechanism of ectopia cordis development includes failure of midline fusion, either total or partial, causing a spectrum of deformities ranging from isolated ectopia cordis to complete ventral evisceration [17, 19–21]. The causes of midline fusion failure are poorly understood nor fully explained but the most suggested theories are:

1. Entanglement of fibrous bands of the amnion to the developing embryo because of a ruptured amniotic membrane, this causes fetal disruption of normal development during gestation and the resulting deformities depend on the site of entanglement and timing of rupture during embryonic life, usual deformities are [22]:
   - Ectopia cordis
   - Midline sternal cleft
   - Frontonasal dysgenesis and mid nasal cleft
   - Limb deformities
     Theories suggest that a rupture insult during the cardiac descent at the third week of gestation is responsible for the development of ectopia cordis [22].
2. Ectopia Cordis cordis can happen in isolation from amniotic rupture and solitary EC differs from EC with rupture, that's why researchers suggest the presence of several other causes of EC including intrauterine exposure to different medications and chemicals [19–23] (Fig. 1).

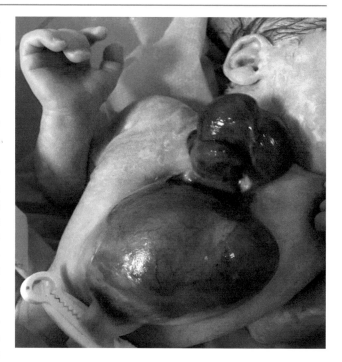

Fig. 1 At Al-Zahra teaching hospital in Najaf city, Iraq. A 30-year-old woman, gravida 5 para 2, had not previously received prenatal care prior to 24 weeks of gestation. During the first ultrasonographic evaluation at 24 gestational weeks of an uneventful pregnancy. There has been no history of congenital anomalies, genetic abnormalities, or ectopia cordis in the family. The mother smoked 15 cigarettes a day while pregnant and she did not take folic acid during pregnancy. And unfavorable prognosis for the fetus was anticipated, this conservative prenatal care was chosen

Classification

Ectopia cordis could be classified into four categories relying on the location of the heart:

1. Thoracic: anterior to the sternum (65%).
2. Thoraco-Abdominal: between the thorax and abdomen (20%).
3. Abdominal: within the abdomen (10%).
4. Cervical: in the neck (5%) [24, 25].

Genetic Basis of EC

Chromosomal disorders, especially trisomy 13,18, and 21, XXY, Turner syndrome, and 17q+ have a close relation to the development of ectopia cordis. It is a sporadic disease with karyotyping that can be normal or abnormal. With this aberration, a chromosomal analysis should be considered [3–7].

Prognosis of EC

Because the heart is exposed and malformed, cervical and thoracic ectopia cordis are usually fatal within days. The absence of intracardiac abnormalities and omphalocele in abdominal ectopia cordis makes this condition carry a better prognosis [26].

The prognosis is often correlated to the congenital anomalies associated with the defect. The more associated anomalies the poorer the prognosis [27].

Differential Diagnosis of EC

- **Pentalogy of Cantrell Sternal:** is a condition that includes the anterior diaphragmatic defect with midline supraumbilical abdominal wall defect and diaphragmatic pericardium defect which is associated with many congenital intracardiac anomalies and lower sternum defect [10].
- **Amniotic band syndrome:** this condition is noticed by many defects such as constriction rings, bands, and amputations [28].
- **Beckwith-Wiedemann syndrome:** this syndrome can be noticed by the enlarged organs, polyhydramnios, and macroglossia with a large omphalocele [29, 30].
- **Limb-body wall complex:** this can be characterized by anomalies of the craniofacial structures, thoracoabdominal wall, extremities, and Columna Vertebralis, and especially the umbilical cord-placental unit [31, 32].

Diagnosis of EC

The diagnosis can be carried out by the following methods:

- **Physical examination by meticulous inspection must be performed at birth to look for specific signs that might include** [33]:
  - Cyanosis of the skin and mucous membranes
  - Polypnea with flail chest
  - An exposed heart covered by the pericardium
  - Open sternum
  - Omphalocele
  - Visible abdominal organs
- **Plain radiograph**

  Frontal chest radiographs can reveal widely spread anterior ribs and the proximal ends of the clavicles on plain chest radiography might indicate sternal cleft. Computed tomography, on the other hand, can provide further detailed information [34].
- **Antenatal ultrasound**

  Ultrasound is frequently used to diagnose this disease, which can occur as early as the first trimester (10–12 weeks). 3D ultrasound and Doppler aid to understand the complex anatomy [35]. When in isolation, the heart is placed in the amniotic cavity with a chest wall defect. The condition may be associated with The Pentalogy of Cantrell, then omphalocele may be seen [33].
- **MR/MDCT**

  The most accurate assessment of ectopia cordis can be achieved through magnetic resonance accompanied by echocardiography in the prenatal period enabling improved prognosis and preoperative planning [36].

  Multidirectional computed tomography can be utilized as an alternative to MR in patients with Cantrell pentalogy. There are different benefits obtained from using MDCT as it provides high resolution, multidirectional views, and fast results without using anesthesia [37].

Management of EC

This complicated and life-threatening abnormality necessitates special care for newborns from the moment they are born. The mother must have a C-section. The endotracheal tube is also beneficial in keeping air moving [38].

Surgery

Surgical repair is the definitive treatment for this anomaly. Cutler and Wilens tried the first ectopia cordis repair in 1925 [39], and Koop (1975) successfully repaired thoracic ectopia cordis in two phases for the first time [35]. "Amato et al. reported on a successful single-stage repair of thoracic ectopia cordis in 1995" [40].

The Procedure of Surgery

Most frequently the repair is done in phases. The surgery takes the following steps:

1. The priority is to provide urgent cover of the exposed heart and abdomen contents with saline-soaked gauze pads or a silastic prosthesis (inactive compounds) to prevent heat loss and desiccation and, if required, hemodynamic palliation.
2. Repair of the defect in the chest wall (either by doing the primary chest wall closures or by using bone or cartilage or artificial prosthesis) [40].
3. The sternal defect is repaired.
4. The initial step includes repair of the related omphalocele, sternal, diaphragmatic, and pericardial abnormalities.
5. The heart is reduced into the left thorax. Surgical repair will be difficult and not tolerated in the neonatal period due to a lack of mediastinal space available to the heart. Due to the extended length of the major arteries and its aberrant course, reducing the heart into the thorax might compress the heart and kink the major arteries, subsequently leading to poor heart-filling and output. If there is hemodynamic instability, palliation might be delayed for a few weeks until the hemodynamic effects of the chest covering have resolved [41]. Reduced pulmonary flow, ventricular septal defect, patent ductus arteriosus, left ventricular diverticulum, and other disorders linked with thoracic ectopia cordis can all be treated with prostaglandin E1. Following tissue covering, these problems can be addressed medically [8, 41].
6. The correction of the intracardiac defects should be postponed until some thoracic cavity growth occurs. This is normally done by the time a child reaches the age of 2 years. At this time, simple stable intracardiac defects including ASD, VSD, LVD, and TOF can be corrected [42]. Furthermore, certain problems, such as ASD or VSD, may have been resolved on their own. Prior to the reduction of the heart into the left thorax and restoration of abdominal contents, intracardiac abnormalities are repaired [43]. The heart is reduced into the thoracic cavity, closed with a skin and muscle flap, and provided with extra strength with the rotation of the lower costochondral cartilage once the intracardiac defect is fixed [41].
7. In coordination with a plastic surgeon, chest wall repair is performed at a later period.
8. Antibiotics and inotropic medicines can be given systemically to prevent infection, support the heart, and enhance blood flow [17, 38, 40, 44].

Outcomes of Surgery

Ectopia cordis with major intracardiac anomalies can live through infancy and receive successful cardiac repair or more definitive palliation for single-ventricle physiology in the absence of significant extracardiac problems [45].

Multiple Choice Questions

1. The prognosis is determined by the following factors except:
   A. Abnormalities associated with the disease
   B. The location of the defect
   C. The length of the limbs
   D. The extent and severity of intracardiac defects
   Answer: C
   The location of the defect, the extent of intracardiac defects, the severity of the intracardiac defects, and the abnormalities connected with it are the four parameters that define the prognosis.
2. Pentalogy of Cantrell has the following lesions, except:
   A. Ectopia cordis
   B. Diaphragmatic defects
   C. Constriction rings, amputations, and bands.
   D. Omphalocele
   Answer: C
   Cantrell pentalogy includes pericardial and diaphragmatic abnormalities, as well as omphalocele and ectopia cordis. Random abnormalities, constriction rings, amputations, and bands describe the amniotic band syndrome.
3. In plain radiograph, the confirmation of the extrathoracic location of the heart is done by:
   A. The anteroposterior view
   B. The lateral view.
   C. The posteroanterior view
   D. None of the above
   Answer: B
   The lateral view is used to confirm the extrathoracic placement of the heart.
4. According to the strategy of repair in the surgical procedure in treating ectopia cordis. One of the following is false:
   A. Urgent coverage to the exposed heart and abdominal contents with saline-soaked gauze
   B. Closure of the chest wall defect
   C. Leave repairing of the associated omphalocele, sternal, diaphragmatic, and pericardial defects to the second phase.
   D. Closure of the sternal defect
   Answer: C
   In the first step, the related omphalocele, sternal, diaphragmatic, and pericardial abnormalities are repaired.

5. According to the strategy of repair in the surgical procedure in treating ectopia cordis. One of the following is false:
   A. Palliation can be postponed for a few weeks if there are hemodynamically significant defects
   B. Urgent coverage to the exposed heart and abdominal contents with saline-soaked gauze
   C. Closure of the chest wall defect
   D. Prostaglandin cannot be used to treat conditions that are associated with thoracic ectopia cordis.
   Answer: D

   Reduced pulmonary flow, ventricular septal defect, patent ductus arteriosus, left ventricular diverticulum, and other problems linked with thoracic ectopia cordis can all be treated with prostaglandin E1.

6. According to the strategy of repair in the surgical procedure in treating ectopia cordis. One of the following is false:
   A. Urgent coverage to the exposed heart and abdominal contents with saline-soaked gauze.
   B. Palliation can be postponed for a few weeks if there are hemodynamically significant defects.
   C. Intracardiac defects are corrected secondly after the reduction of the heart into the left thorax and replacement of abdominal contents.
   D. Prostaglandin can be used to treat conditions that are associated with thoracic ectopia cordis.
   Answer: C

   Prior to the reduction of the heart into the left thorax and replacement of abdominal contents, intracardiac abnormalities are repaired.

7. Non-cardiac defects that are associated with ectopia cordis are all of the following except one:
   A. Encephalocele
   B. Hydrocephalus
   C. Cleft lip
   D. None of the above
   Answer: D

   Encephalocele, hydrocephalus, cleft lip and/or palate abnormalities, and craniorachischisis are all linked to the condition.

   Ectopia cordis may be accompanied with limb abnormalities such as clubfoot, hypodactyly, and the lack of the tibia or radius.

   Gallbladder agenesis and polysplenia are defects in the creation of abdominal organs.

8. According to the strategy of repair in the surgical procedure in treating ectopia cordis. One of the following is false:
   A. Systemic antibiotics and inotropic drugs can be administered to prevent infection and support the heart and improve the blood supply.
   B. Palliation is urgent if there are hemodynamically significant defects.
   C. Prostaglandin can be used to treat conditions that are associated with thoracic ectopia cordis.
   D. Urgent coverage to the exposed heart and abdominal contents with saline-soaked gauze.
   Answer: B

   Palliation can be postponed for a few weeks if there are hemodynamically significant defects

9. Ectopia cordis can be accurately assessed using the following methods:
   A. Echocardiogram and magnetic resonance imaging
   B. Ultrasound
   C. Examination of the body
   D. Plain radiograph
   Answer: A

   In the prenatal period, magnetic resonance imaging combined with echocardiography can provide the most accurate assessment of ectopia cordis, allowing for better prediction and preoperative preparation.

10. According to the prognosis of ectopia cordis which one of the following is false:
    A. Thoracic and cervical ectopia cordis has a better prognosis than other kinds of ectopia cordis.
    B. The prognosis is frequently linked to the congenital malformations that accompany the condition.
    C. The absence of intracardiac abnormalities and omphalocele in abdominal ectopia cordis makes this condition carry a better prognosis.
    D. Because the heart is exposed and malformed, cervical and thoracic ectopia cordis are usually fatal within days.
    Answer: A

    Cervical and thoracic ectopia cordis are frequently lethal within days because the heart is exposed and deformed. Abdominal ectopia cordis has a better prognosis due to the absence of intracardiac anomalies and omphalocele.

    The prognosis is frequently linked to the congenital malformations that accompany the condition. The worse the prognosis, the more related anomalies there are.

References

1. Goncalo FIMD, Ana VRS, Catia FCPM, Ana PDF, Joaquim MDF. Ectopia cordis: caso clinic. Revista Brasileira de Saúde Materno Infantil. 2014;14(3):287–90.
2. Dachlan EG, Cininta N, Pranadyan R, Putri AY, Oktaviono YH, Akbar MI. High maternal neonatal mortality and morbidity in pregnancy with Eisenmenger syndrome. J Pregnancy. 2021;2021:3248850.
3. Malik R, Zilberman M, Tang L, Miller S, Pandian N. Ectopia cordis with a double outlet right ventricle, large ventricular sep-

tal defect, malposed great arteries and left ventricular hypoplasia. Echocardiography. 2014;32(3):589–91.

4. Khoury MJ, Cordero JF, Rasmussen S. Ectopia cordis, midline defects and chromosome abnormalities: an epidemiologic perspective. Am J Med Genet. 1988;30:811–7.

5. King CR. Ectopia cordis and chromosome errors. Pediatrics. 1980;66:328.

6. Soper SP, Roe LR, Hoyme HE, Clemmons JJW. Trisomy 18 with ectopia cordis, omphalocele, and ventricular septal defect: case report. Fetal Pediatr Pathol. 1986;5(3–4):481–3.

7. Say B, Wilsey CE. Chromosome aberration in ectopia cordis (46,XX,17q+). Am Heart J. 1978;95(2):274–5.

8. Morales JM, Patel SG, Duff JA, Villareal RL, Simpson JW. Ectopia cordis and other midline defects. Ann Thorac Surg. 2000;70(1):111–4.

9. Dobell ARC, Williams HB, Long RW. Staged repair of ectopia cordis. J Pediatr Surg. 1982;17(4):353–8.

10. Cantrell JR, Haller JA, Ravitch MM. A syndrome of congenital defects involving the abdominal wall, sternum, diaphragm, pericardium and heart. Surg Gynecol Obstet. 1958;107(5):602–14.

11. Mendaluk T, Mościcka A, Mroziński B, Szymankiewicz M. The incomplete pentalogy of Cantrell—a case report. Pediatr Pol. 2015;90(3):241–4.

12. Correa-Rivas MS, Matos-Llovet I, Garcia-Fragoso L. Pentalogy of Cantrell: a case report with pathologic findings. Pediatr Dev Pathol. 2004;7:649–52.

13. Polat I, Gul A, Aslan H, Cebeci A, Ozseker B, Caglar B, Ceylan Y. Prenatal diagnosis of pentalogy of Cantrell in three cases, two with craniorachischisis. J Clin Ultrasound. 2005;33:308–11.

14. Pivnick EK, Kaufman RA, Velagaleti GV, Gunther WM, Abramovici D. Infant with midline thoracoabdominal schisis and limb defects. Teratology. 1998;58:205–8.

15. Uygur D, Kis S, Sener E, Gunce S, Semerci N. An infant with pentalogy of Cantrell and limb defects diagnosed prenatally. Clin Dysmorphol. 2004;13:57–8.

16. Bittmann S, Ulus H, Springer A. Combined pentalogy of Cantrell with tetralogy of Fallot, gallbladder agenesis, and polysplenia: a case report. J Pediatr Surg. 2004;39:107–9.

17. Jimmy S, Keshav B, Rakesh B. Thoracic ectopia cordis, vol. 2012. BMJ Case Rep; 2012. p. bcr1120115241.

18. Kanagasuntheram R, Verzin JA. Ectopia cordis in man. Thorax. 1962;17:159–67.

19. Kaplan LC, Matsuoka R, Gilbert EF, Opitz JM, Kurnit DM. Ectopia cordis and cleft sternum: evidence for mechanical teratogenesis following rupture of the chorion or yolk sac. Am J Med Genet. 1985;21(1):187–99.

20. Van Allen MI, Myhre S. Ectopia cordis thoracalis with craniofacial defects resulting from early amnion rupture. Teratology. 1985;32(1):19–24.

21. Bieber FR, Mostoufi-zadeh M, Birnholz JC, Driscoll SG. Amniotic band sequence associated with ectopia cordis in one twin. J Pediatr. 1984;105(5):817–9.

22. Ectopia cordis causes, diagnosis, treatment, surgery & survival rate [Internet]. Health Jade. 2022 [cited 14 August 2022]. https://healthjade.net/ectopia-cordis/.

23. Russo R, D'Armiento M, Angrisani P, Vecchione R. Limb body wall complex: a critical review and a nosological proposal. Am J Med Genet. 1993;47(6):893–900.

24. Blatt ML, Zeldes M. Ectopia cordis: report of a case and review of the literature. Am J Dis Child. 1942;63:515.

25. Byron F. Ectopia cordis: report of a case with attempted operative correction. J Thorac Surg. 1949;17:717–22.

26. Achiron R, Shimmel M, Farber B, Glaser J. Prenatal sonographic diagnosis and perinatal management of ectopia cordis. Ultrasound Obstet Gynecol. 1991;1(6):431–4.

27. Gruberg L, Goldstein SA, Pfister AJ, Monsein LH, Evans DM, Leon MB. Cantrell's syndrome: left ventricular diverticulum in an adult patient. Circulation. 2000;101:109–10.

28. Seeds, et al. Br Med J (Clin Res Ed). 1983;286(6369):919–920. 1982.

29. Beckwith JB. Abstract, Western Society for Pediatric Research 1963; Extreme cytomegaly of the adrenal fetal cortex, omphalocele, hyperplasia of kidneys and pancreas, and Leydig-cell hyperplasia: another syndrome? Los Angeles.

30. Wiedemann HR. Complexe malformatif familial avec hernie ombilicale et macroglossia, un syndrome nouveau. J Genet Hum. 1964;13:223–32.

31. Kurosawa K, Imaizumi K, Masuno M, Kuroki Y. Epidemiology of limb-body wall complex in Japan. Am J Med Genet. 1994;51:143–6.

32. Luebke HJ, Reiser CA, Pauli RM. Fetal disruptions: assessment of frequency, heterogeneity, and embryologic mechanism in a population referred to a community-based stillbirth assessment program. Am J Med Genet. 1990;36:56–72.

33. Cabrera A, Rodrigo D, Teresa Luis M, Pastor E, Miguel Galdeano J, Esteban S. Anomalías cardíacas en la ectopia cordis. Rev Esp Cardiol. 2002;55(11):1209–12.

34. Restrepo CS, Martinez S, Lemos DF, et al. Imaging appearances of the sternum and sternoclavicular joints. Radiographics. 2009;29(3):839–59. https://doi.org/10.1148/rg.293055136.

35. Lodhia J, Chipongo H, Chilonga K, Mchaile D, Mbwasi R, Philemon R. Ectopia cordis: a case report of pre-surgical care in resource-limited setting. Int J Surg Case Rep. 2021;83:105965.

36. McMahon CJ, Taylor MD, Cassady CI, et al. Diagnosis of pentalogy of Cantrell in the fetus using magnetic resonance imaging and ultrasound. Pediatr Cardiol. 2007;28:172–5.

37. Santiago-Herrera R, Ramirez-Carmona R, Criales-Vera S, et al. Ectopia cordis with tetralogy of Fallot in an infant with pentalogy of Cantrell: high-pitch MDCT exam. Pediatr Radiol. 2011;41:925–9.

38. Harrison MR, Filly RA, Stanger P, de Lorimier AA. Prenatal diagnosis and management of omphalocele and ectopia cordis. J Pediatr Surg. 1982;17(1):64–6.

39. Cutler GD, Wilens G. Ectopia cordis: report of a case. Am J Dis Child. 1925;30:75.

40. Pius S, Abubakar Ibrahim H, Bello M, Bashir TM. Complete ectopia cordis: a case report and literature review. Case Rep Pediatr. 2017;2017:1–6.

41. Home|Driscoll Children's Hospital [Internet]. Driscoll Children's Hospital. 2022 [cited 14 August 2022]. https://www.driscollchildrens.org/.

42. Pius S, et al. Complete ectopia cordis: a case report and literature review. Case Rep Pediatr. 2017;2017:1858621. https://doi.org/10.1155/2017/1858621.

43. Alphonso N, Venugopal PS, Deshpande R, Anderson D. Complete thoracic ectopia cordis. Eur J Cardiothorac Surg. 2003;23(3):426–8. https://doi.org/10.1016/s1010-7940(02)00811-4.

44. Carmi R, Boughman JA. Pentalogy of Cantrell and associated midline anomalies: a possible ventral midline developmental field. Am J Med Genet. 1992;42(1):90–5.

45. Hornberger LK, Colan SD, Lock JE, Wessel DL, Mayer JE. Outcome of patients with ectopia cordis and significant intracardiac defects. Circulation. 1996;94(9 Suppl):II32–7.

Aortic Stenosis (AS)

Zanyar Qais, Kashmala Qais, and Simrenpreet Dhillon

Abstract

Aortic stenosis (AS) is the most common valvular heart disease affecting 5% of those aged over 65 where severe stenosis occurs in 1–3%. AS can be acquired or congenital. Congenital AS usually shows up early in childhood or early adult life. Acquired AS is rarely seen before the age of 75. The severity of AS is based on valve hemodynamics. The cardinal symptoms of AS are angina, dyspnea, and syncope. The patient is asymptomatic for many years and relatively safe in this latent period. It is when symptoms occur that the mortality increases manyfold, and the prognosis becomes poor. The only curative treatment is to undergo valve replacement. Currently, the preferred method is the surgical approach, however with progression and improvement in the transcatheter method it might become the preferred approach.

Keywords

Aortic stenosis · Valve replacement · Supravalvular stenosis, Subvalvular stenosis · Bicuspid valve Unicuspid valve, transcatheter aortic valve replacement Heart failure

Introduction

The aortic valve is a semilunar valve found between the left ventricle and the aorta. The function of the valve is to provide blood to the systemic circulation without causing leakage back into the ventricle. Aortic stenosis is the term used when there is an obstruction to the outflow from the left ventricle. Even though this condition is usually associated with age-dependent calcification, it is important to know the existence of the various types of aortic stenosis and underlying risk factors which may be present since birth. AS can be divided into valvular, subvalvular, and supravalvular. The obstruction can be either congenital or acquired and most commonly a combination of both as you will read in this chapter.

Epidemiology

Aortic stenosis (AS) is the most common valvular heart disorder and is four times more common in males. The most common cause of aortic stenosis in young and middle-aged adults is almost always due to the calcification of a congenital bicuspid valve. In patients older than 75 years there is usually calcification of a normal tricuspid valve. The prevalence of congenital bicuspid and unicuspid valve is 1–2% respectively. Rheumatic disease is a rare cause of AS in the west, but one of the most common causes in the developing countries and is always associated with mitral dysfunction [1].

Anatomy of the Aortic Valve

It is worth to be familiar with the anatomy of the aortic valve to understand the pathophysiology of the various causes and also the manifestation such as angina. The aortic valve is a tricuspid semilunar valve (not to be confused with the tricuspid valve). The three cusps of the valve have a half moon shape and are called *Right Coronary*, *Left Coronary,* and *Non-coronary*. Some books refer to them as Right, Left, and Posterior or just simply coronary and non-coronary valves. You might have noticed by now that the naming of the valve is relative to the origin of coronary sinus which lies between the ascending aorta and the cusps. The coronary cusps are just proximal to the coronary sinuses. During the course of aortic stenosis, the obstruction itself may limit perfusion to the coronary artery. This is why sometimes symptoms of angina or ischemia may occur without any evidence of atherosclerotic plaque on angiography.

Z. Qais (✉) · K. Qais · S. Dhillon
Medical University of Lublin, Lublin, Poland

G. Tagarakis et al. (eds.), *Clinical and Surgical Aspects of Congenital Heart Diseases*,
https://doi.org/10.1007/978-3-031-23062-2_14

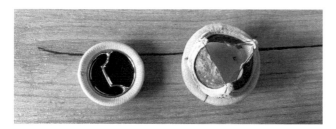

Fig. 1 Picture of mechanical and biological valve

Table 1 Etiology of AS frequencies

Etiology	Approximate frequency
Degenerative	80%
Rheumatic	11%
Post-endocarditis	1%
Congenital	5%
Other	1%

The best place for auscultation is the second left intercostal space. Normally this valve is made up of three leaflets, however valves with only two or one leaflet also exist. Artificial valves are being recreated with various shapes and methods to replace the normal function of the aortic valve (Fig. 1).

Etiology

Valvular Aortic Stenosis

Stenosis of the aortic valve can occur at different levels. The most common type is valvular, and the most common cause is degenerative calcification of a tricuspid and bicuspid valve. AS in elderly patients occurs most commonly due to age-related degenerative calcification of the aortic cusps. The deterioration and calcification of the aortic valve is not a passive process, but rather one that shares many characteristics with vascular atherosclerosis, such as endothelial dysfunction, inflammatory cell activation, lipid accumulation, cytokine release, and upregulation of several signaling pathways. Many patients with VAS also have coronary artery disease. Rheumatic disease of the aortic valves causes commissural fusion, which can result in a bicuspid valve. This, in turn, makes the leaflets more vulnerable to damage, eventually leading to fibrosis, calcification, and further stenosis. By the time the obstruction to left ventricular (LV) outflow causes substantial clinical dysfunction, the valve is usually a rigid calcified mass. The valve does not open properly nor close and therefore aortic regurgitation (AR) presents concurrently. Rheumatic AS is always associated directly with mitral valve dysfunction and aortic regurgitation [2].

Younger patients with AS typically have a congenital defect, a bicuspid or unicuspid valve. Due to this defect, they are more prone to degenerative processes than a normal tricuspid valve. Bicuspid valve is a far more common defect than a unicuspid valve. The production of fibrous material

and the deposition of lime in the valve system is a gradual process. The manifestation presents itself in adulthood and rarely in childhood.

Supravalvular

Supravalvular aortic stenosis (SVAS) is an uncommon cause of AS. The obstruction in this type lies above the valve where there is a diffuse narrowing of the ascending aorta. The most common form is where the ascending aorta takes the form of an hourglass. The defect is due to a systemic elastin arteriopathy which may present in nonsyndromic or syndromic state. It is usually part of William syndrome which is characterized by mental retardation, growth delay, and elf-like facies. William syndrome occurs due to the deletion of the gene at chromosome 17 which produces elastin. This protein is responsible for the distensibility in tissues, especially the arteries. These patients also tend to present with stenosis of other vessels, the pulmonary, renal, and coronary arteries. Similar to valvular stenosis the patient remains asymptomatic for a long time and the symptoms usually occur when there is severe stenosis. These patients develop symptoms much earlier in life around their 20s. When symptoms occur, they are similar to those of valvular type. Note however that on auscultation different findings may be present (Table 1).

Subvalvular

Subvalvular aortic stenosis (SAS) is an uncommon congenital disorder seen in infants. The cause of the obstruction is usually a muscular membranous outgrow in the left ventricle just proximal to the aortic valve which obstructs the outflow. Similar to SVAS it is highly associated with syndromes but also with other congenital heart diseases such as ventricular septal defect, coarctation of aorta, and bicuspid aortic valve. The progression is gradual and the symptoms usually appear in the first decade of life. The definitive treatment for a symptomatic patient is surgery (Table 2).

Table 2 Etiology of AS regarding to age

Age of onset	Etiology of AS
30–70	Calcification of congenital bicuspid valve
75+	Calcification of normal tricuspid aortic valve

Table 3 Criteria for lesion severity: ACC/AHA/ASE Guidelines 2014

Indicator	Mild	Moderate	Severe
Jet velocity	<3.0 m/s	3.0–4.0	>4.0 m/s
Mean gradient	<25 mmHg	25–40	>40 mmHg
Valve area	>1.5 cm^2	1.0–1.5	<1.0 cm^2

Pathophysiology

Normally there is free flow between the valve and aorta during systole. When the aortic valve becomes stenotic, it causes resistance to systolic ejection and the formation of a systolic pressure gradient over the left ventricle and the aorta. This outflow blockage raises the systolic pressure of the left ventricle (LV). As a compensatory mechanism to decrease LV wall stress, LV wall thickness increases via parallel sarcomere replication, resulting in concentric hypertrophy. It is worth mentioning that not every patient presents with hypertrophy, even in severe stages of stenosis. In the early stages of AS the chamber is not dilated, and ventricular function is intact, while diastolic compliance is diminished. However, as LV end-diastolic pressure (LVEDP) rises, pulmonary capillary arterial pressures rise as well, resulting in a decrease in cardiac output due to diastolic dysfunction. Myocardium contractility may start to decline after a while, resulting in a decrease in cardiac output due to systolic dysfunction. Heart failure develops as a result [3].

Despite a higher LV systolic pressure, most individuals with aortic stenosis have sustained LV systolic function and cardiac output for many years. Although cardiac output is normal at rest, it frequently fails to increase correctly during exercise, leading to exercise-induced symptoms. Patients often mistake these exertional symptoms to be due to deconditioning.

Adult Presentation

The clinical presentation in an adult is usually asymptomatic until there is mild to moderate stenosis. AS is a chronic and slow-progressing disease in which the ventricles attempt to compensate by developing myocardial hypertrophy. As a result, we will usually see symptoms in the late stages of disease [4].

The three cardinal symptoms of aortic stenosis are exertional dyspnea, near syncope or syncope and angina. One very interesting thing about AS is that it has a long latent period where morbidity and mortality are low. When AS patients start to become symptomatic the mortality increases manyfold. There is no single parameter which can alone define the severity of AS. The severity depends on clinical symptoms, pressure gradient between the ventricle and valve area. Table 3 shows the criteria made by the AHS for lesion severity. The rate at which progression of AS from asymptomatic to symptomatic is hard to predict and varies for every patient. Thus, it is very important with regular follow-up in patients with recognized AS, even if it is asymptomatic and mild. In severe stenosis, death occurs within 2–3 years if no measures are taken to treat it surgically (Table 3).

Dyspnea is usually the first and only symptom to occur in AS. It occurs due to a hypertrophic and stiff heart which leads to backflow and pulmonary congestion. Increased filling pressure, myocardial ischemia, and the need to overcome pressure gradient from left ventricle to aorta are all the factors that contribute to dyspnea. Tachyarrhythmias and physical activity can aggravate dyspnea as well.

Angina is caused by a concurrent increase in oxygen demand by the hypertrophic myocardium and a decrease in oxygen supply because of a decreased coronary flow reserve, lower diastolic perfusion pressure, and relative subendocardial myocardial ischemia. Many risk factors are shared by aortic stenosis and coronary heart disease, and up to half of the patients evaluated for aortic valve surgery have substantial coronary stenosis.

Syncope

Syncope can be caused by either tachyarrhythmias, AV-block, bradyarrhythmia, or due to a fall in blood pressure.

Neonatal Presentation

AS does not always have a latent period and is sometimes present as early as in the first days of life. 10–15% may present the symptoms before the age of 1. The etiology of AS then is most probably all other congenital causes except for congenital bicuspid valve since these tend to present in young adulthood, such as subvalvular stenosis and supravalvular. Pediatric patients with severe stenosis can present with signs of heart failure, shock, and poor growth rate in the neonatal period. These patients are in critical need of intervention and are dependent on the patency of PDA to survive. The first priority in the management is to keep the ductus patent to maintain adequate perfusion to vital organs. Further evaluation should then be done to estimate if the ventricle size of the neonate allows for intervention in the form of balloon dilation. If the ventricle size does not allow balloon dilation the surgeon needs to perform surgical valvotomy.

Diagnosis

Both physical examination and echocardiogram play an important role in the diagnosis of AS. The most common presentation is a murmur or incidental abnormal findings on echocardiography. Physical examination is both sensitive and specific and has an important role as echocardiogram. As we discussed earlier there are several causes of AS. With the help of echocardiography, we can visualize the type of obstruction and also to what degree. It also can assist in the assessment of the pressure gradient which helps in determining the severity of the disease and potential surgery in the future. Since valvular AS is the most common form, we are going to focus on this type further in this chapter [4].

Physical Examination

The main components of the clinical examination are palpation of the peripheral pulses, auscultation, and to look for signs of heart failure. The peripheral pulse should be assessed and especially the carotids. One should note the amplitude of the pulse. In AS the patient has pulsus parvus and tardus which means the pulse is weak and slow to rise. This is due to the fact that there is an obstruction at the valvular level which causes the contraction in the ventricle to slower translate into a pulse in the carotids (Fig. 2).

ECG

ECG is unreliable as a diagnostic test. In AS hypertrophy is a normal finding, however not everyone will have it. Even patients with severe stenosis may have a normal ECG and even if there are no abnormal findings, it does not exclude severe stenosis. Atrial fibrillation is also a common finding in AS [5].

Echocardiography

Echocardiography is the gold standard for assessing and diagnosing AS. By looking at the structure of the valve and its surrounding, such as the number of cusps and the presence of calcification we can find out the etiology and potentially coexisting lesions. This diagnostic test does not only allow us to visualize the structure but also to find out the severity of the obstruction by measuring the velocity, mean gradient over the valve. The left ventricle function is also assessed, and we can see if there is hypertrophy (Fig. 3).

Stress Test
Exercise testing is a contraindication in symptomatic patients. This test is mainly done on asymptomatic patients who present with severe stenosis.

Auscultation
- During auscultation, we can hear a low pitched, harsh early systolic murmur called crescendo and decrescendo. The murmur is heard in early systole when AS is mild, but as the disease progresses it is heard in mid systole. The sound is produced due to the turbulent blood flow passing through the valve. The murmur is best heard over the second intercostal space and radiates to the right carotid artery.
- Ejection click is a sound produced in early systole due to the abrupt opening of the valve. The sound comes from the valve being mobile, which in advanced stage is no longer the case and therefore may be absent. In severe cases the aortic sound of the S2 is diminished and we only hear the closure of the pulmonic valve. This is due to the aortic valve not being mobile.

Fig. 2 Pulse presentation of AS

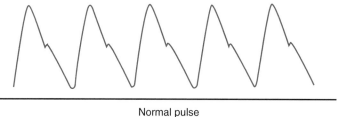

Normal pulse

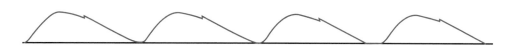

Pulsus parvus et tardus (Delayed peak)

Fig. 3 Echo of stenotic valve

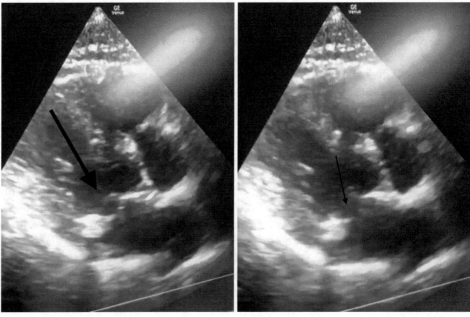

Fig. 4 Heart sound
presentation of AS

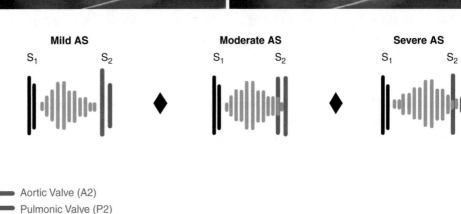

- Physiologically there is splitting of the two components of S2, the aortic valve closes first and then the pulmonic valve, this is known as splitting. During inspiration, the venous return is increased to the heart resulting in more blood volume being pumped across the right part of the heard and consequently later closure of the pulmonic valve. This leads to a greater delay between the two sounds of S2. However, in AS we have the opposite. Due to the obstruction in the valve the aortic valve closes later than the pulmonic valve and the aortic tone of the S2 comes after the pulmonic. During inspiration, the pulmonic valve delays its closure and leads to a narrowing of the S2 sound. This is called the paradoxical splitting of the S2. Normal splitting of the S2 can exclude severe obstruction.
- If the patient develops diastolic heart failure, we can hear an S4 heart sound. This sound is caused by the atria contracting blood against a stiff hypertrophic ventricle. For the S4 sound to be present the atria should be contracting normally. Note however that we can never hear S4 in atrial fibrillation, a rhythm which is common in AS (Fig. 4).

Findings on Auscultation

Ejection click (Systolic)

- *Crescendo–Decrescendo murmur*
- *Soft S2 or single S2*
- *Paradoxal splitting of S2*
- *S4 sound due to diastolic failure*

Management

The main goal of the treatment of AS is to control the symptoms of heart failure. It is not possible to cure AS with medications, the definitive curative treatment of aortic stenosis is surgically. The choice of treatment is a multidisciplinary task. Factors to be considered are age of onset, type of aortic stenosis, severity of symptoms, and surgical risks. Treatment of symptomatic AS medically has a poor prognosis and holds no value in curative treatment, but rather as palliative and symptomatically. All patients with recognized aortic stenosis should receive prophylaxis for endocarditis [6].

As mentioned earlier in this chapter children born with congenital bicuspid valves are at higher risk for development of aortic stenosis, but children with tricuspid aortic valve can also develop this condition. If the symptoms are severe, surgery is needed with balloon dilatation of the valve. As a rule, it is expected that patients who have been operated in childhood need reoperation within the next 10–15 years.

Medical Management

Treatment with medications serves only as symptomatic relief and does not stop the underlying process, nor decrease mortality. It mainly aims to treat the heart failure and the arrhythmias associated with it. The aim is usually to stabilize the patient in anticipation of surgery or as palliative treatment. AS and coronary artery disease (CAD) share the same risk factors and one would think that the use of statins would be beneficial. However, studies have shown them not to be effective in stopping the progression of AS alone. Since CAD often occurs together with AS it may still be beneficial with statins for the patient. Even though it does not prevent AS directly, it can prevent coronary events [7].

- *Heart Failure* Use of ACE inhibitor may be useful if the patient has heart failure or hypertension but should be used with caution. Start with a low dose to prevent hypotension. Beta-blockers should generally be avoided in AS to prevent LV dysfunction. Digitalis may also be used.
- *Symptomatic* Diuretics may be used in the case of dyspnea due to pulmonary edema. Nitrates may be used with caution in patients with pulmonary congestion.

Surgical Management

Indications for Operation Patient with severe aortic stenosis and who are symptomatic should undergo aortic valve replacement (AVR), a procedure where the valve is excised and replaced with a prosthetic valve. Asymptomatic patients with AS are relatively safe and it is important to recognize the right indication for intervention in this group of patients to not put the patient under unnecessary surgical risk, however in some circumstances it might be necessary. Patients who are asymptomatic and have a poor ventricular function measured as low ejection fraction should also be referred for surgery. In Table 3 you can see the indications for AVR in asymptomatic patients.

For patients who are eligible and candidates for aortic valve replacement there are two options, either open or percutaneous. replacement. The choice of method depends on the surgical risk and comorbidities of the patient. The stan-

dard choice of method is open-heart surgery, especially in younger patients [8, 9].

Percutaneous Valve Replacement Since the introduction of transcatheter aortic valve replacement (TAVR) it has given patients who were not able to tolerate surgery a good alternative treatment. These valves are biological which are expanded in the place of the old valve through a catheter. The valve can be either self-expanding or expanded with the help of a balloon. TAVR is mainly reserved for patients who are at high operative risk. Due to it potentially causing paravalvular leakage, AV blocks, and other challenges, the use is limited to those who do not tolerate open surgery. In recent times there has been improvement in the methods of TAVR and may even become the standard choice in the future, even for those at low surgical risk. Recent studies are also starting to show comparable results between the two methods [10].

Prosthetic Valve There are two options for prosthetic valves, biological or mechanical. Both have advantages and disadvantages and the best choice is relative to the circumstance of the patient. For example, biological valve does not require anticoagulation and is a good choice for young fertile female. However, these valves tend to have a lifespan of 10–15 years and therefore can be a good choice in elderly patients who are not expected to live beyond the lifetime of the valve. Mechanical valve on the other hand lasts lifelong and good biomechanical properties but requires long-life anticoagulation use and is not suitable for women of childbearing age (Fig. 5).

Percutaneous Aortic Valvuloplasty (PAV) is reserved for patients with severe comorbidities which does not allow them to undergo AVR, such as patients with cardiogenic shock. If no contraindication is present AVR should be performed over PAV, even if the patient is of older age. In most cases restenosis usually occurs within months. The life expectancy of an adult patient treated with balloon valvulo-

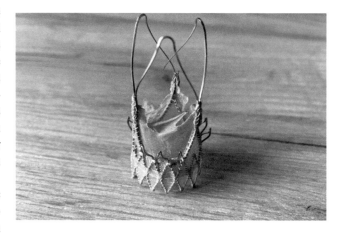

Fig. 5 Picture of biological transcatheter valve

Fig. 6 Indications for surgery

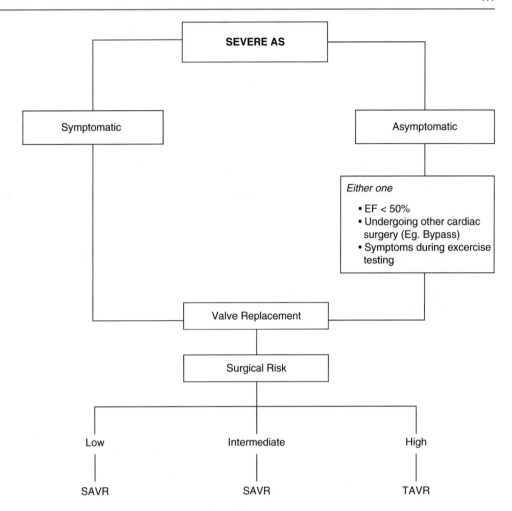

plasty is the same as those not treated and nowadays this method is mainly reserved for young children and adults who are hemodynamically unstable to undergo AVR (Fig. 6).

Multiple Choice Questions
1. What is the most common cause of AS in the elderly?
   A. Congenital
   B. Rheumatic
   C. Degenerative
   D. Bicuspid valve
2. What are the cardinal symptoms of AS?
   A. Angina, hypertension, dyspnea
   B. Angina, dyspnea, syncope
   C. Heart failure, hypertension, syncope
   D. None of the above
3. What syndrome is supravalvular AS commonly associated with?
   A. Down syndrome
   B. Angelman syndrome
   C. William syndrome
   D. Marfan syndrome

4. Patient with severe asymptomatic AS and EF 30%, treatment of choice?
   A. Refer patient to heart team for valve replacement
   B. Patient is asymptomatic and does not need surgery.
   C. Wait and observe
   D. None of the above
5. What medication should be used carefully in patients with AS
   A. Beta-blockers
   B. Diuretics
   C. Ace inhibitors
   D. All the above
6. Which of these are not typical findings in severe stenosis during auscultation?
   A. Crecendo-Decrecendo systolic murmur
   B. Ejection click
   C. Increased splitting of S2 during inspiration
   D. Single/decreased S2 sound
7. Which statement is false about TAVR
   A. TAVR is preferred over SAVR
   B. TAVR is used when the patient is at low surgical risk

C. TAVR is used when the patient cannot undergo SAVR due to high surgical risk

D. A + B

8. What is commonly the first and only symptom in AS?
   A. Exertional angina
   B. Exertional dyspnea
   C. Edema
   D. Syncope

9. A young patient presents with symptoms of AS. After further diagnostic evaluations, the diagnosis of AS is confirmed. What is the most likely cause of AS in this patient?
   A. Supravalvular
   B. Degenerative calcification
   C. Rheumatic AS
   D. Bicuspid valve

10. What are the complications associated with TAVI
    A. AV block
    B. Valve regurgitation
    C. A + B
    D. Pulmonary valve regurgitation

Answers

1. C

   The most common cause of AS in patients older than 65 is the calcification of a tricuspid valve. The most common cause in those younger than 65 is the calcification of a congenital bicuspid valve.

2. B

   The cardinal symptoms of AS are exertional angina, dyspnea, and syncope.

3. D

   William syndrome. The syndrome in which the deletion of the elastin leads to systemic arteriopathy and narrowing of the ascending aorta.

4. A

   This patient should be referred to a heart team for AVR. Patients who are asymptomatic and have severe stenosis with EF lower than 50% have indication for AVR.

5. D

   All of the above should be given with care. ACE inhibitors should be started at low dose to decrease the risk of sudden hypotension which can further exacerbate the condition. Beta-blockers are usually avoided in AS

patients to prevent left ventricular dysfunction. While giving diuretics reduces the pulmonary congestion it is important to realize that the patient is dependent on adequate filling pressure to maintain optimal cardiac output.

6. C

   This is a physiological mechanism. During AS we usually have paradoxical splitting where the splitting is decreased during inspiration. The absence of paradoxical splitting excludes severe stenosis.

7. D

   TAVR is usually only considered when the patient is a high-risk patient for surgery.

8. D

   Dyspnea is usually the first and only symptom of AS.

9. D

   The most common cause of AS in those under 65 is the calcification of a bicuspid valve.

10. C

    Regurgitation and AV blocks are some of the complications which occur today when treating with TAVR. AV block can occur due to the over or underestimation of the necessary valve size which may compress the AV node when put in place.

References

1. Kang D-H, et al. Early surgery or conservative care for asymptomatic aortic stenosis. N Engl J Med. 2020;382(2):111–9.
2. Makkar RR, et al. Association between transcatheter aortic valve replacement for bicuspid vs tricuspid aortic stenosis and mortality or stroke. JAMA. 2019;321(22):2193–202.
3. Pawade T, et al. Why and how to measure aortic valve calcification in patients with aortic stenosis. JACC Cardiovasc Imaging. 2019;12(9):1835–48.
4. Bing R, et al. Imaging and impact of myocardial fibrosis in aortic stenosis. JACC Cardiovasc Imaging. 2019;12(2):283–96.
5. Strange G, et al. Poor long-term survival in patients with moderate aortic stenosis. J Am Coll Cardiol. 2019;74(15):1851–63.
6. Everett RJ, et al. Extracellular myocardial volume in patients with aortic stenosis. J Am Coll Cardiol. 2020;75(3):304–16.
7. Pawade T, et al. Computed tomography aortic valve calcium scoring in patients with aortic stenosis. Circulation. 2018;11(3):e007146.
8. Alkhouli M, et al. Contemporary trends in the management of aortic stenosis in the USA. Eur Heart J. 2020;41(8):921–8.
9. Généreux P, et al. Staging classification of aortic stenosis based on the extent of cardiac damage. Eur Heart J. 2017;38(45):3351–8.
10. Lancellotti P, Vannan MA. Timing of intervention in aortic stenosis. N Engl J Med. 2020;382(2):191–3.

Atrioventricular Septal Defect

Kiran Shafiq Khan and Irfan Ullah

Abstract

"The term atrioventricular septal defect (AVSD) is characterized by a common atrioventricular junction with coexisting atrioventricular septation defect with the incidence of 4–5.3 per 10.000 live births". Most of the cases are associated with Down syndrome and a large number of cases are accompanied by aortic valve regurgitation. The majority of patients present with central cyanosis although murmur could not be appreciated at a younger age. With the advancement in the surgical era, the mortality rate has been reduced significantly. Patients with preoperative regurgitation or any associated cardiac or extracardiac issue may experience problems postoperatively or required reoperation otherwise they may live a healthy life. Patient education and understanding regarding the defect and procedure are very important.

Keywords

Atrioventricular septal defect · Atrioventricular valve Central cyanosis · Murmur · Embryogenesis · AVSD

Introduction

The term atrioventricular defect (AVSD) is defined as a deficiency of the atrioventricular septum above or below the atrioventricular valve [1] with an incidence of 4–5 per 10,000 lives birth [2]. It is also named ostium primum atrial septal defects (ASDs), AV canal defects, endocardial cushion defects, and AV commissure [3]. Around 7% of congenital heart diseases are AVSD and 30–40% of cases are associated with Down syndrome [3–7]. The morphogenesis is still controversial. The main problem that arises is right to left shunt at atrial and ventricular levels. In the majority of cases, these defects are accompanied by AV valve abnormality which may lead to aortic regurgitation. Before surgical treatment, the mortality rate was 50% [8]. Now, the goal of surgical repair is to preserve and improve the AV valve function with a good long-term outcome [6]. This chapter summarizes the anatomy, embryogenesis, types, treatment plan, and associated pathologies.

Pathophysiology

Incomplete AVSD: In 10% of the population moderate to severe left AV valve regurgitation occur. It is often directed to the right atria therefore, it is typically called left ventricular to right atrial shunt [2]. This term is a misnomer because the shunt can also go from left ventricular to left atrium due to an increase in left ventricular shunting magnitude [9].

Complete AVSD: These patients usually present earlier in life because of both atrial and ventricular level shunting [2]. They usually present with congestive heart failure. In a study, it has been reported that 90% of the patients with untreated and complete AVSD develop the pulmonary vascular disease by age 1 year due to bigger left to right shunt that may be worsened by AV regurgitation [9].

Types

AVSD is of two types

1. Complete AVSD
2. Incomplete AVSD/partial AVSD

Complete AVSD includes ostium primum defect at atrial septum level and defect in the inlet portion of the ventricular septum. This type may have one AV annulus and a common AV valve. This common AV valve mostly comprises superior

K. S. Khan
Dow Medical College, Karachi, Pakistan

I. Ullah (✉)
Kabir Medical College, Gandhara University, Peshawar, Pakistan

and inferior leaflets across the ventricular septum [10]. In this type of AVSD shunting take place at atrial as well as ventricular level. Mostly an isolated atrial component is present in complete AVSD that bridges the leaflet attached to the ventricular septum with one annulus. This results in two orifices and shunting occur at the atrial level [10].

In partial AVSD (isolated ventricular component) is less commonly found incomplete AVSD, where the leaflets are partially fused and attached to the atrial septum. This AVSD is related to inlet ventricular septal defect clinically [5].

Of note, the intermediate also known as transitional AVSD includes ostium primum defect and a restrictive VSD just below the AV valves with two separate AV orifices because of bridging leaflets [10]. Besides, some authors and IPCCC neither support this classification nor acknowledged it as an AVSD type because of 2 annuli [11]. IPCCC defines AVSD with unequal and unbalanced ventricular and AV valve positions with some degree of ventricular hypoplasia [10].

Anatomy

Morphologically, "AVSD is described by the presence of a common atrioventricular junction, a defect in the muscular and membranous atrioventricular septum, and an ovoid shape of the common atrioventricular junction with displaced left ventricular outflow tract" [2]. Normally, the inlet and outlet dimensions of the left ventricle are equal but in AVSD a disparity in outlet dimension is found [12].

Incomplete AVSD: The incomplete AVSD is due to the continuousness of the left superior and inferior leaflet. The commissure between them forms the cleft of the left AV valve therefore most incomplete AVSD has no ventricular shunting [12]. This continuity of tissues forms a bridge that obliterates the shunting below the leaflets level [2].

Complete AVSD: Incomplete AVSD, there is a space between the bridging leaflets therefore the AV orifices are common. The left-to-right shunting is because of the attachment of bridging leaflets with the atrial septum and ventricular septum. The shunting tendency in a complete AVSD depends upon the position and extension of leaflets that may increases from type A to C according to Rastelli classification [2], where type A leaflet is divided by an interventricular septum and attached to the VSD crest. Type B and C fibers extend to the right ventricle [2].

Valvular dysfunction is another important feature of AVSD, which is due to dysplasia of the AV valve of a lateral leaflet [13]. There are some abnormalities found in the heart conduction system specifically in AVSD patients [14]. Right bundle branch block, first degree AV block and more rarely second and third degree AV block all are present in AVSD patients [15, 16]. AV node is positioned more posteriorly, this defines the presence of a long non-branching bundle of His [16].

In all types of AVSD, there is a common orifice with different extension and fusion of leaflets with the atrial or ventricular septum with the difference in conducting system. Therefore, it is very essential to appreciate the importance of leaflets even in post-surgical patients [17].

Embryology

Typically, cardiac septation occurs in the first 9 weeks of embryogenesis. Splanchnic mesoderm forms the primary heart tube. In addition, the second pool of mesoderm tissue formed the arterial and venous side of the fetal heart. The inner endocardial layers form first then the outer myocardial layer. These two layers are separated by cardiac jelly [18]. During the later stage of heart development, four endocardial cushions form the AV valve. Initially, an opening is present between the septum primum and AV canal. To complete the AV septation these two structure fuses later on with the vestibular spine [19]. The superior and inferior endocardial cushion forms the leaflets of the tricuspid valve and mitral valve [20]. The right lateral cushion forms the anterior and posterior leaflets [20].

The insufficient looping and fusion of the endocardial cushion and mesenchymal cap result in abnormal development of the heart. Also, the heterogeneous mutation in GATA4 [21] and NR2F2 [22] in the mouse can result in partial (ASD1) or complete AVSDs. This mutation is because of deficient endocardial cushions development thus resulting in complete AVSD [23]. Whereas, the mutation in (SHF specific) Shh [24] and Pdgfr-a [25] reduces the DMP formation and leads toward partial AVSD. It has been reported that abnormal AV septation affects the development of the heart conduction system [26]. In AVSD the anterior and posterior AV node fails to fuse which defines the posterior position of the AV node in patients with AVSD [27].

Clinical Presentation

The clinical picture of AVSD depends upon the morphology and type of defect present.

Incomplete AVSD: Clinically 10% of the patient present with moderate to severe AV valve regurgitation. The presenting symptoms are pulmonary congestion and infection, dyspnea, tachycardia, and failure to thrive [28]. Medically uncontrolled congestive heart failure and presentation at early age indicates the need for early surgical intervention. This may be due to the presence of left-sided anomalies such as LV hypoplasia, LV outflow tract obstruction, and aortic arch obstruction [2].

Complete AVSD: The patent with complete AVSD is usually present in infancy. The signs and symptoms are worsened by AV regurgitation [29]. On physical examination, hyperactive pericardium with thrill is found. A systolic murmur at the left sternal border, mid-diastolic flow murmur across the AV valve, and a high-pitched murmur at apex due to AV regurgitation can be appreciated on auscultatory examination [28]. A split first heart sound can be heard due to pulmonary vascular resistance [2].

Infants with complete AVSD are likely to develop congestive heart failure within starting months of life. Due to significant regurgitation coarctation of the aorta or ventricular imbalance, cardiac failure, Eisenmenger's syndrome may occur much earlier than the expected timeline [2]. Around 25% of untreated or undiagnosed AVSD patients can die during infancy [28]. Newborn with AVSD may present with central cyanosis due to bidirectional shunting in the presence of increased pulmonary vascular resistance [29].

Diagnosis

Prenatal Diagnosis

The AVSD can be detected in utero with the help of fetal echocardiography till 12 weeks of gestation [30]. The sensitivity in detecting AVSD in routine screening is 27% [31]. It has been reported that with the advanced training and protocols the detection rate on routine screening has raised to 67% for balanced AVSD and 93% for unbalanced AVSDs [11]. To get better with the detection ratio atrial to ventricular ratio [32] and level of linear insertion [33] have been added in detection findings. Due to the negative prognosis, elective termination of pregnancy has been suggested [7, 34]. Cardiac anomalies, extra-cardiac abnormalities, and aneuploidy specifically Down syndrome in 40–50% of cases have been reported [35]; therefore, early invasive testing is recommended, i.e., array comparative genomic hybridization to detect the presence of copy number variations [36].

Postnatal Diagnosis

Clinically the patient may present with central cyanosis, congestive heart failure, severe AV regurgitation, and Eisenmenger syndrome if left untreated [37]. The partial AVSD can remain asymptomatic for years [10]. Following imaging studies can be used to detect the abnormality.

Imaging Studies

Chest Radiography
Mild cardiomegaly and prominent pulmonary vascular margins can be seen in patients with incomplete AVSD, whereas in complete AVSD significant cardiomegaly and vast change in pulmonary marking are noticed. It may also indicate levocardia and a left-sided aortic arch [37].

Doppler Echocardiography
Doppler echocardiography is a diagnostic tool; in incomplete AVSD atrial defect with absent ventricular shunting can be seen [38]. While incomplete AVSD atrial and ventricular shunting along with valve abnormality can be noticed [38]. It has been reported that 3D echocardiography can show additional findings that may play an additive role in surgical planning [39]. Moreover, the use of intraoperative transesophageal echocardiography decreases the rate of reoperation [40] and regurgitation [41].

The four-chamber view is mostly used in antenatal screening ultrasound anomaly scans. This view can detect the AVSD easily. Diagnostic features are obstetric four-chamber view of the heart in the presence of a common atrioventricular valve [42]. The detection of anomalies plays a vital role in deciding for surgeons as well as for parents. An accurate indication of the outcome can be given [2]. The mortality rate is higher in a patient with other associated cardiac anomalies such as left atrial isomerism, congenital complete heart block. It may have a very poor prognosis and result in fetal loss [43].

Electrocardiography
The characteristic finding on ECG is the superior orientation of the frontal QRS loop [37]. Left axis deviation with prominent p wave presenting atria enlargement and a prolonged PR interval is noted in incomplete AVSD. Whereas, biventricular hypertrophy is an additional finding of incomplete AVSD [44].

Diagnostic Procedures

Cardiac Catheterization
Cardiac catheterization is indicated in an adult population with incomplete AVSD. Due to decreased pulmonary artery flow, a high fraction of inspired oxygen (FiO_2) is required in these patients. Whereas incomplete AVSD is allowed in young patients as well even patients under 1-year-old [45].

Treatment

Medical Therapy

Patients with incomplete AVSD rarely required medical treatment whereas complete AVSD patients were treated promptly with medical therapy [46]. Complete AVSD patients usually present with congestive heart failure, therefore, required diuretics or volume overload, digoxin can be used as an inotropic agent and angiotensin-converting enzyme (ACE) inhibitors use to reduce that afterload effects [38]. The associated issues such as feeding difficulty and calories deficit can be managed with a nasogastric tube and added calories [10].

Surgical Therapy

It is the method of choice for AVSD repair. Younger patients and a good functioning AV valve provide the best outcome postoperatively [47]. Multiple surgical techniques are used for repairs such as single-patch technique, two-patch technique, and modified single-patch technique [48]. In a single patch, one prosthetic material is used to close both atrial and ventricular defects [38]. In the double or two-patch technique, two patches are used to close the defect separately whereas in the modified patch technique common valve is stitched to the ventricular septum and the atrial defect closes separately with a patch [38]. Most of the time, incomplete AVSD closes with a single patch technique and complete AVSD closes with two patch techniques. Choice of technique depends upon the condition of the patient and extend of the defect but all of them provide the same surgical outcome [38].

Because of the high mortality rate due to pulmonary vascular resistance, AVSD repair is recommended at 3 months of age [38, 49]. According to a literature search, the median age of AVSD repair varies from 1.8 [50] to 7.9 years [51]. It has been reported that surgical repair at an early age is associated with LAVV regurgitation [49]. Likewise, surgical repair at an older age has less morbidity and mortality ratio [51].

Follow-Up

Patients with AVSD are recommended to have lifelong follow-up at least every 2–3 years [52] because a displaced and angulated anterolateral papillary muscle has been found in patients with AVSD repair [53]. 3D echocardiography should be done to rule out further complications [54] such as subaortic stenosis and left atrioventricular regurgitation. Antibiotic prophylaxis is recommended in case of subacute endocarditis [54].

The 10-year survival percentage has been raised to 70% [55]. The incidence of postoperative arrhythmias ranges between 0.5 and 7.5% [56, 57], mostly in patients with complete AVSD repair.

Postoperative Complications, Outcome, and Prognosis

In 10–15% of patients, postoperative AV regurgitation has been noticed [58] that may lead to reoperation. Postoperative heart block may be because of trauma to AV node or bundle of His. In a study, 22% of cases reported right bundle branch block [58].

Previously, repair at a young age under 2 years was supposed to be a major factor for mortality in patients with AVSD but in a recent report, it has been found that age has no relation with the mortality rate and disease outcome [59, 60]. Only good preoperative management is necessary, it may reduce the mortality risk and improve the outcome [61]. Preoperative AV regurgitation, associated trisomy 21, Tetralogy of Fallot (TOF), and unbalanced AVSD provided the worse outcome [62].

Pregnancy and AVSD: A close and detailed examination is required inpatient with partial AVSD who wants to get pregnant. In the presence of severe pulmonary hypertension pregnancy should be avoided [63]. While a patient with corrected AVSD can tolerate pregnancy and its physiological changes very well. Some women experienced few complications during pregnancy. 17% of women with corrected AVSD have AVV regurgitation, 19% experienced arrhythmias during their pregnancy [64]. Around 10–12% recurrence rate of AVSD was reported in the offspring of a mother with AVSD [64, 65].

Conclusion

Early diagnosis and prompt management are necessary for a patient with AVSD. Timely plans for surgical intervention provide the best results with a low mortality rate. A long-term follow-up prevents further complications. The patient should watch for atrioventricular valve function, left ventricular outflow tract obstruction, and dysrhythmia.

Multiple Choice Questions

1. The most common presentation of AVSD is:
   A. Central cyanosis
   B. Peripheral cyanosis
   C. Jaundice
   D. Syncope
      Answer: A
2. The following type present earlier with AVSD
   A. Complete AVSD
   B. Incomplete AVSD

C. Partial AVSD

D. Transitional AVSD

Answer: A

3. In complete AVSD the primary defect locates at:
   A. Ostium secundum
   B. Ostium primum
   C. Sinus venosus
   D. Lower portion of ventricle

   Answer: B

4. In AVSD the left ventricle dimensions are
   A. Equal inlet and outlet dimensions
   B. Unequal inlet dimensions but equal outlet dimensions
   C. Unequal inlet and outlet dimensions
   D. Equal outlet dimensions, unequal inlet dimensions

   Answer: C

5. Shunting tendency depends upon:
   A. Position of leaflet only
   B. Dimensions of inlet and outlet
   C. Extension of leaflet only
   D. Both extension and position of leaflet

   Answer: D

6. Cardiac septation occurs in which week of gestation:
   A. 5
   B. 6
   C. 9
   D. 12

   Answer: C

7. Prenatal diagnosis of AVSD can be done till which week of gestation?
   A. 11
   B. 13
   C. 12
   D. 20

   Answer: C

8. Which of the following is the diagnostic tool?
   A. Chest x-ray.
   B. Echocardiography
   C. ECG
   D. Doppler ultrasound

   Answer: B

9. Which view can detect AVSD on ultrasound?
   A. 2 chamber view
   B. 3 chamber view
   C. 4 chamber view
   D. None

   Answer: C

10. What percentage can be found in the offspring of patient with AVSD?
    A. 10%
    B. 17%
    C. 20%
    D. 8%

    Answer: A

References

1. Egbe A, Lee S, Ho D, Uppu S, Srivastava S. Prevalence of congenital anomalies in newborns with congenital heart disease diagnosis. Ann Pediatr Cardiol. 2014;7(2):86.
2. Craig B. Atrioventricular septal defect: from fetus to adult. Heart. 2006;92:1879–85.
3. Asani M, Aliyu I, Also U. Pattern of congenital heart diseases among children with Down syndrome seen in Aminu Kano Teaching Hospital, Kano, Nigeria. Niger J Basic Clin Sci. 2013;10(2):57.
4. Hoffman JI, Kaplan S, Liberthson RR. Prevalence of congenital heart disease. Am Heart J. 2004;147:425–39.
5. Reller MD, Strickland MJ, Riehle-Colarusso T, et al. Prevalence of congenital heart defects in metropolitan Atlanta, 1998-2005. J Pediatr. 2008;153:807–13.
6. Loffredo CA, Hirata J, Wilson PD, et al. Atrioventricular septal defects: possible etiologic differences between complete and partial defects. Teratology. 2001;63:87–93.
7. Christensen N, Andersen H, Garne E, et al. Atrioventricular septal defects among infants in Europe: a population-based study of prevalence, associated anomalies, and survival. Cardiol Young. 2013;23(4):560–7.
8. Garcia-Canadilla P, Dejea H, Bonnin A, Balicevic V, Loncaric S, Zhang C, et al. Complex congenital heart disease associated with disordered myocardial architecture in a midtrimester human fetus. Circulation. 2018;11(10):e007753.
9. Carabuena JM. Atrioventricular septal defect, AV canal. In: Consults in obstetric anesthesiology. Cham: Springer; 2018. pp. 81–82.
10. Calkoen EE, Hazekamp MG, Blom NA, Elders BB, Gittenberger-de Groot AC, Haak MC, et al. Atrioventricular septal defect: from embryonic development to long-term follow-up. Int J Cardiol. 2016;202:784–95.
11. Cetta F, Minich LL, Edwards WD, et al. Atrioventricular septal defect. In: Allen HD, Driscoll DJ, Shaddy R, Feltes TF, editors. Moss and Adams' heart disease in infants, children and adolescents. Philadelphia: Lippincott William and Wilkins; 2008. p. 648.
12. Briggs LE, Kakarla J, Wessels A. The pathogenesis of atrial and atrioventricular septal defects with special emphasis on the role of the dorsal mesenchymal protrusion. Differentiation. 2012;84(1):117–30.
13. Hoohenkerk GJ, Wenink AC, Schoof PH, et al. Results of surgical repair of atrioventricular septal defect with double-orifice left atrioventricular valve. J Thorac Cardiovasc Surg. 2009;138:1167–71.
14. Desai AR, Branco RG, Comitis GA, et al. Early postoperative outcomes following surgical repair of complete atrioventricular septal defects: is down syndrome a risk factor? Pediatr Crit Care Med. 2014;15:35–41.
15. Okada Y, Tatsuno K, Kikuchi T, et al. Complete atrioventricular septal defect associated with tetralogy of Fallot: surgical indications and results. Jpn Circ J. 1999;63:889–92.
16. Thiene G, Wenink ACG, Frescura C, et al. Surgical anatomy and pathology of the conduction tissues in atrioventricular defects. J Thorac Cardiovasc Surg. 1981;82:928–37.
17. Penkoske PA, Neches WH, Anderson RH, et al. Further observations on the morphology of atrioventricular septal defects. J Thorac Cardiovasc Surg. 1985;90:611–22.
18. Person AD, Klewer SE, Runyan RB. Cell biology of cardiac cushion development. Int Rev Cytol. 2005;243:287–335.
19. Webb S, Brown NA, Anderson RH. Formation of the atrioventricular septal structures in the normal mouse. Circ Res. 1998;82:645–56.
20. de Lange FJ, Moorman AF, Anderson RH, et al. Lineage and morphogenetic analysis of the cardiac valves. Circ Res. 2004;95:645–54.
21. Rajagopal SK, Ma Q, Obler D, et al. Spectrum of heart disease associated with murine and human GATA4 mutation. J Mol Cell Cardiol. 2007;43:677–85.

22. Al TS, Manickaraj AK, Mercer CL, et al. Rare variants in NR2F2 cause congenital heart defects in humans. Am J Hum Genet. 2014;94:574–85.

23. Tian Y, Yuan L, Goss AM, et al. Characterization and in vivo pharmacological rescue of a Wnt2-Gata6 pathway required for cardiac inflow tract development. Dev Cell. 2010;18:275–87.

24. Goddeeris MM, Rho S, Petiet A, et al. Intracardiac septation requires hedgehog-dependent cellular contributions from outside the heart. Development. 2008;135:1887–95.

25. Bax NA, Bleyl SB, Gallini R, et al. Cardiac malformations in Pdgfralpha mutant embryos are associated with increased expression of WT1 and Nkx2.5 in the second heart field. Dev Dyn. 2010;239:2307–17.

26. Blom NA, Gittenberger-de Groot AC, Deruiter MC, et al. Development of the cardiac conduction tissue in human embryos using HNK-1 antigen expression: possible relevance for understanding of abnormal atrial automaticity. Circulation. 1999;99:800–6.

27. Blom NA, Ottenkamp J, Deruiter MC, et al. Development of the cardiac conduction system in atrioventricular septal defect in human trisomy 21. Pediatr Res. 2005;58:516–20.

28. Berger TJ, Blackstone EH, Kirklin JW, et al. Survival and probability of cure without and with operation in complete atrioventricular canal. Ann Thorac Surg. 1979;27:104–11.

29. Tubman RJ, Shields MD, Craig BG, et al. Congenital heart disease in Down's syndrome: two year prospective early screening study. BMJ. 1991;302:1425–7.

30. Jansen FA, Calkoen EE, Jongbloed MR, et al. Imaging the first trimester heart: ultrasound correlation with morphology. Cardiol Young. 2014;24 Suppl 2:3–12.

31. Jacobs JP, Burke RP, Quintessenza JA, et al. Congenital heart surgery nomenclature and database project: ventricular septal defect. Ann Thorac Surg. 2000;69:S25–35.

32. Machlitt A, Heling KS, Chaoui R. Increased cardiac atrial-to-ventricular length ratio in the fetal four-chamber view: a new marker for atrioventricular septal defects. Ultrasound Obstet Gynecol. 2004;24:618–22.

33. Adriaanse BM, Bartelings MM, van Vugt JM, et al. The differential and linear insertion of the atrioventricular valves: a useful tool? Ultrasound Obstet Gynecol. 2014;44(5):568–74.

34. Beaton AZ, Pike JI, Stallings C, et al. Predictors of repair and outcome in prenatally diagnosed atrioventricular septal defects. J Am Soc Echocardiogr. 2013;26:208–16.

35. Berg C, Kaiser C, Bender F, et al. Atrioventricular septal defect in the fetus—associated conditions and outcome in 246 cases. Ultraschall Med. 2009;30:25–32.

36. Jansen FA, Blumenfeld YJ, Fisher A, et al. Array comparative genomic hybridization and fetal congenital heart defects: a systematic review and meta-analysis. Ultrasound Obstet Gynecol. 2015;45:27–35.

37. Silverman NH, Zuberbuhler JR, Anderson RH. Atrioventricular septal defects: cross-sectional echocardiographic and morphologic comparisons. Int J Cardiol. 1986;13:309–31.

38. Fleishman CE, Marx GR. Atrioventricular canal defects. In: Crawford MH, DiMarco JP, Paulus WJ, editors. Cardiology. 3rd ed. Philadelphia: Elsevier; 2010. p. 1561–71.

39. Kutty S, Smallhorn JF. Evaluation of atrioventricular septal defects by three-dimensional echocardiography: benefits of navigating the third dimension. J Am Soc Echocardiogr. 2012;25:932–44.

40. Lee HR, Montenegro LM, Nicolson SC, et al. Usefulness of intraoperative transesophageal echocardiography in predicting the degree of mitral regurgitation secondary to atrioventricular defect in children. Am J Cardiol. 1999;83:750–3.

41. Jacobstein MD, Fletcher BD, Goldstein S, et al. Evaluation of atrioventricular septal defect by magnetic resonance imaging. Am J Cardiol. 1985;55:1158–61.

42. Ter Heide H, Thompson JDR, Wharton GA, et al. Poor sensitivity of routine fetal anomaly scanning ultrasound screening for antenatal detection of atrioventricular septal defect. Heart. 2004;90:916–7.

43. Huggon IC, Cook AC, Smeeton NC, et al. Atrioventricular septal defects diagnosed in fetal life: associated cardiac and extra-cardiac abnormalities and outcome. J Am Coll Cardiol. 2000;36:593–601.

44. Sulafa AK, Tamimi O, Najm HK, Godman MJ. Echocardiographic differentiation of atrioventricular septal defects from inlet ventricular septal defects and mitral valve clefts. Am J Cardiol. 2005;95:607–10.

45. Haworth SG. Pulmonary vascular bed in children with complete atrioventricular septal defect: relation between structural and hemodynamic abnormalities. Am J Cardiol. 1986;57:833–9. c Pulmonary vascular structural changes in AVSD increase with age in parallel with pulmonary artery pressure and resistance.

46. Kirk R, Dipchand AI, Rosenthal DN, et al. The International Society of Heart and Lung Transplantation guidelines for the management of pediatric heart failure: executive summary. J Heart Lung Transplant. 2014;33:888–909.

47. Bharati S, Kirklin JW, McAllister HA Jr, et al. The surgical anatomy of common atrioventricular orifice associated with tetralogy of Fallot, double outlet right ventricle and complete regular transposition. Circulation. 1980;61:1142–9.

48. Pan G, Song L, Zhou X, et al. Complete atrioventricular septal defect: comparison of modified single-patch technique with two-patch technique in infants. J Card Surg. 2014;29:251–5.

49. Kogon BE, Butler H, McConnell M, et al. What is the optimal time to repair atrioventricular septal defect and common atrioventricular valvar orifice? Cardiol Young. 2007;17:356–9.

50. Minich LL, Atz AM, Colan SD, et al. Partial and transitional atrioventricular septal defect outcomes. Ann Thorac Surg. 2010;89:530–6.

51. Bowman JL, Dearani JA, Burkhart HM, et al. Should repair of partial atrioventricular septal defect be delayed until later in childhood? Am J Cardiol. 2014;114:463–7.

52. Buratto E, McCrossan B, Galati JC, et al. Repair of partial atrioventricular septal defect: a 37-year experience. Eur J Cardiothorac Surg. 2015;47(5):796–802.

53. Calkoen EE, Roest AA, Kroft LJ, et al. Characterization and improved quantification of left ventricular inflow using streamline visualization with 4DFlow MRI in healthy controls and patients after atrioventricular septal defect correction. J Magn Reson Imaging. 2015;41(6):1512–20.

54. Takahashi K, Mackie AS, Thompson R, et al. Quantitative real-time three-dimensional echocardiography provides new insight into the mechanisms of mitral valve regurgitation post-repair of atrioventricular septal defect. J Am Soc Echocardiogr. 2012;25(11):1231–44.

55. Lacour-Gayet F, Bonnet N, Piot D, et al. Surgical management of atrio ventricular septal defects with normal caryotype. Eur J Cardiothorac Surg. 1997;11:466–72.

56. Kaza AK, Colan SD, Jaggers J, et al. Surgical interventions for atrioventricular septal defect subtypes: the pediatric heart network experience. Ann Thorac Surg. 2011;92:1468–75.

57. Vohra HA, Chia AX, Yuen HM, et al. Primary biventricular repair of atrioventricular septal defects: an analysis of reoperations. Ann Thorac Surg. 2010;90:830–7.

58. Myers PO. Heart valve repair in children. Doctoral dissertation, University of Geneva; 2014.

59. Morimoto K, Hoashi T, Kagisaki K, Kurosaki K, Shiraishi I, Ichikawa H. Post-operative left atrioventricular valve function after the staged repair of complete atrioventricular septal defect with tetralogy of Fallot. Gen Thorac Cardiovasc Surg. 2014;62(10):602–7.

60. Spray TL, Lewis M. Tetralogy of fallot with complete atrioventricular canal. In: Surgery of conotruncal anomalies. Cham: Springer; 2016. pp. 163–172.

61. Miller A, Siffel C, Lu C, Riehle-Colarusso T, Frías JL, Correa A. Long-term survival of infants with atrioventricular septal defects. J Pediatr. 2010;156(6):994–1000.

62. Arunamata A, Balasubramanian S, Mainwaring R, Maeda K, Tierney ESS. Right-dominant unbalanced atrioventricular septal defect: echocardiography in surgical decision making. J Am Soc Echocardiogr. 2017;30(3):216–26.

63. Baumgartner H, Bonhoeffer P, De Groot NM, et al. ESC guidelines for the management of grown-up congenital heart disease (new version 2010). Eur Heart J. 2010;31:2915–57. [107] Erik.

64. Drenthen W, Pieper PG, van der Tuuk K, et al. Cardiac complications relating to pregnancy and recurrence of disease in the offspring of women with atrioventricular septal defects. Eur Heart J. 2005;26:2581–7.

65. Burn J, Brennan P, Little J, et al. Recurrence risks in offspring of adults with major heart defects: results from first cohort of British collaborative study. Lancet. 1998;351:311–6.

Bicuspid Aortic Valve

Kiran Shafiq Khan and Irfan Ullah

Abstract

"The bicuspid aortic valve affects 1–2% of the total population. Majority of patients with bicuspid aortic valves are asymptomatic". Therefore, it remains undetected until infection and calcification disturbs the valve. Antibiotic prophylaxis is recommended for patients with infective endocarditis. Diagnosis is based on echocardiographic changes. In the pre-surgical era, the diagnosis and treatment of BAV were difficult with a high mortality rate. Now, with the advancement in medicine field, valve replacement is the mainstay for treatment.

Keywords

Bicuspid aortic valve · Congenital heart disease Bicommissural valve · Aortic stenosis · Aortic regurgitation · Ascending aortic dilation · Systolic ejection murmur · William's syndrome · Aortopathy Interrupted aortic arch

Introduction

The bicuspid aortic valve (BAV), also called bicommissural, is regarded as the most common congenital heart disease. It consists of 2 unequal-sized leaflets or cups with one line of coaptation [1]. It may lead to multiple pathologies, i.e., valvular dysfunction, aortic stenosis, aortic regurgitation, infective endocarditis, coarctation of the aorta, aortic dissection, and ascending aortic dilation and aneurysm formation [1, 2]. It affects 1–2% of the total population [1, 2]. This chapter includes the background, anatomy, clinical presentation, and complications associated with the bicuspid aortic valve.

Background

Around 500 years back, the first detailed illustration of BAV was drawn by Leonard do Vinci [2]. In 1844, it was first described as a pathological interest by Paget. In 1858, Peacock identified BAV obstructive lesions [3]. In 1886, Sir William Osler recognized BAV as the most common congenital heart valve disease [4]. In a study, 18 cases of BAV were studied in which the tendency of valve to develop infective endocarditis was discussed [5]. In 1950, it has been reported that isolated calcification of BAV is due to the intrinsic property of the valve rather than an effect of rheumatic fever [6, 7]. Wauchope et al., in their autopsy report, regarded it as a commonest congenital anomaly of the heart [8, 9]. The first association of BAV with aortic dissection was discovered in 1927 by Abbott [2]. The risk factor associated with the development of aortic dissection in patients with BAV was first described by Larson and Edward in 1984 [10]. With the advancement in the field of medicine, etiology, morphology, and other aspects of BAV are well defined [1, 2].

Embryology

Normally, during the development of the heart, the embryonic spiral conotruncal septum divided the truncus arteriosus [2] Right and left aortic leaflet or cups formed at the junction of ventricular and arterial ends of the conotruncal channel. The posterior or non-septal cusp forms from other conotruncal channel tissue. Mesenchymal outgrowth, also known as cardiac cushion gives rise to the semilunar valve [2]. Any abnormalities during development in this area lead to incomplete septation of valve tissue, thus, results in a bicuspid aortic valve [11].

In contrast, the histological assessment of hamsters done by Sans-Coma and his colleagues revealed that fusion of right and left valve cushion is the key factor that results in the

K. S. Khan
Dow Medical College, Karachi, Pakistan

I. Ullah (✉)
Kabir Medical College, Gandhara University, Peshawar, Pakistan

© The Author(s), under exclusive license to Springer Nature Switzerland AG 2023
G. Tagarakis et al. (eds.), *Clinical and Surgical Aspects of Congenital Heart Diseases*,
https://doi.org/10.1007/978-3-031-23062-2_16

development of bicuspid aortic valve [12–14]. Other researchers suggested that abnormal valvulogenesis could be because of abnormal molecular mixing of extracellular matrix protein that helps in cell differentiation and cusp formation [15, 16]. In another study, Lee and colleagues claimed that lacking endothelial nitric oxide synthase could result in BAV formation. Any mutation in this protein may disturb the intracellular signaling pathways [17].

Bicuspid Aortic Valve Morphology

Anatomically, BAV consists of 2 leaflets, usually of unequal size. This could be due to the fusion of two cusps resulting in the formation of one larger cusp [2] with a raphe or false commissure [18]. The larger leaflet also called the conjoined leaflet is mostly identified in BAV patients [19]. Two commissures partially fused at the hinge point forms a high raphe that eventually predisposed toward stenosis in half of the patients. Histologically, no valve tissue was found in raphe providing no plane of attachment to the two commissures [20]. For that reason, they never extend to free margins of the conjoined cusp [21].

The orientation and anatomy of valve leaflets vary the most. The right and left with true commissure oriented anterior and posterior in positions, it may be in anteroposterior orientation [18]. Generally, right and left coronary leaflets fused to form larger, fused leaflet. Other non-coronary leaflets are separated by true commissure. BAV's free edge is usually rounded rather than straight contributing to its limited mobility [18]. In a recent study, a conjoined leaflet was found in 76% of specimens [22]. Out of these, 86% have fused raphe between right and left cusps while left and non-coronary cusp fusion was noticed in 3% of specimens [22].

Different BAV alignments manifest different pathophysiological outcomes [23]. BAV without raphe is a true BAV while the presence of raphe makes it more vulnerable to more aggressive forms of the disease [23]. It has been reported that its absence accelerates the aortic dilation [23] and the patient presents at an early age with more complications [23, 24]. On the contrary, in a recent study found that patients with raphe compared with 237 patients with BAV without raphe, results show poor prognostic effects of raphe in patient with BAV [25]. Therefore, it remains controversial that different morphologies of BAV can predict prognostic outcomes [25, 26].

BAV is usually asymptomatic and diagnosed as an incidental finding in children and young adults on echocardiogram [27]. In a recent study, a review of the echocardiograms was conducted among 1135 children with BAV which revealed the most found morphologic variant, i.e., right-coronary and left-coronary leaflet fusion in 70% of cases. It has also been noticed that fusion of the right-coronary and non-coronary leaflet, was more likely to be associated with aortic stenosis or regurgitation pediatrics group whereas, a fusion of the left coronary and non-coronary cusps was the least common morphologic variant found in the study [2].

Epidemiology

Bicuspid aortic valves affect 1–2% of the total population [2]. According to autopsy and echocardiographic studies, 0.5–2.0% cases have been reported [1]. Normal functioning BAV prevalence is around 0.6–0.9% [1]. In a recent retrospective study based on 85 confirmed necropsy cases of BAV, 13 of them showed no association with any complication, i.e., stenosis, regurgitation, or underlying structural heart disease giving an estimated result of 0.9% population with normal functioning BAV. If the affected population was added the percentage will rise to 2% of the population [3].

Formerly, Osler noted 7 cases of normal functioning BAV out of 800 necropsy studies giving the prevalence of 1.3% [28]. Similar results were detected by Lewis and Grant's study with the prevalence of 1.39% [29]. A recent report suggests a lower incidence rate in African-Americans [30].

The male-to-female ratio is 2:1 [30] or 3:1 [31, 32]. It is more common among the Caucasian population [10]. In a recent echocardiographic screening of 817 asymptomatic children, BAV was found in 4 of them with 3 of them were male [33].

Clinical Presentation and Diagnosis

The majority of patients with BAV are asymptomatic and have normal functioning valves throughout their lives, few of them may develop progressive calcification and other complications such as stenosis or regurgitation [34]. "Clinically, BAV presented with aortic ejection click with or without ejection systolic murmur on routine physical examination" [35]. The aortic ejection click defines as a short sound heard well at the apex with the diaphragm of the stethoscope, it is less distinct and of medium pitch, heard throughout expiration and inspiration just after the first heart sound (S1). Its duration and sound velocity may vary with certain maneuvers (e.g., hand-grip, Valsalva, squatting) [36]. In the presence of ejection click, subtle valve insufficiency can also be heard, high pitched sound at the third intercostal space with a diaphragmatic stethoscope [36].

"2D-echocardiography is recommended as a screening tool for the progeny and first-degree relatives especially males because of the high recurrence rate, i.e., 12–17% has been confirmed in quite a few families" [37].

Laboratory studies: It has been reported that a high level of low-density lipoprotein (LDL) cholesterol accelerates sclerosis of the bicuspid aortic valve [38]. Patients with a family history of hypercholesterolemia and early coronary artery disease should get tested for lipid profile [38].

Imaging Studies

Chest X-Ray

The plain film chest x-ray provides multiple clues that point toward BAV presence. Lung field and pulmonary arteries may look completely normal in case of aortic stenosis. Commonly, aortic root dilation is noted, it doesn't correlate with the valve functional capacity [39–41]. On lateral projection, aortic valve calcification can be easily identified [42, 43]. An enlarged cardiac silhouette and aortic enlargement are often present in chronically regurgitate BAV. A plain film can also identify other associated congenital lesions especially COA. Rib notching and convexity of descending aorta can be identified easily [43]. But it is not regarded as the best screening tool for BAV.

Echocardiography

Two-dimensional echocardiography provides the best results. Therefore, it is the most accurate tool for confirming BAV [44]. 2D-echo shows BAV in multiple planes. Most of the information can be gathered from parasternal long-axis and short-axis views [2].

In parasternal long-axis view, systolic doming due to limited valve opening and eccentric valve closure are the distinctive features of BAV presence. During peak systole, appropriate valve orifice diameter can be measured [2, 45].

In patients with asymmetrical bicuspid leaflets and raphe, the valve may appear tricuspid in the diastole phase. The leaflets become more fibrosed and thickened with age. Due to extensive calcification with age, valve doming disappears and is no longer noted in the short-axis view. Thus, it becomes very difficult to distinguish it from tricuspid aortic valve (TAV) calcific stenosis [2]. In that case, the opening pattern of the aortic valve is very helpful. BAV false-positive results can be because of incomplete demonstration of all 3 valve closure lines. The bicuspid valve can be missed if a high raphe is detected with valve closure [2].

However, it has been reported that BAV diagnosis may become difficult in severe stenosis and after cusp fusion secondary to inflammation. Then, a definitive diagnosis can be made by a histological examination after the excision of the valve [46].

Angiography

Angiography is not the primary method to diagnose BAV. The valve is best viewed at the anteroposterior 30° right anterior oblique (RAO) with systolic doming due to incomplete opening of the valve [47].

Transesophageal Echocardiography

It provides information regarding valve commissures and vegetation which is very necessary to obtain in adolescents and young adults especially in symptomatic patients [47]. Transesophageal echocardiography has a sensitivity and specificity of 78% and 96% for identification of BAV [48]. Espinal and colleagues reported a high degree of sensitivity and specificity of transesophageal echocardiography for assessing valve morphology especially in multiple planes [48].

Treatment Plans (Medical, Surgical, Diet, Activity)

The initial plan to manage the BAV is to maintain a healthy diet by controlling the lipid profile. Risk factors like hypercholesterolemia and coronary artery disease increase sclerosis and deterioration of BAV. Therefore, it is very important to maintain a healthy diet especially in patients with recognizable risk factors. The fat diet should be no more than 30% of total calories and not more than 10% from saturated fat [38, 49]. Other risk factors that accelerate calcification include age, arterial hypertension, dyslipidemia, diabetes, and smoking [50].

It has been reported in a study conducted by Michelena et al. that presence of raphe and dyslipidemia may increase the vale degeneration of BAV [51]. Hence, the use of statins and control over cardiovascular risk factors may reduce BAV degeneration [19].

Patients with normal functioning BAV don't need any intervention other than dietary changes. They can take part in any strenuous activities or sports after valve clearance and assessment for aortic dilation by echocardiogram [52]. But patients with valve insufficiencies are restricted from doing strenuous exercise and activities such as weight lifting, rope climbing, and pull-ups [53]. Thus, a regular follow-up is necessary for early diagnosis and avoidance of any complication, i.e., valve insufficiency, valve stenosis, and progressive aortic root dilation [53, 54].

The most appropriate and definitive treatment of deteriorating BAV is valve replacement. 30% of the individuals develop complications such as valve insufficiency, valve stenosis, progressive aortic root dilatation, and possible bacterial endocarditis [22, 55, 56]. Surgery is indicated in symptomatic patients, patients with abnormal left ventricle function and valvular dysfunction. In the former patients, early valve surgery is recommended [46]. Patients with isolated aortic regurgitation are the candidate for early valve repair, it can save them from long-term consequences and the need for anticoagulation [46]. Around 50–75% of the patients of BAV undergo valve replacement during their lifetime [57]. Most aortic surgeries are performed for dilation of the aortic root or ascending aorta, and rarely for aortic dissection [57, 58].

Postoperatively, patients with BAV not required prophylaxis antibiotics for any invasive and dental procedures [59]. It is recommended only if the patient developed endocarditis. No special recommendation is required in patients with uncomplicated BAV other than bacterial endocarditis [59].

In a pre-surgery era, 19% of the patients with BAV died because of complications, commonly due to coarctation [60]. Presently, this number has been reduced.

Associated Pathologies and Their Outcome

The overall complication rate varies in patients with BAV [3]. In a mean 13-year follow-up 39% had at least one cardiac event [61]. Pathologies associated with the bicuspid aortic valve are aortic stenosis, aortic regurgitation, and infective endocarditis [62] (Table 2).

In 20% of the cases, BAV is usually an isolated defect, while in 50% BAV may be associated with multiple other cardiovascular problems [2].

Aortic Stenosis

BAV is most frequently accompanied by aortic stenosis and a large number of patients need surgery because of stenosis development. Patients with severe stenosis develop premature calcium deposition, fibrosis, and stiffening, it all leads toward abnormal functioning valve [35] but it could be age-related [47, 63]. It has been reported that people with asymmetrical cusps may have worse and progress more rapidly toward severe stenosis [35, 64, 65].

In the second decade, BAV sclerosis begins and calcification becomes more prominent in the fourth decade [66]. Patients with coronary risk factors such as smoking, high LDL levels, and low HDL levels experience valve abnormality at an earlier age. The rheumatic fever appeared as the most common cause of aortic stenosis. In developed countries, the bicuspid aortic valve remains the most common cause of aortic stenosis due to the declining graph in rheu-

matic fever cases [66], whereas in developing countries rheumatic fever is still the main problem for the development of aortic stenosis. The aortic valve damage due to rheumatic fever can only be confirmed by the presence of Aschoff bodies [66].

A recent report showed that most of the patient's valvular calcification started by the age of 20 and almost every one of them showed calcified valve by the age of 30 years and required aortic valve replacement [65] (Table 3).

Aortic Regurgitation

Patients with BAV develop aortic regurgitation due to cusps prolapse, fibrotic retraction, and dilation of the sino-tubular junction. Isolated regurgitation develops in younger patients [67]. Endocarditis seems to be the most common and earlier complication in patients with BAV plus regurgitation [67]. According to reports the incidence of aortic regurgitation in the presence of BAV is 1.5–3% [68, 69]. It can be present with aortic root dilation, coarctation of the aorta, or infective endocarditis [70, 71] (Table 3).

Patent Ductus Arteriosus

Patent ductus arteriosus (PDA) usually presents as an isolated pathology. In the pediatric population, BAV is found to be associated with PDA [72, 73]. It is recommended that adults with treated PDA should get a further evaluation for the assessment of BAV [72, 73].

Supravalvular AS and William's Syndrome

"William's syndrome is characterized by elfin facies, short stature, stellate iris, peripheral pulmonic stenosis, arterial hypertension, COA, and renal artery stenosis" [39]. The diagnosis is usually made during childhood. Around 60% of the patients with supravalvular aortic stenosis have this syndrome, and 35% of patients have BAV [74]. The patient usually presents with exertional chest pain during their adulthood and 56% of patients required reoperation as compared to the 19% of individuals with normal functioning valves [75].

Ventricular Septal Defect

It is the most common congenital heart defect. It may be found as an isolated defect or in connotation with their multifarious lesions [2]. In 30% of the cases, VSD is associated with BAV [76, 77]. It could be due to partial prolapse of an aortic leaflet. In addition, reconstructive surgeries for VSD may cause aortic insufficiencies as well [2]. Therefore, determination of BAV is necessary before correcting perimembranous VSD [2].

Bacterial (Infective) Endocarditis

Around 10–30% of the patient with BAV are at risk of developing infective endocarditis during their lifetime. In 25% of infants and children, BAV is the second most common etiology for IE [78]. As discussed above, infective endocarditis complicates 50% of aortic regurgitation in patients with BAV [2], and 43% and 60% cases of cusps perforation have been reported [78, 79] with a significant 9% mortality rate [71].

Moreover, BAV-associated endocarditis occurs usually in young adults of 38–53 years of age and predominates in 73% of males [71, 80]. The most common organisms responsible for the development of endocarditis are Staphylococci and viridans streptococci [81]. They have been accounted for ¾ of the cases. If not treated at an earlier stage, they may result in heart failure, valvular or myocardial abscess [81]. Due to the development of the these complications, surgery is recommended beforehand [71].

The Bicuspid Aortic Valve and Aortic Wall Abnormalities

Following the aortic wall, abnormalities are associated with BAV [2]:

1. Coarctation of the aorta (50% to 80%)
2. Aortic dissection (36%)
3. Aortic aneurysm

The development of cystic medial necrosis is the mainstay for the development of aortic wall abnormalities [2]. Pachulski et al. found that patients with BAV have significantly larger aortic diameter than normal individuals [82]. Dissolution of aortic elastic tissue in the upper aortic ring causes root dilatation [83].

Coarctation of the Aorta (COA)

Around 85% of cases of coarctation of the aorta are associated with BAV and 27% have interrupted aortic arch [78, 84]. The ignorance of these associations may lead to myocardial infractions [85]. It has been reported that untreated, inadequate treatment, and recurrent COA may increase the chances of aortic stenosis, aortic regurgitation, or dissection of the aorta [35].

Coarctation of the aorta is classified as a simple or complex defect. The former is associated with intracardiac and extracardiac defects [2]. Patients with COA associated with bicuspid aortic valve undergo treatment at an earlier age. Around 11-14% of patients required long-term follow-up after surgical correction [85]. In a report, a large group of patients 41% undergo reoperation due to valvular indication [86]. As a result, these patients undergo long-term follow-up with echocardiographic assessment and modification of avoidable risk factors [2].

Aortic Root Dissection

Post-stenotic dilation and abnormal elastic fibers are the two main aggravating factors [87]. The association with Marfan syndrome is also because of abnormally developed and broken elastic fibers [87] (Table 3).

A retrospective cohort study conducted among 416 patients over a follow-up of 16 years reported a low incidence of aortic dissection in BAV patients 2 of 416 [87]. Another study reported nine times higher risk of dissection in BAV patients [11]. A 7–13% unselected cases also reported aortic dissection in BAV patients [35, 54]. Morphogenic studies show less elastic tissue concentration in BAV patients than normal functioning valves [88]. Aortic dissection can also occur in normal functioning valves but usually with stenosed valves and require valve replacement at an earlier age [35].

Aortopathy

The prevalence of aortopathy in BAV patients ranges from 20 to 80% [53, 89]. Aortopathy defines as the progressive dilation of ascending aorta, root, tubular part, the aortic arch, or less commonly descending aorta. The risk of acute complications such as aortic rupture and dissection is eight times higher than normal individuals [90]. To prevent these acute aortic events, surgery is recommended [23]. In several community studies, it has been observed that 20 years after diagnosis of aortic dilation another kind of cardiovascular disease surgery is required [88, 91]. A recent meta-analysis claimed a ten times higher risk of aortic dilation development in patients with AVR surgery [92].

In a recent study, the aortic root was found to be dilated in 34% of cases, and ascending aorta in 76% of the cases. A large number of controversial data exist that define aortic dilation threshold and BAV morphology [90]. Aortic stenosis and aortic regurgitation both are associated with aortic dilatation but AR is independently associated [35]. It has been found that the younger population specifically males had a high prevalence of root dilation [35].

Survival Rate

Despite multiple complications, 2 larger series have claimed that there is no change in life expectancy in patients with BAV disease. In asymptomatic patients the 10-year rate of valve function varies from 96.1 to 96.5% [47], in symptomatic patients, it ranges up to 90.3% for 20 years of survival [47].

Conclusion

Subsequently, the survival rate of patients with BAV is good. Reviews and reports suggest that the course of life is fairly good and long but numerous serious problems will occur if care were not taken properly or prompt treatment was not given due to valve tear and over workload. Routine and regular follow-up is required.

Patient and family education is important regarding the accelerated aging process, i.e., progressive stenosis and diet changes. The development of infective endocarditis should be explained in detail and it should be emphasized that BAV is the potential source for its development, therefore good oral and dental hygiene is important. The patient should know that no physical restriction is required unless any stenosis or regurgitation developed. At least one simple examination is required before participating in a sports competition.

MCQS

1. The male-to-female ratio in the bicuspid aortic valve is
   A. 1:2
   B. 2:1
   C. 3:4
   D. 1:3
      Answer: B
2. The bicuspid aortic valve has ____ leaflets
   A. 2 unequal size leaflets
   B. 2 equal size leaflets
   C. 3 equal size leaflets
   D. 3 unequal size leaflets
      Answer: A
3. The presence of raphe makes BAV more____
   A. The presence of raphe indicates good prognosis
   B. The absence of raphe indicates good prognosis
   C. The presence of raphe has no impact
   D. The absence of raphe indicates poor prognosis
      Answer: B
4. Clinically patients with BAV present with what symptoms?
   A. Ejection systolic murmur heard well at the apex with the diaphragm of the stethoscope
   B. Diastolic murmur heard well at the apex with the diaphragm of the stethoscope
   C. Ejection clicks at sternal boarder

D. Ejection systolic murmur heard well at the apex with the belt of the stethoscope
      Answer: A
5. The lipid profile of BAV patients shows:
   A. High LDL and high HDL
   B. High LDL and high TAG
   C. High HDL and low LDL
   D. High LDL and low HDL
      Answer: D
6. The best modality tool for BAV is
   A. Chest X-ray (PA view)
   B. Echocardiography
   C. Transesophageal echocardiography
   D. Angiography
      Answer: B
7. Risk factor for BAV include all except:
   A. Age
   B. Arterial hypertension
   C. Dyslipidemia
   D. Exercise
      Answer: D
8. What percent of patient needs surgical intervention due to the development of complication?
   A. 40%
   B. 30%
   C. 90%
   D. 45%
      Answer: B
9. Supravalvular aortic stenosis is usually associated with which syndrome?
   A. Down syndrome
   B. Edward syndrome
   C. William's syndrome
   D. Marfan syndrome
      Answer: C
10. Which of the following factor aggravates aortic root dilation in patients with BAV?
    A. Post-stenotic dilation and abnormal elastic fibers
    B. Pre-stenotic dilation and abnormal microfibrils
    C. Post stenotic dilation and abnormal smooth muscle fibers
    D. Pre-stenotic dilation and abnormal fibrous tissue
       Answer: A

References

1. Cripe L, Andelfinger G, Martin LJ, Shooner K, Benson DW. Bicuspid aortic valve is heritable. J Am Coll Cardiol. 2004;44(1):138–43.
2. Braverman AC, Güven H, Beardslee MA, Makan M, Kates AM, Moon MR. The bicuspid aortic valve. Curr Probl Cardiol. 2005;30(9):470–522.
3. Roberts WC. The congenitally bicuspid aortic valve: a study of 85 autopsy cases. Am J Cardiol. 1970;26(1):72–83.

4. Çakar MA, Aydın E. Diagnosis and treatment of bicuspid aortic valve disease. Erciyes Med J. 2015;37(1).

5. PerloV JK. Congenital heart disease in adults. In: Braunwald E, editor. Heart disease, a textbook of cardiovascular medicine. 5th ed. Philadelphia: WB Saunders; 1997. p. 969.

6. Campbell M, Kauntze R. Congenital aortic valvular stenosis. Br Heart J. 1953;15(2):179.

7. Bacon A, Matthews M. Congenital bicuspid aortic valves and the aetiology of isolated aortic valvular stenosis. Q J Med. 1959;28:545–60.

8. Mills P, Leech G, Davies M, Leathan A. The natural history of a non-stenotic bicuspid aortic valve. Heart. 1978;40(9):951–7.

9. Wauchope GM. The clinical importance of variations in the number of cusps forming the aortic and pulmonary valves. QJM. 1928;83:383–99.

10. Larson EW, Edwards WD. Risk factors for aortic dissection: a necropsy study of 161 cases. Am J Cardiol. 1984;53(6):849–55.

11. Evangelista A, Gallego P, Calvo-Iglesias F, Bermejo J, Robledo-Carmona J, Sánchez V, et al. Anatomical and clinical predictors of valve dysfunction and aortic dilation in bicuspid aortic valve disease. Heart. 2018;104(7):566–73.

12. Soto-Navarrete MT, López-Unzu MÁ, Durán AC, Fernández B. Embryonic development of bicuspid aortic valves. Prog Cardiovasc Dis. 2020;63(4):407–18.

13. Fernández B, Soto-Navarrete MT, López-García A, López-Unzu MÁ, Durán AC, Fernández MC. Bicuspid aortic valve in 2 model species and review of the literature. Vet Pathol. 2020;57(2):321–31.

14. Piccoli G, Slavich G, Gianfagna P, Gasparini D. Cleft bicuspid aortic valve: the Achilles' heel of echocardiography? Eur Heart J. 2010;31(17):2140.

15. Camenisch TD, Runyan RB, Markwald RR. Molecular regulation of cushion morphogenesis. In: Heart development and regeneration. Academic; 2010. pp. 363–387.

16. Fedak PW, Verma S, David TE, et al. Clinical and pathophysiological implications of a bicuspid aortic valve. Circulation. 2002;106:900–4.

17. El Accaoui RN, Gould ST, Hajj GP, Chu Y, Davis MK, Kraft DC, et al. Aortic valve sclerosis in mice deficient in endothelial nitric oxide synthase. Am J Phys Heart Circ Phys. 2014;306(9):H1302–13.

18. Hickey EJ, Caldarone CA, McCrindle BW. Left ventricular hypoplasia: a spectrum of disease involving the left ventricular outflow tract, aortic valve, and aorta. J Am Coll Cardiol. 2012;59(1S):S43–54.

19. Fernandes SM, Khairy P, Sanders SP, Colan SD. Bicuspid aortic valve morphology and interventions in the young. J Am Coll Cardiol. 2007;49(22):2211–4.

20. Tanaka K, Sata M, Fukuda D, Suematsu Y, Motomura N, Takamoto S, et al. Age-associated aortic stenosis in apolipoprotein E-deficient mice. J Am Coll Cardiol. 2005;46(1):134–41.

21. Roberts WC, Janning KG, Ko JM, Filardo G, Matter GJ. Frequency of congenitally bicuspid aortic valves in patients≥ 80 years of age undergoing aortic valve replacement for aortic stenosis (with or without aortic regurgitation) and implications for transcatheter aortic valve implantation. Am J Cardiol. 2012;109(11):1632–6.

22. Sievers HH, Schmidtke C. A classification system for the bicuspid aortic valve from 304 surgical specimens. J Thorac Cardiovasc Surg. 2007;133(5):1226–33.

23. Kari FA, Beyersdorf F, Siepe M. Pathophysiological implications of different bicuspid aortic valve configurations. In: Cardiology research and practice. 2012.

24. Kong WK, Delgado V, Poh KK, Regeer MV, Ng AC, McCormack L, et al. Prognostic implications of raphe in bicuspid aortic valve anatomy. JAMA Cardiol. 2017;2(3):285–92.

25. Fernández B, Durán AC, Fernández-Gallego T, Fernández MC, Such M, Arqué JM, Sans-Coma V. Bicuspid aortic valves with different spatial orientations of the leaflets are distinct etiological entities. J Am Coll Cardiol. 2009;54(24):2312–8.

26. Habchi KM, Ashikhmina E, Vieira VM, Shahram JT, Isselbacher EM, Sundt TM, et al. Association between bicuspid aortic valve morphotype and regional dilatation of the aortic root and trunk. Int J Cardiovasc Imaging. 2017;33(3):341–9.

27. Andreassi MG, Della Corte A. Genetics of bicuspid aortic valve aortopathy. Curr Opin Cardiol. 2016;31(6):585–92.

28. Bryant R. Congenital heart defects that include cardiac valve abnormalities. In: Heart valves. Boston: Springer; 2013. pp. 45–72.

29. Kiyota Y, Della Corte A, Vieira VM, Habchi K, Huang CC, Della Ratta EE, et al. Risk and outcomes of aortic valve endocarditis among patients with bicuspid and tricuspid aortic valves. Open Heart. 2017;4(1):openhrt-2016.

30. Khan W, Milsevic M, Salciccioli L, Lazar J. Low prevalence of bicuspid aortic valve in African Americans. Am Heart J. 2008;156(3):e25.

31. Verma S, Siu SC. Aortic dilatation in patients with bicuspid aortic valve. N Engl J Med. 2014;370:1920–9.

32. Tutar E, Ekici F, Atalay S, Nacar N. The prevalence of bicuspid aortic valve in newborns by echocardiographic screening. Am Heart J. 2005;150(3):513–5.

33. Nistri S, Basso C, Marzari C, Mormino P, Thiene G. Frequency of bicuspid aortic valve in young male conscripts by echocardiogram. Am J Cardiol. 2005;96(5):718–21.

34. Azevedo CF, Nigri M, Higuchi ML, Pomerantzeff PM, Spina GS, Sampaio RO, et al. Prognostic significance of myocardial fibrosis quantification by histopathology and magnetic resonance imaging in patients with severe aortic valve disease. J Am Coll Cardiol. 2010;56(4):278–87.

35. Tzemos N, Therrien J, Yip J, Thanassoulis G, Tremblay S, Jamorski MT, et al. Outcomes in adults with bicuspid aortic valves. JAMA. 2008;300(11):1317–25.

36. Head CEG, Thorne SA. Congenital heart disease in pregnancy. Postgrad Med J. 2005;81(955):292–8.

37. Rabuş MB, Kayalar N, Sareyyüpoğlu B, Erkin A, Kıralı K, Yakut C. Hypercholesterolemia association with aortic stenosis of various etiologies. J Card Surg. 2009;24(2):146–50.

38. Steiner RM, Reddy GP, Flicker S. Congenital cardiovascular disease in the adult patient: imaging update. J Thorac Imaging. 2002;17:1–17.

39. Gatzoulis MA, Webb GD, Daubeney PE. Diagnosis and management of adult congenital heart disease e-book. Elsevier Health Sciences; 2010.

40. Diller GP, Gatzoulis MA. Pulmonary vascular disease in adults with congenital heart disease. Circulation. 2007;115(8):1039–50.

41. Takeda H, Muro T, Saito T, Hyodo E, Ehara S, Hanatani A, et al. Diagnostic accuracy of transthoracic and transesophageal echocardiography for the diagnosis of bicuspid aortic valve: comparison with operative findings. Osaka City Med J. 2013;59(2):69–78.

42. Malaisrie SC, Carr J, Mikati I, Rigolin V, Yip BK, Lapin B, McCarthy PM. Cardiac magnetic resonance imaging is more diagnostic than 2-dimensional echocardiography in determining the presence of bicuspid aortic valve. J Thorac Cardiovasc Surg. 2012;144(2):370–6.

43. Cognet T, Séguéla PE, Thomson E, Bouisset F, Lairez O, Hascoët S, et al. Assessment of valvular surfaces in children with a congenital bicuspid aortic valve: preliminary three-dimensional echocardiographic study. Arch Cardiovasc Dis. 2013;106(5):295–302.

44. Hillebrand M, Koschyk D, Ter Hark P, Schüler H, Rybczynski M, Berger J, et al. Diagnostic accuracy study of routine echocardiography for bicuspid aortic valve: a retrospective study and meta-analysis. Cardiovasc Diagn Ther. 2017;7(4):367.

45. McMahon C. 30 left ventricular outflow obstruction: aortic valve stenosis, subaortic stenosis, supravalvar aortic stenosis, and bicuspid aortic valve. In: Pediatric cardiovascular medicine. 2012. p. 406.

46. Shen M, Tastet L, Capoulade R, Arsenault M, Bédard É, Clavel MA, Pibarot P. Effect of bicuspid aortic valve phenotype on pro-

gression of aortic stenosis. Eur Heart J Cardiovasc Imaging. 2020;21(7):727–34.

47. Michelena HI, Desjardins VA, Avierinos JF, Russo A, Nkomo VT, Sundt TM, et al. Natural history of asymptomatic patients with normally functioning or minimally dysfunctional bicuspid aortic valve in the community. Circulation. 2008;117(21):2776–84.

48. Franchi E, Cantinotti M, Assanta N, Viacava C, Arcieri L, Santoro G. State of the art and prospective for percutaneous treatment for left ventricular outflow tract obstruction. Prog Pediatr Cardiol. 2018;51:55–61.

49. Taylor AP, Yadlapati A, Andrei AC, Li Z, Clennon C, McCarthy PM, et al. Statin use and aneurysm risk in patients with bicuspid aortic valve disease. Clin Cardiol. 2016;39(1):41–7.

50. Stefani L, Galanti G, Toncelli L, Manetti P, Vono MC, Rizzo M, Maffulli N. Bicuspid aortic valve in competitive athletes. Br J Sports Med. 2008;42(1):31–5.

51. De Mozzi P, Longo UG, Galanti G, Maffulli N. Bicuspid aortic valve: a literature review and its impact on sport activity. Br Med Bull. 2008;85(1):63–85.

52. Ngow HA, Wan Khairina WMN. Undiagnosed bicuspid aortic valve: a silent danger. IIUM Med J Malaysia. 2012;11(2):45–8.

53. Mordi I, Tzemos N. Bicuspid aortic valve disease: a comprehensive review. Cardiol Res Pract. 2012;2012:196037.

54. Michelena HI, Khanna AD, Mahoney D, Margaryan E, Topilsky Y, Suri RM, et al. Incidence of aortic complications in patients with bicuspid aortic valves. JAMA. 2011;306(10):1104–12.

55. Skillington PD, Mokhles MM, Takkenberg JJ, Larobina M, O'Keefe M, Wynne R, Tatoulis J. The Ross procedure using autologous support of the pulmonary autograft: techniques and late results. J Thorac Cardiovasc Surg. 2015;149(2):S46–52.

56. Borger MA, David TE. Management of the valve and ascending aorta in adults with bicuspid aortic valve disease. In: Seminars in thoracic and cardiovascular surgery, vol. 17, no. 2. WB Saunders; 2005. pp. 143–147.

57. Siu SC, Silversides CK. Bicuspid aortic valve disease. J Am Coll Cardiol. 2010;55(25):2789–800.

58. Roberts WC, Vowels TJ, Ko JM, Filardo G, Hebeler RF Jr, Henry AC, et al. Comparison of the structure of the aortic valve and ascending aorta in adults having aortic valve replacement for aortic stenosis versus for pure aortic regurgitation and resection of the ascending aorta for aneurysm. Circulation. 2011;123(8):896–903.

59. Rodrigues I, Agapito AF, de Sousa L, Oliveira JA, Branco LM, Galrinho A, et al. Bicuspid aortic valve outcomes. Cardiol Young. 2017;27(3):518–29.

60. Novaro GM, Katz R, Aviles RJ, Gottdiener JS, Cushman M, Psaty BM, et al. Clinical factors, but not C-reactive protein, predict progression of calcific aortic-valve disease: the cardiovascular health study. J Am Coll Cardiol. 2007;50(20):1992–8.

61. Thiene G, Basso C. Pathology and pathogenesis of infective endocarditis in native heart valves. Cardiovasc Pathol. 2006;15(5):256–63.

62. Halpern EJ, Gupta S, Halpern DJ, Wiener DH, Owen AN. Characterization and normal measurements of the left ventricular outflow tract by ECG-gated cardiac CT: implications for disorders of the outflow tract and aortic valve. Acad Radiol. 2012;19(10):1252–9.

63. Sudhakar P, Jose J, George OK. Contemporary outcomes of percutaneous closure of patent ductus arteriosus in adolescents and adults. Indian Heart J. 2018;70(2):308–15.

64. Sawaimoon SK, Jadhav MV, Rane SR, Sagale M, Khedkar B. Aortic dissection and bicuspid aortic valve: an autopsy study. Indian J Pathol Microbiol. 2006;49(3):327–9.

65. Collins RT II, Kaplan P, Somes GW, Rome JJ. Long-term outcomes of patients with cardiovascular abnormalities and Williams syndrome. Am J Cardiol. 2010;105(6):874–8.

66. Vohra HA, Whistance RN, De Kerchove L, Punjabi P, El Khoury G. Valve-preserving surgery on the bicuspid aortic valve. Eur J Cardiothorac Surg. 2013;43(5):888–98.

67. Thakkar H, Sebastian M. Partial anomalous pulmonary venous connection presenting as Eisenmenger's syndrome. Heart Lung Circulation. 2017;26:S325–6.

68. Minette MS, Sahn DJ. Ventricular septal defects. Circulation. 2006;114(20):2190–7.

69. Eleyan L, Khan AA, Musollari G, Chandiramani AS, Shaikh S, Salha A, et al. Infective endocarditis in paediatric population. Eur J Pediatr. 2021;180(10):3089–100.

70. Fishbein GA, Fishbein MC. Pathology of the aortic valve: aortic valve stenosis/aortic regurgitation. Curr Cardiol Rep. 2019;21(8):1–9.

71. Panico BS, Panico AF, Dieter RS. Inflammatory and connective tissue disorders of the aorta. In: Diseases of the aorta. 2019. pp. 231–258.

72. Yener N, Oktar GL, Erer D, Yardimci MM, Yener A. Bicuspid aortic valve. Ann Thorac Cardiovasc Surg. 2002;8(5):264–7.

73. Mubarik A, Law MA. Bicuspid aortic valve. 2018.

74. Hernesniemi JA, Heiskanen J, Ruohonen S, Kartiosuo N, Hutri-Kähönen N, Kähönen M, et al. Aortic sinus diameter in middle age is associated with body size in young adulthood. Heart. 2018;104(9):773–8.

75. Eichhorn JG, Ley S, Kropp F, Fink C, Brockmeier K, Loukanov T, Ley-Zaporozhan J. Aortic coarctation a systemic vessel disease—insights from magnetic resonance imaging. Thorac Cardiovasc Surg. 2019;67(S4):e1–e10.

76. Lis P, Lyzwa P, Walczewski R, Mozenska O, Kosior DA. Bicuspid aortic valve–state-of-the-art. J Adv Cardiol Res. 2017;1(1).

77. Lee MG, Babu-Narayan SV, Kempny A, Uebing A, Montanaro C, Shore DF, et al. Long-term mortality and cardiovascular burden for adult survivors of coarctation of the aorta. Heart. 2019;105(15):1190–6.

78. Ma L, Gu Q, Ni B, Sun H, Zhen X, Zhang S, Shao Y. Simultaneously surgical management of adult complex coarctation of aorta concomitant with intracardiac abnormality. J Thorac Dis. 2018;10(10):5842.

79. Jayendiran R, Campisi S, Viallon M, Croisille P, Avril S. Hemodynamics alteration in patient-specific dilated ascending thoracic aortas with tricuspid and bicuspid aortic valves. J Biomech. 2020;110:109954.

80. Schattner A. Diagnostic errors in thoracic aortic dissection. QJM. 2021;114(10):687–8.

81. Yim ES. Aortic root disease in athletes: aortic root dilation, anomalous coronary artery, bicuspid aortic valve, and Marfan's syndrome. Sports Med. 2013;43(8):721–32.

82. Subbaraj SS. Coarctation of aorta with aberrant right subclavian artery presenting as Dysphagia lusoria and the impact of bicuspid aortic valve. Univ J Med Med Special. 2016;2(6).

83. Roberts WC, Vowels TJ, Ko JM. Natural history of adults with congenitally malformed aortic valves (unicuspid or bicuspid). Medicine. 2012;91(6):287–308.

84. Choudhary P, Canniffe C, Jackson DJ, Tanous D, Walsh K, Celermajer DS. Late outcomes in adults with coarctation of the aorta. Heart. 2015;101(15):1190–5.

85. Eleid MF, Forde I, Edwards WD, Maleszewski JJ, Suri RM, Schaff HV, et al. Type A aortic dissection in patients with bicuspid aortic valves: clinical and pathological comparison with tricuspid aortic valves. Heart. 2013;99(22):1668–74.

86. Cecconi M, Nistri S, Quarti A, Manfrin M, Colonna PL, Molini E, Perna GP. Aortic dilatation in patients with bicuspid aortic valve. J Cardiovasc Med. 2006;7(1):11–20.

87. Goudot G, Mirault T, Bruneval P, Soulat G, Pernot M, Messas E. Aortic wall elastic properties in case of bicuspid aortic valve. Front Physiol. 2019;10:299.

88. Della Corte A, Bancone C, Buonocore M, Dialetto G, Covino FE, Manduca S, et al. Pattern of ascending aortic dimensions predicts the growth rate of the aorta in patients with bicuspid aortic valve. JACC Cardiovasc Imaging. 2013;6(12):1301–10.

89. Laforest B, Nemer M. Genetic insights into bicuspid aortic valve formation. In: Cardiology research and practice. 2012.

90. Antequera-González B, Martínez-Micaelo N, Alegret JM. Bicuspid aortic valve and endothelial dysfunction: current evidence and potential therapeutic targets. Front Physiol. 2020;11:1015.

91. Girdauskas E, Borger MA, Secknus MA, Girdauskas G, Kuntze T. Is aortopathy in bicuspid aortic valve disease a congenital defect or a result of abnormal hemodynamics? A critical reappraisal of a one-sided argument. Eur J Cardiothorac Surg. 2011;39(6):809–14.

92. Chandra S, Lang RM, Nicolarsen J, Gayat E, Spencer KT, Mor-Avi V, Hofmann Bowman MA. Bicuspid aortic valve: inter-racial difference in frequency and aortic dimensions. JACC Cardiovasc Imaging. 2012;5(10):981–9.

Cardiomyopathies

Mohamad Dawood

Abstract

Cardiomyopathies are a group of diseases which affect the muscle of the heart, impairing its function and interfering with the normal systolic ejection fraction. They can be classified into three major groups which differ by etiology and outcome. Dilated cardiomyopathy "DCM," is the most common form, it can be primary or idiopathic accounting for more than 50% of cases or secondary due to underlying etiology as in cases of alcohol consumption, inflammatory diseases of the myocardium (myocarditis), and metabolic/endocrine diseases. On echocardiography there can be detected enlargement of the myocardium and decrease of the EF; treatment is based on symptomatic management of congestive heart failure together with the treating of underlying etiology. Restrictive cardiomyopathy is (RSV) another form of cardiomyopathy which is way less common than DCM, characterized by infiltration of the myocardium by different substances such as amyloid and fibrotic infiltrates. However, the EF is preserved in RSV and echocardiography detects a decrease in the ventricular filling. Arrhythmogenic right ventricle cardiomyopathy (ARVC) is characterized by impairment of the right ventricle of the heart because of the fibrotic infiltrate which leads to dysfunction of the right part of the heart and subsequently the left part and congestive heart failure.

Keywords

Cardiomyopathy · Dilated cardiomyopathy Restrictive cardiomyopathy · Hypertrophic obstructive cardiomyopathy · Loeffler and eosinophilic endocarditis Stress-induced cardiomyopathy · Peripartum cardiomyopathy · Myocarditis · Amyloidosis

Introduction

Cardiomyopathies represent a group of heterogenous diseases that can progress often to congestive heart failure, with high mortality and morbidity. This disease is classified into some other group based on the etiology, pathology manifestations, and management.

This disease in most of its cases is asymptomatic early in life and slowly it can progress and present with clinical manifestations of the underlying disease; manifestations as dyspnea, edema peripheral or pulmonary, fatigue, paroxysmal nocturnal dyspnea, and other electrical abnormality. Diagnostics such as ECG, echocardiography, and endocardial muscle biopsy can be used and management is based on lifestyle change as the first step together with medical and various surgical interventions to limit the progression of the disease and relieve various symptoms and signs.

Groups of cardiomyopathies are:

1. Dilated cardiomyopathy.
2. Restrictive cardiomyopathy.
3. Hypertrophic obstructive cardiomyopathy.

Dilated Cardiomyopathy

The disease of heart muscle is characterized by enlargement of ventricular chambers one or both and abnormality of the contractile function; it is a progressive disease asymptomatic initially but leads to decompensated heart failure mostly later, classified as primary(idiopathic) or secondary due to underlying etiology [1].

M. Dawood (✉)
Kharkiv National Medical University, Kharkiv, Ukraine

Epidemiology

The prevalence of this disease is estimated to be 36 per 100,000 in the population in the united states; more common in men than in women.

Etiology (Table 1)

Genetic Causes of DCM

Recent studies have shown a strong relation between mutation in some genes (more than 60) and development of DCM. Titin (TTN) gene mutation is very important and DCM is detected in more than 25% of the population expressing this mutation, although its mutation is not obligatory associated with DCM and the patient may be phenotypically normal due to other gene modifier effects. Diagnostics using echocardiography should be done for the family members who are at high risk to develop DCM along with genetic tests for early diagnosis of DCM; screening should be routinely every 2–3 years since the risk is age-dependent.

The predominant mode of inheritance of DCM is autosomal recessive to be more than X-linked or mitochondrial-related, although some of the mutated genes can be related to X chromosome as Duchenne muscular dystrophy(dystrophin).

Other genetic causes also predispose to DCM autosomal dominant diseases, as for diseases which affect actin, desmin, and lamin proteins present in cardiomyocytes.

Histological examination of the heart in DCM shows typically interstitial and perivascular fibrosis also necrosis of the subendocardial cells.

Clinical Manifestations

The course of the disease varies from person to person but in general a slow course of progression is dominant in DCM, patients at the early stage are usually asymptomatic, at the late stages with the progression of the disease DCM may present with signs and symptoms of congestive heart failure such as dyspnea, peripheral edema, and jugular vein distention. The patient should be treated conservatively as treating patient with CHF due to any other etiology as coronary heart disease… [2].

On physical examination, a S3 sound may be heard on auscultation of the heart together with enlargement of heart border (cardiomegaly). Laboratory and instrumental diagnostics may show elevated brain natriuretic peptide (BNP) secreted from the left atrium which indicates heart failure (it may be normal at the early stages), ECG may show left bundle branch block and ventricular enlargement; chest x-ray may show cardiomegaly.

Diagnosis

ECG
Not specifically diagnostic and is used as first-line for any patient with any heart abnormality to rule out ischemic coronary diseases. ECG in DCM may show tachycardia, left ventricle enlargement, and some electrical conduction abnormalities as LBBB due to fibrotic changes in the heart. Tachycardia is seen only in 20–30% of patients having DCM.

Echocardiography
Echocardiography in DCM shows enlargement and dilation of the left ventricle, shows a decrease in the EF, and also

Table 1 Etiologies and diagnostics of dilated cardiomyopathy

Cause	Example	Diagnosis
Idiopathic	• Mutations of TTN gene, encoding for the intrasarcomeric protein titin (connectin) • Mutations of MYH7 gene, encoding for the beta-myosin heavy chain	Family history
Infiltrative/ inflammatory	• Hemosiderosis, sarcoidosis • SLE, dermatomyositis	ESR, CRP, history + clinical features, biopsy is the gold standard
Pregnancy		History + signs and features of heart failure in the last trimester of pregnancy + echocardiography
Toxins	Alcohol, amphetamines, cocaine…	History of the patient + urine toxicology screening
Infections	Coxsackie A and B/HIV/CMV/parvovirus B19/chagas disease	Serology test for the infection suspected
Metabolic/ endocrine	Electrolyte disturbances hypocalcemia, hypophosphatemia Endocrine disorder (pheochromocytoma, Cushing…)	Blood electrolytes, blood metanephros's level, hormone level of suspected disease

shows valvular abnormality as mitral and tricuspid regurgitation; however, echocardiography cannot distinguish between the cause predisposed for DCM either it is idiopathic or secondary.

Cardiac Magnetic Resonance Imaging

This procedure is more specific and can differentiate between ischemic and non-ischemic heart dilation. In cardiomyopathy due to ischemic coronary heart disease it usually shows late gadolinium enhancement (LGE), extending transmurally to epicardium; however, DCM may show features of absence of LGE.

Myocarditis and DCM

Viral myocarditis in its chronic form has a bad outcome on the myocardium and it can be a major cause of DCM. Virus such as coxsackie b, CMV, HIV are common viruses that can progress to DCM in their chronic form to cardiomyopathy; however, recent studies have shown that patient with chronic form of myocarditis and those who have developed DCM can still benefit from anti-viral medication such as interferon β-1 and it has proven by consequent biopsies taken from a patient with chronic myocarditis where appeared clearance of the virus and improvement of the features of DCM. Early treatment and preventing the chronic form of myocarditis is of high value however there are no enough studies about the efficiency of anti-viral medication.

Endomyocardial biopsy (EMB) is considered as the gold standard for the diagnosis of DCM due to myocarditis. The procedure should be guided with MRI target area to decrease the risk of complications. Biopsies are taken for histological exam and they show myocardial fibrosis.

Peripartum Cardiomyopathy (PPCM)

PPCM is a rare form of cardiomyopathy that develops in a pregnant woman during her last trimester or during the 5 months postpartum. The full etiology of this form of cardiomyopathy is not fully understood but it is assumed to be related due to cleavage of protein and oxidative stress peri/postpartum. PPCM is a diagnosis of exclusion after excluding all other causes that can predispose the patient to cardiomyopathy and heart failure, PPCM is considered during the last trimester or within 5 months postpartum; features are those in a patient with congestive heart failure as dyspnea, edema. Treatment is different from other etiologies because some drugs are teratogenic or should not be prescribed for lactating women [3].

Stress-Induced Cardiomyopathy

Also called takotsubo cardiomyopathy after the Japanese cardiologist takotsubo.

Etiology of this form is related to a history of stress or physical activity along with dyskinesia in the left part of the heart seen on imaging. ECG shows ST elevation which resembles the elevation in acute MI however the elevation here is reversible and transient. Coronary angiography is used to rule out obstructive causes of coronary artery diseases. Etiology suggested to be a high level of catecholamines secreted during emotional and physical stress, contractile abnormality, and LV dyskinesia are noted on imaging, imaging such as ECG (shows transient and reversible ST elevation), echocardiography demonstrating LV hypokinesis and enlargement together with a decrease in EF, and cardiac MRI which is the best imaging in detecting such cardiomyopathy by demonstrating dyskinesia in the LV.

Drug-Induced Cardiomyopathy

Many drugs have been implicated in cardiotoxicity in their chronic courses for treatment, and these drugs have a remodeling outcome on the myocardium even though applied in a proper way. Some of these drugs are anti-tumor medications such as anthracyclines. These drugs are highly cardiotoxic, and their forms are acute and subacute which manifest in a short time after beginning treatment as myocarditis and pericarditis or in chronic forms which begins in late-onset years after beginning treatment. Diagnostics such as echocardiography are highly suggestive in confirming the diagnosis and should be done routinely in patient on an antineoplastic treatment for early diagnosis. Management, when heart failure has developed, consists of treatment of systolic heart failure with β-blockers, ACE inhibitors, spironolactone in NYHA III and IV, and amiodarone is also used for arrhythmia.

Management

There is no specific treatment for DCM. Treatment is based on treating chronic heart failure and complications coming from it, together with eliminating the underlying cause which predisposed to DCM as in cases of an alcoholic by abstinence from alcohol or drug-induced DCM by eliminating the drug. Treatment of heart failure consists of drugs such as β-blockers and ACE inhibitors, diuretics such as furosemide in case of volume overloads, effusions in decompensated heart failure, and also amiodarone and different antiarrhythmic drugs in case of any arrhythmia detected.

Invasive approach has significant importance in patients with recurrent ventricular fibrillation and desynchrony. Implantable cardioverter defibrillator "ICD" has shown an important outcome by decreasing rates of sudden cardiac death caused by DCM by a rate of 31% according to a meta-analysis study.

In patients with extremely dilated heart and features of heart failure, the option of ventricular remodeling and reconstruction together with mitral annuloplasty should be considered apart from the etiology as either ischemic or idiopathic has led to DCM [4].

Although stem cell transplantation has shown a good outcome in ischemic DCM, it is still not confirmed if it is with good outcome in idiopathic DCM.

Restrictive Cardiomyopathy "RSC"

RSC is a disease of the myocardium characterized by impaired filling of the ventricles due to interstitial fibrosis and calcification of one ventricle and is called non-diffuse RSC or both ventricles and called diffuse form RSC. It could be classified as primary where the etiology is unknown as idiopathic RSC and Loffler's endocarditis or secondary due to infiltrative diseases such as sarcoidosis, amyloidosis, or storage diseases as hemochromatosis. Unlike the other cardiomyopathies, the abnormality in RSC is hemodynamic related more than morphological as the case in DCM and diastolic function is impaired not systolic which may be increased in this case. The disease is progressive and begins with reduced ventricular filling and ventricular stiffness which later progress to reduced systolic function and signs of heart failure.

Etiology (Table 2)

Idiopathic RSC is a rare form of cardiomyopathy which manifest mainly in children and adults. Assumed to be a genetic related to autosomal dominant inheritance encoding sarcomere proteins such as troponin T, alpha cardiac actin, and beta-myosin heavy chain.

RSV of idiopathic form manifested mainly in children who require high systolic pressure for maintenance of output, with reduced output in RSV of idiopathic form systolic

Table 2 Restrictive cardiomyopathy, examples of primary and secondary causes

Etiology	Examples
Primary/ idiopathic	Endomyocardial fibrosis Loeffler eosinophilic endomyocardial disease
Secondary	Sarcoidosis, hemochromatosis, progressive systemic sclerosis, radiation, glycogen storage diseases such as Fabry disease and Gaucher

dysfunction appear and manifest with signs and symptoms of congestive heart failure. Studies have shown that children with poor left ventricle function despite a normal diastolic function could be a hallmark of restrictive heart disease.

Loeffler Endocarditis

Defined as the eosinophilic infiltrate of the myocardium due to any cause (allergic, parasitic, idiopathic.) described by W. Loeffler in 1936.

Divided into idiopathic, primary, and secondary.

Idiopathic which is the most common cause characterized by idiopathic eosinophilia, primary has been associated with an underlying myeloproliferative and stem cells disorders like leukemia and lymphoma, and secondary which is reactive to underlying non-neoplastic causing crises of eosinophils levels as allergic reaction, parasitic infections.

The pathophysiology of Loeffler endocarditis is not well understood. Some suggest that the eosinophils infiltrating the heart secrete protein granules damaging the endocardium and myocardium by producing some toxins which later activate platelets. Platelets by their turn form intracavitary and intravascular thrombi damage the endocardium.

Biopsy of the endocardium demonstrates fibrosis and thickening of ventricles leading to a decrease in ventricular size. On a light microscope degranulated eosinophils and eosinophilic infiltration are seen.

Patient's clinical symptoms are variable from heart failure' symptoms as dyspnea, palpitations, chest pain, cough, and fatigue to others as pericarditis (4% of patients with Loeffler endocarditis) 0.38% of patients may develop congestive heart failure. Eosinophils infiltration may cause valvular abnormality (42% of cases are detected with mitral insufficiency, aortic stenosis and regurgitation are as well detected (4%).

Diagnostics of Loeffler endocarditis is done with:

ECG (may show T wave inversion, left atrial enlargement, and left ventricle hypertrophy.)

Echocardiogram (it may show left ventricle hypertrophy, endomyocardial thickening, mitral valve stenosis, or any other valvular abnormality.)

Cardiac magnetic resonance (more specific and sensitive, shows cardiac fibrosis and thickening.)

And the gold standard with endomyocardial biopsy.

Treatment and Management

Regarding treatment of primary RSC, there is no specific treatment, the main thing is to treat symptomatically by managing congestive heart failure with diuretics, ACE inhibitors, and anticoagulant as well as valvuloplasty and other interventions aiming to treat valvular abnormalities.

The treatment of Loeffler endocarditis consists of correctly identifying the condition before the end-stage fibrosis occurs. Medical therapy with corticosteroids, cytotoxic agents, and interferon to suppress the intense eosinophilic infiltration of the myocardium.

Endomyocardectomy and cardiac transplantation are also other advanced interventions in advanced RSC.

Amyloidosis

Light chain amyloidosis is consequent on a clonal plasma cell proliferative disorder in which misfolded immunoglobulin light chains are deposited as amyloid fibrils in multiple organs, including heart. In about half of cases heart is frequently involved but other organs and systems may be involved such as as renal and respiratory.

Early diagnosis is not frequent. Patients usually come with late stages of disease, when patients present with signs and symptoms of right-side heart failure such as jugular vein distention, dyspnea, peripheral edema, and others.

First type of cardiac amyloidosis is cardiac transthyretin amyloidosis associated with the inherited dominant syndromes of familial amyloid neuropathy and familial amyloid cardiomyopathy.

Second is wildtype transthyretin amyloidosis referred to senile systemic amyloidosis increasing in the aging population.

Third type is hereditary transthyretin amyloidosis; transthyretin gene (TTR) gene is located on chromosome 18, many mutations usually occur in this gene but only specific mutation is responsible for the development of this disease. Inheritance is autosomal dominant.

Diagnostics

Diagnosis usually requires biopsy and histologic examination for confirmation of cardiac amyloidosis.

Some serum markers such as natriuretic peptide, troponin, and others should increase the suspicion of cardiac amyloidosis in a patient with senile patients and with known plasma cell dyscrasia and should prompt other diagnostics.

ECG

It may show in progressed disease right ventricular hypertrophy, left heart hypertrophy or both, as well as leads voltages are decreased in all leads. Infarctions and arrhythmias are also common and because of the infiltration AV block may occur.

Echocardiography

Thick-walled ventricles, small left ventricular chamber volume, valve thickening atrial enlargement.

Interventricular septum thickness > 12 mm in absence of hypertension or controlled hypertension.

Cardiovascular Magnetic Resonance (CMR)

It has a high specificity and sensitivity especially with the use of gadolinium-based contrast agent, especially useful in patients with increased left ventricular wall thickness.

Treatment

Supportive treatment with salt and fluid restriction, together with restriction of medications managing heart failure including beta blockers, ACE inhibitors, and ARB, since this medication are poorly tolerated in amyloidosis because they decrease cardiac output.

Chemotherapy directed toward amyloidosis is the mainstay of treatment as bortezomib which is a proteasome inhibitor used with other agents or alone and associated with hematological response in up to 90%.

Stem cell transplantation is associated with the most durable remission.

Therapeutic antibodies have the potential to target amyloid deposit directly. Liver transplantation as well is a good variant in some forms of amyloidosis.

Hypertrophic Cardiomyopathy (HOCM)

HOCM is a genetic disease that affects heart cells causing hypertrophy in an abnormal disorganized, asymmetric way with fibrosis/scarring in between cells. Mitral valve can be affected and it may cause obstruction of blood flow from the left part of the heart.

The disease prevalence is 1 in 500, although some patients remain not diagnosed. Individuals undergo normal life longevity since the majority of patients are asymptomatic. Symptomatic patients may have chest pain, dyspnea, and fatigue. Some patients with HOCM are at risk of developing sudden cardiac death, especially during physical exam.

Pathogenesis

HOCM is autosomal dominant, men and women have the same chance of inheriting this disease, and not all patients who inherit the disease may show signs and symptoms of the disease.

In HOCM, the muscular wall of the left ventricle becomes thickened, most often increasing thickness of the upper part of the septum.

Increased thickness of the septum may cause obstruction of blood ejection from the left ventricle causing increasing pressure in the left ventricle. Impairing of the mitral valve function leads to mitral regurgitation together with other complications related to HOCM.

Mutations in genes coding for β-myosin heavy chain and myosin binding protein C as HCM, MYH7, MYBPC3 are the most commonly mutated genes involved in developing HOCM. Mutations in genes responsible for storage disease such as Gaucher is also involved in the development of HOCM.

Clinical Manifestations

Most of the patients have no or few symptoms. Commonly seen in puberty after hypertrophy of the heart, the most common symptoms in patients:

- Dyspnea,
- Chest pain during rest or exertion,
- Fainting or syncope,
- Palpitations,
- Light shades when standing or sitting up,
- Peripheral edema.

Diagnosis

Whenever HOCM because of genetic predisposition or clinical symptoms is suspected different diagnostics methods from ECG, Echocardiography, or cardiac magnetic resonance together with biopsy and genetic testing should be done to confirm the HOCM.

ECG performed as the first choice may show enlargement of one ventricle or both, or electrical activity abnormalities.

Echocardiography: It detects the size of the chambers of the heart as well as valvular functions and motions and ejection fraction of the heart and can detect the thickness of the interventricular septum. Highly rerecommended in patient with family genetic predisposition to HOCM.

Arrhythmia evaluation by using Holter monitoring recording patient ECG for 24 or 48 h: It detects arrhythmia and the cause for which arrhythmia has occurred.

Cardiovascular magnetic resonance: It detects the thickness of the septum and thickened area which could not be detected by the echocardiography as well as valves motions abnormalities.

Cardiac catheterization: It detects the pressure of blood in different chambers of the heart usually done before surgery to detect any obstruction at the coronary artery levels.

Evaluation of first-degree relatives is recommended whenever HOCM is diagnosed.

Treatment

Treatment in HOCM is aimed to reduce symptoms and complications and to prevent sudden cardiac death. There is no specific treatment for HOCM.

Treatment is targeted to relieve symptoms of heart failure, and to prevent arrhythmia and sudden cardiac death.

People with HOCM are recommended to avoid dehydration and compensate immediately for any cause leading to dehydration to avoid hypovolemia. Patients with HOCM are also recommended to avoid competitive sports which need high energy and eventually need high oxygen compensation of different tissues of the body which the heart in HOCM cannot afford and may lead to sudden cardiac death which is the most common death in adults with this form of cardiomyopathy [5].

Beta blockers, calcium channel blockers, and other antiarrhythmic drugs are used to reduce the risk of complications of HOCM. They increase the filling of the left ventricle, decrease oxygen need, and favor oxygen supply to cardiomyocytes and eventually decrease the risk of arrhythmia and sudden cardiac death. Avoiding inotropic drugs is also with significant value and should be avoided together with sympathomimetics and glycosides such as digoxin.

Patient should cover also all the risk factors which can predispose to coronary artery diseases and should control blood pressure with anti-hypertensive drugs (ACE inhibitors, ARB, diuretics). He should reduce all forms of lipid intake and control the level of lipids with drugs which decrease lipids level in the blood (statins).

All patient is advised to maintain normal oxygen level and prevent hypoxia and treat it immediately in case has occurred by controlling COPD exacerbation and preventing smoking.

Other invasive procedures are considered in patients who fail to preserve heart function with conservative and medical treatments and in patients with severe obstruction of the aortic outflow and thickened septum. Procedure such as septal myectomy which is a surgical procedure is performed only under specialized operators (class I recommendations of 2011 ACCF/AHA) to remove the excess muscular tissue in the septum causing obstruction and preventing normal outflow from the left part of the heart. Some precautions should be considered in patients with septal myectomy according to the 2011 ACCF/AHA recommendations III:

- Avoidance of this procedure in asymptomatic patients with HOCM.
- Mitral valve replacement is not an alternative treatment to septal myectomy.
- Avoidance of alcohol septal ablation in patients who are candidates for septal myectomy in whom septal myectomy can be performed (pediatric patients <21 y.o, patients with comorbidities, and patients >40 y.o).

Mitral Valve Replacement

Reserved for patients with severe mitral regurgitations, particularly in patients who developed congestive heart failure.

Pacemaker Implantation

To maintain atrioventricular synchrony and prevent sudden cardiac death, it has shown some good impacts on decreasing the level of left ventricular outflow obstruction and increasing the quality of life in HOCM patients.

2011 ACCF/AHA recommends avoiding this procedure in patients, candidates for septal myectomy, and in asymptomatic patients as well.

Catheter Septal Ablation

Transvenous catheter ablation of the septal region using selective arterial ethanol infusion to destroy myocardial tissues lead to remodeling of the septum and significant decrease of the septum thickness. It has shown great outcomes since 1990 and is still performed as the main invasive procedure in many medical centers.

Alcohol Septal Ablation

Superior over septal myectomy in some areas as it does not require surgical incision, recovery is shorter and used in elderly populations with comorbidities which are not candidate for invasive procedures.

Indicated for patients with drug refractory treatments, and not indicated in patients with thickness of septum >30 mm. postoperative complications may include AV block and the need for permanent pacemaker.

Implantable Cardioverter Defibrillator (ICD)

Sudden cardiac death in HOCM is approximately 1% each year. Individual with high risk may benefit from ICD to prevent SCD due to Vfib.

Cardiac Transplantation

Recommended in patients according to American college of cardiology foundation/American heart association (ACCF/AHA) patients with advanced heart disease and NYHA class III and IV, symptoms which are refractory to managing.

Multiple Choice Questions

1. All of the following are considered as etiologies for congestive dilated cardiomyopathy except:
   A. Metabolic.
   B. Peripartum.
   C. Ischemic.
   D. hemochromatosis.
2. Amyloid and sarcoid are considered what type of cardiomyopathy?
   A. Infiltrative.
   B. Restrictive.
   C. Congestive.
   D. Dilated.
   E. Hypertrophic.
3. Which of the following is a common echo finding in patients with restrictive cardiomyopathy?
   A. Left ventricle dilation.
   B. Asymmetric septal hypertrophy.
   C. Pericardial effusion.
   D. Right ventricle dilation.
   E. Normal left atrial size.
4. Patients with advanced symptoms from having a dilated cardio might benefit from all the following except:
   A. MV replacement.
   B. Intra-aortic balloon pump.
   C. LV assist device.
   D. Heart transplant.
5. In what type of restrictive cardiomyopathy eosinophilic infiltration of the myocardium is found under microscope?
   A. Sarcoidosis.
   B. Hemochromatosis.
   C. Loeffler endocarditis.
   D. Amyloidosis.
6. In a hypertrophic obstructive cardiomyopathy patient with comorbidities which is not a candidate for surgical procedure what is the best next step?
   A. Alcohol septal ablation.
   B. Mitral valve replacement.
   C. Septal myectomy.
   D. Implantable cardioverter defibrillator.
7. In a 27 y.o patient practicing some kind of sport and suddenly lost conscious and lost pulse despite many chest compressions cycles. He presents to the hospital and died, this patient's most common cause of death is:
   A. Constrictive cardiomyopathy.
   B. Restrictive cardiomyopathy,
   C. Aortic dissection.
   D. Hypertrophic obstructive cardiomyopathy.

8. Regarding diagnostic interventions in different variants of cardiomyopathies the least informative variants to detect such abnormality is:
   A. Endomyocardial biopsy.
   B. Echocardiography.
   C. Cardiac magnetic resonance.
   D. ECG.

9. In a patient with gastric adenocarcinoma undergoing chemotherapy presents with signs of heart failure, after cardiac follow-up with echocardiography dilated cardiomyopathy is suggested as preliminary diagnosis, what is the most common cause of DCM?
   A. Viral myocarditis.
   B. Myocardial ischemia.
   C. Drug-induced cardiomyopathy.
   D. Alcohol-induced cardiomyopathy.

10. The most common type of cardiomyopathy is:
   A. Dilated cardiomyopathy.
   B. HOCM.
   C. Restrictive cardiomyopathy.
   D. Arrhythmogenic type.

Answers

1. D.

   Explanation: Dilated cardiomyopathy has different etiologies either primary or secondary due to underlying causes, causes as metabolic as hypocalcemia, thyrotoxicosis, and other causes as ischemic as CAD may cause cardiomyopathy and lead to CHF; however, hemochromatosis is an underlying cause of cardiomyopathy but restrictive form where deposition of iron and ferritin is diagnostic.

2. A.

   Explanation: Although deposition of amyloid and sarcoid in the myocardium is considered a form of restrictive cardiomyopathy, this form does not develop until a later stage and is considered as infiltrative cardiomyopathy in the early presentation.

3. C.

   Explanation: On echocardiography, the most common specific sign suggesting restrictive cardiomyopathy besides decreased ejection fraction and signs of heart failure is pericardial effusion because of deposition of substances such as amyloid in the myocardium.

4. A.

   Explanation: In patients with advanced heart failure according to NYHA stage III or IV interventions such as valvuloplasty and mitral valve replacement are not con-

sidered beneficial however interventions to decrease mortality such as IVD are considered.

5. C.

   Explanation: Loeffler endocarditis is considered a major etiology of restrictive cardiomyopathy, and under endomyocardial microscopic biopsy eosinophilic infiltration is seen, other causes such as sarcoidosis, hemochromatosis may also lead to RSC but other findings are seen.

6. A.

   Explanation: This patient with HOCM is not a candidate for surgery and has many comorbidities and noninvasive procedures should proceed due to the high risk of complications. The best step is to go with alcohol septal ablation which is noninvasive and with a low risk of postoperative complications. Septal myectomy is invasive and should be avoided. (choice B) Although mitral valve is abnormal and mostly regurgitate blood and should be displaced is not the first step for HOCM. ICD should be considered in patients presenting with arrhythmia.

7. D.

   Explanation: This patient mostly has HOCM, which is the most common cause of death among adults, physical activity should be avoided by such patients because it increases the oxygen demand of heart which cannot be accomplished in HOCM leading eventually to arrhythmia and sudden cardiac death.

8. D.

   Explanation: ECG is the first-line diagnostic in patients with chest pain, is not specific to diagnose any type of cardiomyopathy, and is just a first-line intervention to exclude myocardial infarction and angina. It can detect some abnormalities such as AV block, LV hypertrophy, and others and further diagnostics should be done to put diagnosis. Endomyocardial biopsy is the gold standard diagnostic for cardiomyopathy.

9. C.

   Explanation: Drug-induced cardiomyopathy is the most common cause in this patient. Anthracyclines which are widely used as antineoplastic agents have a high degree of cardiotoxicity and cause a cardiac characteristic form of dose-dependent toxic cardiomyopathy. It should be suspected in all patients with suspected cardiomyopathy who are undergoing chemotherapy.

10. A.

   Explanation: Dilated type cardiomyopathy is the most common type of cardiomyopathy among all types.

References

1. Izzy M, et al. Redefining cirrhotic cardiomyopathy for the modern era. Hepatology. 2020;71(1):334–45.
2. Schultheiss H-P, et al. Dilated cardiomyopathy. Nat Rev Dis Primers. 2019;5(1):1–19.
3. Jia G, Hill MA, Sowers JR. Diabetic cardiomyopathy: an update of mechanisms contributing to this clinical entity. Circ Res. 2018;122(4):624–38.
4. Beesley SJ, et al. Septic cardiomyopathy. Crit Care Med. 2018;46(4):625–34.
5. Smith ED, et al. Desmoplakin cardiomyopathy, a fibrotic and inflammatory form of cardiomyopathy distinct from typical dilated or arrhythmogenic right ventricular cardiomyopathy. Circulation. 2020;141(23):1872–84.

Complete Heart Block (CHB)

Ali Talib Hashim, Qasim Mehmood, and Shoaib Ahmad

Abstract

"Complete heart block, also called third-degree heart block, is a condition in which no signals can pass from atria to ventricles." It is considered as the most severe heart block and is relatively rare. Common causes of this pathological condition include coronary ischemia leading to progressive degeneration of the conducting system of heart, congenital causes which are mostly linked to SLE, Lyme disease causing Lyme carditis, certain drugs like quinidine, and hyperkalemia which decreases the conductivity of the heart. An acute MI can also present with a complete AV block requiring the insertion of a permanent pacemaker. Symptoms include chest pain, dizziness, palpitations, and syncope. Treatment may be medicinal or surgical. Although insertion of pacemaker is the definitive treatment option, drugs like atropine, dopamine, or epinephrine may be helpful.

Keywords

Complete heart block · Third-degree heart block
SA node · AV node · Conducting system · Pacemaker
Atropine

Introduction

Heart block is also referred to as atrio-ventricular block (AV block). A heart block occurs when the electrical activity pathway which originates from the sino-atrial node (SA node) to the AV node becomes partially or completely blocked [1]. Throughout this chapter, complete heart block will be discussed. Complete heart block as the name entails occurs when no electrical activity passes from the atria to the ventricles as the SA node cannot propagate to the ventricles. As will be discussed in the "Physiology" section below; as a compensatory mechanism to this blockage the ventricles try to generate their own impulses by generating an accessory pacemaker [1]. Complete heart block is also known as third-degree heart block [2].

Physiology

As mentioned above, AV CHB is a type of arrhythmia where the signal is completely blocked when moving from the atria to the ventricles since the AV node is not conducting the signals from the SA node. This results in the SA node to work independently from the ventricles. CHB is principally the endpoint of either Mobitz I or Mobitz II AV block [2, 3]. CHB is in fact considered to be the most pathological and severe heart block and is also referred to as third-degree AV block. In CHB, it is important to note that even if the atria are going at a normal rate of 60 beats per minute (bpm) as if everything was normal, none of these signals make it down to the ventricles [3]. As a compensatory mechanism, the ventricles try to generate their own impulses by generating an accessory pacemaker. This accessory pacemaker is generated from either the bundle of His, or the right and/or the left bundle or the ventricular muscle itself depending on where the level of block is. This phenomenon is known as an escape rhythm [4]. In fact, on an ECG rhythm escape beats at very slow rates are normally visible. These escape rhythms are normally around 30 beats per minute. Also, the PR Interval is variable since there is no relationship between the atria and the ventricles and they are both working independently but regularly from each other [5].

A. T. Hashim (✉)
Golestan University for Medical Sciences, Gorgan, Iran

Q. Mehmood
King Edward Medical University, Lahore, Pakistan

S. Ahmad
Department of Pediatrics, District Head Quarters Teaching Hospital, Faisalabad, Pakistan

Epidemiology

Although other AV blocks are not uncommon, CHBs are relatively rare [1]. In 2005, the global annual incidence of CHB was estimated to be 430,000 [2]. Eighty percent of these estimates were reported in low/middle-income countries with only 20% of patients being under treatment. The incidence of CHB seems to vary according to etiology; in the healthy asymptomatic population, the reported incidence was 0.001% [3]. Nonetheless, this incidence increases in individuals with greater disease burden, with an incidence of 0.6% in individuals with hypertension and 1.1% in those with diabetes [4]. The only and sole treatment of CHB is pacemaker, and the number of pacemaker implantation is on the rise [5]. It has been reported that CHB 5-years mortality without pacemaker is as high as 68% [2], which adds on the economic burden related to the disease.

Etiology

As will be mentioned in this section, numerous conditions can result in third-degree heart block, yet the most common cause is coronary ischemia [6]. Coronary ischemia can lead to a progressive degeneration of the heart's electrical conduction system which can result in first-degree AV block, second-degree AV block, bundle branch block, or bifascicular block and finally leading to third-degree heart block [7].

It is also important to note that an acute myocardial infarction (MI) may also present with a complete AV block. An MI in the inferior wall may result in AV node damage causing CHB. In this case, the pathology is usually transitory. Numerous studies have shown how in the case of an inferior wall MI a CHB which may have occurred usually resolves within 2 weeks of its onset [7].

An anterior wall MI may also result in a complete AV block by causing damage to the distal conductive system. The damage caused is typically so extensive that it results in permanent damage to the conduction system resulting in the need of the insertion of a permanent pacemaker [8].

Congenital causes of complete AV block have also been reported. The main congenital cause has been linked to the presence of systemic lupus erythematosus (SLE). SLE may cause heart damage to the fetus by antibodies from the mother which may cross the placenta during gestation and attack the fetus's heart [9].

Hyperkalemia can also decrease conduction through the His-Purkinje bundle system inducing the formation of a complete heart block distal to the AV node junction. Lyme disease causes Lyme carditis which may also lead to heart block.

Borrelia burgdorferi, the spirochete which causes Lyme disease, damages the heart directly by either causing direct invasion and/or stimulating an exaggerated immune response of the body to the disease [10].

History and Physical Examinations

AV blocks severity, and symptoms vary from person to person according to their degree. The first-degree cases are mainly asymptomatic, second-degree cases from one hand can be either asymptomatic or associated with fainting, feeling dizzy, chest pain, heart palpitations, nausea, and pre-syncope/syncope. Symptoms of third-degree cases, on the other hand, are similar to the previous one. Nevertheless, they are more intense and severe due to the slow heart rate [11].

The initial clinical evaluation of a symptomatic person has an objective to identify an obvious diagnosis and stratify the patient risk according to severity as high or medium. At first, it is necessary to perform a detailed interrogation with the patient and his surroundings. This examination aims at clarifying four key elements listed as follows:

- The age; since AVB is increasingly seen in the elderly population.
- The family history in case of a sudden death, considering any possible existence of heart diseases.
- The personal history of heart disease in a middle-aged person.
- The types of medication, such as beta-blockers, calcium channel blockers, antiarrhythmic drugs, or digoxin [12].

It is noteworthy that expert must clarify the posture at the time of the onset of symptoms (standing, sitting, lying, etc.) according to the patient's activity (effort or rest), in addition to specifying any abnormal movements or other symptoms and their duration, considering that momentary amnesia can mislead the patient on the exact duration, the mode of awakening (sudden or progressive, with or without a post-critical phase, and the presence of nausea, vomiting, profuse sweating, a feeling of cold or urinary loss).

It is sometimes impossible to know whether the loss of consciousness was really complete or not, especially when it is very brief. Thus, it is necessary to know how to give up collecting this information, especially in the elderly population [13].

Diagnoses

First of all, we can see the severe bradycardia and the hypotension. If left untreated for a long while and/or in severe cases hemodynamic instability may also occur [14]. The ECG will show P waves with a regular P-to-P interval (in other words, a sinus rhythm). This represents the first rhythm. The ECG will also show QRS complexes with regular R-R interval. This represents the second rhythm. The PR interval will be variable, as the hallmark of complete heart block is that the P waves and the QRS complex occur independent of each other and there is no relationship between them [15].

Congenital third heart block may be detected during pregnancy using an ultrasound scan to measure the fetal heartbeat. An abnormally slow heartbeat may signify a heart block. An echocardiogram before or after birth may also be used to confirm congenital third-degree heart block [16].

Differential Diagnosis

CHB identification is usually confusing so it must not be mixed with other disorders like high-grade AV block and AV dissociation due to similarity in symptoms. In CHB, atrial impulses cannot be conducted to ventricles while in AV dissociation, atrial impulses will capture the ventricles if temporal opportunity and non-refractory tissue permit [17]. It may often occur that second-degree heart block and high-degree heart block mistaken for CHB but regular repetitive ECG is helpful in identifying CHB, minimizing the chance of error [17].

Complications and Prognosis

Patients who are suffering from complete heart block are at increased risk of experiencing symptomatic bradycardia and decreased cardiac output. Both these factors lead to decreased organ's perfusion. Thus, patients with CHB may be at increased risk of syncope leading to falls and head injuries. Additionally, decreased perfusion may lead to decreased organ perfusion leading to organ injury and less oftenly cardiac arrest [18].

Long-term prognosis of third-degree AV block is not well studied. Its occurrence is unpredictable and its incidence varies depending on the presence or absence of risk factors.

Patients with third-degree AV block are rarely asymptomatic, frequently presented with severe symptoms such as bradycardia, hypotension syncope, and sometimes hemodynamic instability. These CHB's patients have then a poor prognosis without any pacemaker implantation, especially if the patient has exhibited syncopal symptoms [19].

A sudden death in some patients whose cause can often be tachyarrhythmias secondary to the change in ventricular repolarization (prolongation of the QT interval) and sudden changes in frequency might be the result of this type of block.

A person with complete atrioventricular block compared to a person of the same age who does not present with a block has a survival rate during the first year of less than 50% [20].

As previously mentioned, it is difficult to predict the prognosis of these cases. Thus, a pacemaker should be implanted using the endocardial or epicardial approach in order to avoid any fatal evolution.

To sum up, the prognosis in atrioventricular (AV) block is directly linked to its degree. Individuals with AV block who are not treated with permanent pacing remain at risk for syncope and sudden cardiac death, especially cases with underlying structural heart disease [21].

Although pacemaker is the definitive treatment for patients in third-degree AV block, a recent study showed that a heart failure might be one of the most frequent consequences of pacemaker implantation [22].

Treatment/Management

The incipient management of bradycardic patients with symptoms is atropine according to advanced cardiac life support recommendations 2021 [23]. Epinephrine and dopamine are second-line drugs in treating bradycardia in third-degree heart block which are not responding to atropine (see Table 1). Transcutaneous pacing is more rapid, although both electrical and mechanical capture must be assured [24].

"If transcutaneous pacing is not successful, a transvenous pacemaker would be necessary. In cases of drug toxicity, transcutaneous pacing is not successful unless the underlying cause is treated" [24].

Table 1 Dosage of drugs used in complete heart block

Name of drugs	Atropine	Epinephrine	Dopamine
Dosing	1 mg	1 mg	400 mg
Time	3–5 min	2–10 mcg/min	5–20 mcg/kg/min

Multiple Choice Questions

1. Complete heart block is also called:
   A. First-degree heart block.
   B. Second-degree heart block.
   C. Third-degree heart block.
   D. Fourth-degree heart block.
   E. None of these.
2. Congenital complete-degree heart block is commonly linked to
   A. Down's syndrome.
   B. Systemic lupus erythematosus.
   C. Turner's syndrome.
   D. Hydrocephalus.
   E. All of these.
3. Which of the following drugs leads to complete degree heart block?
   A. Quinidine.
   B. Flecainide.
   C. Beta-blockers.
   D. Amiodarone.
   E. All of these.
4. Most common cause of complete degree heart block is:
   A. Coronary ischemia.
   B. Pneumonia.
   C. Thromboembolism.
   D. Sore throat.
   E. All of these.
5. Borrelia burgdorferi can cause.
   A. Lyme disease.
   B. Lyme carditis.
   C. Syphilis.
   D. Sore throat.
   E. Both A and B.
6. Complete degree heart block may be linked to:
   A. Hyperkalemia.
   B. Hypermagnesemia.
   C. Hyponatremia.
   D. Hypokalemia.
   E. None of these.
7. Risk factors of third-degree heart block include.
   A. Young age.
   B. Old age.
   C. Positive family history.
   D. Both B and C.
   E. All of these.
8. Definitive treatment for complete degree heart block is:
   A. Heart transplant.
   B. Beta-blockers.
   C. Artificial pacemaker.
   D. Chemotherapy.
   E. None of these.
9. Which drug prove promising in case of third-degree heart block?
   A. Atropine.
   B. Dopamine.
   C. Epinephrine.
   D. Beta-blockers.
   E. A, B, and C.
10. Patients with complete degree heart block are at increased risk of:
   A. Symptomatic bradycardia.
   B. Symptomatic tachycardia.
   C. Lung cancer.
   D. Pneumonia.
   E. All of these.

Answers

1. C.
2. B.
3. E.
4. A.
5. E.
   Explanation: Borrelia burgdorferi causes Lyme disease which can lead to Lyme carditis.
6. A
   Explanation: Hyperkalemia decreases the conduction velocity of the heart leading to complete-degree heart block.
7. D
   Explanation: Old age and positive family history are usually linked to complete-degree heart block.
8. C.
   Explanation: Definitive management option for complete degree heart block is insertion of pacemakers.
9. E.
   Explanation: Antimuscarinic drugs (atropine) and beta-adrenergic agonists (dopamine and epinephrine) may be helpful in managing complete degree heart block.
10. A

References

1. Vogler J, Breithardt G, Eckardt L. Bradyarrhythmias and conduction blocks. Rev Esp Cardiol. 2012;65(7):656–67.
2. Merchant FM, Hoskins MH, Musat DL, Prillinger JB, Roberts GJ, Nabutovsky Y, Mittal S. Incidence and time course for developing heart failure with high-burden right ventricular pacing. Circ Cardiovasc Qual Outcomes. 2017;10(6):e003564.
3. Eronen M, et al. Short-and long-term outcome of children with congenital complete heart block diagnosed in utero or as a newborn. Pediatrics. 2000;106(1):86–91.

4. Sholler GF, Walsh EP. Congenital complete heart block in patients without anatomic cardiac defects. Am Heart J. 1989;118(6):1193–8.

5. Groves AM, Allan LD, Rosenthal E. Outcome of isolated congenital complete heart block diagnosed in utero. Heart. 1996;75(2):190–4.

6. Cardiac Electrophysiology | PDF | Vagus Nerve | Cardiac Muscle [Internet]. Scribd. 2022 [cited 14 August 2022]. https://www.scribd.com/doc/154451030/Cardiac-Electrophysiology-1

7. Thambo J-B, et al. Detrimental ventricular remodeling in patients with congenital complete heart block and chronic right ventricular apical pacing. Circulation. 2004;110(25):3766–72.

8. Boutjdir M. Molecular and ionic basis of congenital complete heart block. Trends Cardiovasc Med. 2000;10(3):114–22.

9. Brucato A, et al. Risk of congenital complete heart block in newborns of mothers with anti-Ro/SSA antibodies detected by counterimmunoelectrophoresis: a prospective study of 100 women. Arthritis Rheum. 2001;44(8):1832–5.

10. Chandler SF, Fynn-Thompson F, Mah DY. Role of cardiac pacing in congenital complete heart block. Expert Rev Cardiovasc Ther. 2017;15(11):853–61.

11. Donofrio MT, et al. Congenital complete heart block: fetal management protocol, review of the literature, and report of the smallest successful pacemaker implantation. J Perinatol. 2004;24(2):112–7.

12. Jayaprasad N, Johnson F, Venugopal K. Congenital complete heart block and maternal connective tissue disease. Int J Cardiol. 2006;112(2):153–8.

13. Brucato A, et al. Normal neuropsychological development in children with congenital complete heart block who may or may not be exposed to high-dose dexamethasone in utero. Ann Rheum Dis. 2006;65(11):1422–6.

14. Pollack C. Differential diagnosis of cardiopulmonary disease. Cham: Springer; 2019.

15. Hutter D, Silverman ED, Jaeggi ET. The benefits of transplacental treatment of isolated congenital complete heart block associated with maternal anti-Ro/SSA antibodies: a review. Scand J Immunol. 2010;72(3):235–41.

16. Eronen M, Heikkilä P, Teramo K. Congenital complete heart block in the fetus: hemodynamic features, antenatal treatment, and outcome in six cases. Pediatr Cardiol. 2001;22(5):385–92.

17. Olshansky B, Chung M, Pogwizd S, Goldschlager N. Bradyarrhythmias—conduction system abnormalities. Arrhythm Essent. 2017:28–86.

18. Eronen M, et al. Relationship of maternal autoimmune response to clinical manifestations in children with congenital complete heart block. Acta Paediatr. 2004;93(6):803–9.

19. Ho A, et al. Isolated complete heart block in the fetus. Am J Cardiol. 2015;116(1):142–7.

20. Buyon JP, et al. Anti-Ro/SSA antibodies and congenital heart block: necessary but not sufficient. Arthritis Rheum. 2001;44(8):1723–7.

21. Ayyildiz P, et al. Evaluation of permanent or transient complete heart block after open heart surgery for congenital heart disease. Pacing Clin Electrophysiol. 2016;39(2):160–5.

22. Lin M-C, et al. Congenital complete heart block. Acta Paediatrica Taiwanica. 2001;42(1):42–5.

23. Yoshida H, et al. Treatment of fetal congenital complete heart block with maternal administration of beta-sympathomimetics (terbutaline). Gynecol Obstet Investig. 2001;52(2):142–4.

24. Knabben V, Chhabra L, Slane M. Third-degree atrioventricular block. [Updated 2022 May 22]. In: StatPearls [Internet]. Treasure Island, FL: StatPearls Publishing; 2022. https://www.ncbi.nlm.nih.gov/books/NBK545199/

Dextrocardia

Ibad Ur Rehman, Khadija Iqbal, and Irfan Ullah

Abstract

Dextrocardia is the first cardiac malposition that was described in the early seventeenth century. It can be explained as a right-sided heart with a base apex axis pointed toward the right side. It occurs very rarely and has 1 in 12,000 incidences. It occurs during development due to a defect in cardiac looping or laterality determination. Even though its cause has not been identified some association have been made with a defect in dynein or ciliary motility.

Patient suffering from dextrocardia can either be asymptomatic or present with a variety of symptoms, most of which can be attributed to the associated anomaly it presents with. In order to make a correct and accurate diagnosis, patients must undergo a thorough physical examination, imaging like X-ray, CT abdomen, ECG, echocardiogram, and cardiac catheterization. Interventions in these patients are comparatively difficult and require a different approach. Treatment in patients of dextrocardia majorly includes managing the underlying problems and anomalies. Special consideration must be given to associated cardiac anomalies before doing any cardiac surgery in such patients. Supportive treatment and counseling of patients and their attendants can be helpful in managing such patients in the long run.

Keywords

Dextrocardia · X-ray · Cardiac surgery · ECG Echocardiogram · Cyanosis · Sepsis · Dextroposition

Introduction

The human heart is aptly poised within the pericardial sac in the inferior part of the middle mediastinum typically residing on the left side of the thoracic cavity with its apex located deep to fifth intercostal space. Location of the heart anywhere but its usual position would be termed as a cardiac malposition [1]. Such a malposition may include surrounding organs and vessels or may be limited to the heart itself. Described first in 1606 by Fabricius, dextrocardia is believed to be the first cardiac malposition explained [2]. Dextrocardia (From Latin dexter meaning "right" and Greek kardia meaning "heart") is an uncommon congenital disorder in which the heart lies on the right side of the thoracic cavity instead of its usual position on the left. It is a malposition intrinsic to the heart and may happen in association with other congenital abnormalities [3]. Depending on the time of malformation, dextrocardia may present with situs solitus (dextrocardia with thoracoabdominal structures in their normal position), situs inversus (thoracoabdominal structures are mirrored from their normal position), or isomerism (heterotaxy syndrome) [4, 5].

Definitions

Before starting the discussion about dextrocardia, it is important to understand some definitions relevant to the disease [5–7] (Tables 1 and 2).

I. U. Rehman (✉)
Shifa College of Medicine, Shifa Tameer e Millat University, Islamabad, Pakistan

K. Iqbal
Al Nafees Medical College, Isra University, Islamabad, Pakistan

I. Ullah
Kabir Medical College, Gandhara University, Peshawar, Pakistan

148 I. U. Rehman et al.

Table 1 Shows different terms relevant to dextrocardia

Term	Description
Dextrocardia	Right-sided position of the heart in the thoracic cavity regardless of the cause
Levocardia	Left-sided position of the heart in the thoracic cavity
Mesocardia	When the heart is located in the midline
Situs solitus	Normal position of the visceral organs (liver and stomach)
Situs inversus	Left to right reversal in position of visceral organs (stomach on right and liver on left)
Situs inversus totalis	Dextrocardia in combination with situs inversus Also called as true dextrocardia/mirror image dextrocardia
Isolated dextrocardia	Dextrocardia in combination with situs solitus
Dextroposition	Pathology in which an anatomically correct heart is displaced to the right in the thoracic cavity

Table 2 Signs of BAV

Five components for diagnosing dextrocardia
1. Physical examination
2. Chest X-ray
3. ECG
4. Echocardiogram
5. Cardiac catheterization selective cineangiography

Epidemiology

The exact incidence of dextrocardia is unbeknown. Most of the population-based studies suggest that it is a rare disease with an incidence of 1 in 12,000 pregnancies [8–10]. It occurs in equal frequency in both male and female genders and has no predilection in terms of ethnicity or origin.

No of cases of situs solitus, situs inversus, and isomerism are found to be equal. On the other hand, associated cardiac malformations are found to be more common in the isomerism and situs inversus group and more severe in both situs solitus and isomerism group [9, 10].

As for its incidence in some of the associated malformations almost 50% of patients of primary ciliary dyskinesia present with situs inversus totalis and hence kartagener syndrome. Comparatively only 0.6% of patients having primary ciliary dyskinesia present with situs solitus [11–13].

Etiology

The etiology of dextrocardia depends on whether the pathology is primary or secondary [13]. Primary dextrocardia is always congenital while secondary dextrocardia can be both acquired and congenital. The exact reason for the heart pointing toward the right side instead of the left side of the chest

is unknown but it is thought to be secondary to the abnormal position of other organs during development [9, 11, 13, 14].

Some patients having dextrocardia with situs inversus totalis have issues with cilia responsible for filtering the air entering their air passage ways (primary ciliary dyskinesia). Kartagener syndrome is a subset of primary ciliary dyskinesia and represents the triad of paranasal sinusitis, situs inversus totalis, and primary ciliary dyskinesia. A defect in left-right dynein is seen in the syndrome and since dynein is involved in left-right asymmetry, it can cause dextrocardia [15].

In another type of dextrocardia, the abnormal position of the heart is accompanied by the abnormal assembly of other organs in thorax and abdominal region (heterotaxy). It is called the heterotaxy syndrome and is a sequalae of disrupted left-right axis orientation. It is a very serious condition associated with a high number of abdominal and cardiac defects including asplenia, abnormal gallbladder system, problem with lungs, and severe heart and blood vessel defects like anomalous pulmonary venous connections and systemic venous abnormalities [15, 16].

Pathophysiology

The precursor cells required for the development of the heart arise from the epiblast and migrate through the primitive streak into the splanchnic layer of mesoderm [17]. A cluster of cells forms the endocardial heart tubes. After the folding of embryo in the cranial and lateral directions, the change in position of the heart and fusion of tubes takes place to form a single tube on the ventral surface of the embryo into the pericardial cavity.

After the formation of heart tubes, the next step is the looping of heart tube which demarcates the relative positions of various chambers of heart.

The research shows that one of the causes of dextrocardia, in which the position of heart changes from left to right is abnormal looping of heart. Dextrocardia may be associated with a change in the position of viscera, i.e., situs inversus [17–20]. The critical period for developing laterality defects like dextrocardia is day 15–16. Faulty Bulbo ventricular looing may lead to L and D dextrocardia in hemithorax.

The second common cause for these defects is loss of ciliary motility as seen in Kartegners syndrome. In these cases association of respiratory infections with laterality defects is also seen. During gastrulation the fate mapping of embryo determining the right and left sides of the embryo is also the main cause predicted by the researchers. The key factor regulating the mechanism is serotonin (5-HT). During pregnancy, the intake of antidepressants of the selective serotonin inhibitors class can lead to an increase in heart defects [17–21] (Flow Chart 1).

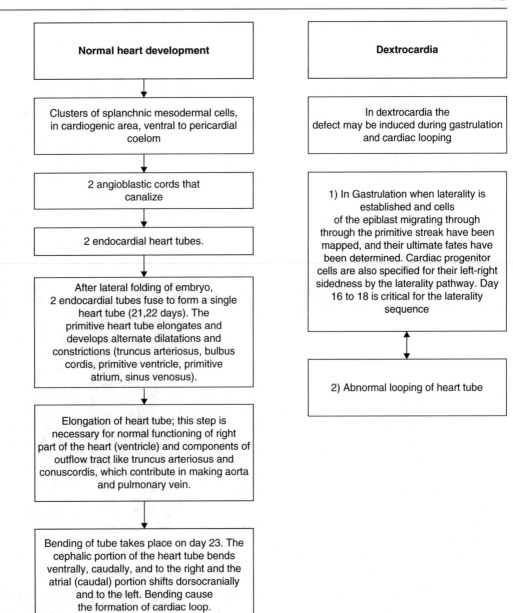

Flow Chart 1 Development of a normal heart versus dextrocardia [10–21]

Clinical Presentation

Clinical features in a patient with dextrocardia vary according to its type and whether it is isolated or happening in association with situs inversus totalis or as a subset of primary ciliary dyskinesia in the form of kartagener syndrome [22–24].

The simplest dextrocardia (without any association) is asymptomatic [22–26].

Symptoms

Patient might present with [27–29]

- Complaints of bluish discoloration (cyanosis).
- Breathing difficulties (dyspnea).
- Difficulties in growth (failure to thrive).
- Fatigue and tiredness.
- Yellow discoloration of skin and eyes (jaundice).
- Decreased exercise tolerance.

- Respiratory infections including repeated sinus or lung infections.
- Headache.
- Intestinal obstruction.

Sign

The detailed physical examination of a patient with dextrocardia can help in narrowing down the cause and type of dextrocardia. The patient may have following signs on examination [29–32]

- Cyanosis.
- Clubbing.
- Pulsations (apex beat on the right side).
- Palpation of apex beat on the right side of the chest.
- Heart sounds audible on the right side of the chest.

Evaluation of Physical Examination

In order to evaluate and diagnose dextrocardia patient's history of symptoms and physical examination including percussion and palpation are of utmost importance [33–36].

A detailed examination starts with a general physical examination in order to evaluate the patient's growth assessment and vitals including heart rate and pulse. Followed by inspection of all the abovementioned signs and symptoms especially pallor, skin discoloration, and signs of clubbing [29–32].

The next part is the examination of the precordium including inspection, palpation, and auscultation. Even though in a patient with dextrocardia heart would be on the right side instead of the left, the approach to the examination would be the same. The patient will be inspected for visible pulsations and prominent veins. It will be followed by palpation for apex beat, starting from the lower part of the right side of the chest instead of the left, then along the right parasternal border, and finally upper part of the left side of the chest. The examiner will look for the site and character of apex beat, parasternal heave, and palpable heart sound. In the last part, patients' heart will be auscultated and assessed for normal heart sounds, any other sounds or clicks, and murmurs (may present in patients having associating cardiac anomalies) [29–36].

Assessment on Investigations

In terms of prenatal diagnosis of dextrocardia, a wide spectrum of complex cardiac defects makes it very difficult to diagnose it on prenatal ultrasound. A comparatively newer method known as fetal intelligent navigation echocardiography (FINE) has proven to be a rapid and reliable method of detection of congenital heart diseases including dextrocardia [33].

1. Imaging studies.

In adults, imaging studies like an X-ray, CT scan, echocardiography (ECHO), MRI, and cardiac catheterization may all be used to assess and diagnose dextrocardia and even classify it.

- *Chest X-ray;* Its diagnosis on X-ray is mostly incidental in routine radiological examination revealing that the heart is not in its usual position. Chest radiography might show a right-sided cardiac silhouette which can also be seen in Figs. 1 and 2 [34–38].
- *CT Abdomen:* A CT abdomen might help to assess the position of visceral organs and further differentiate dextrocardia. In situs inversus totalis, liver will be seen on the left side and spleen on the right side [37–39].

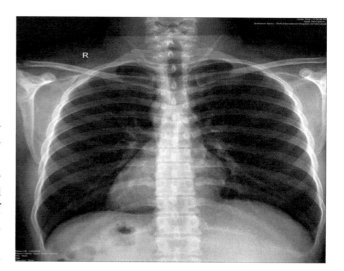

Fig. 1 X-ray of a patient with dextrocardia

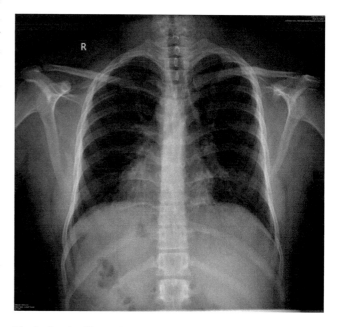

Fig. 2 Another X-ray of a patient with dextrocardia

- *Echocardiography*: Echocardiography is used to assess the structural defects and provide an analysis of the situs, connections, and anatomy of the heart. Color-flow echocardiography is more important than traditional echocardiography because it can help evaluate complex congenital heart defects associated with dextrocardia [39, 40].
2. Cardiac catheterization:

    Catheterization is not the study of choice for a patient with dextrocardia but when the heart anatomy is difficult to be evaluated by echocardiography it may be used [39, 40].
3. Electrocardiogram (ECG):

    The major features of dextrocardia on ECG are:
    - Right-axis deviation.
    - Negative P wave, QRS complex, and T wave in lead I.
    - Positive QRS complex in aVR.
    - Reversal of R-wave progression in the precordial leads.

It is important to note that in order to differentiate between human errors such as opposite limb electrode placement from situs inversus totalis R-wave progression should be traced. In situs inversus totalis, it would be absent [39, 40].

For testing and screening associated conditions like kartagener syndrome, some additional tests like nasal brush biopsy and nasal nitric oxide can be used. For confirmation of the diagnosis of underlying conditions of said syndrome (primary ciliary dyskinesia), genetic testing and electron microscopy can be used [37–41].

Treatment and Management

In terms of treatment and management of dextrocardia, interventions are not needed in the majority of the patients since they are asymptomatic, especially if there are no associated anomalies (cardiac or otherwise).

In patients who do present with symptoms or other congenital anomalies, interventions can be done. Although, medicines will be required before patients are ready for surgical intervention [42–44].

Medical

Medical treatment has no direct effect in managing dextrocardia however it can alleviate some of the symptoms these patients may present with. This treatment depends on the associated condition the patient has,

- Antibiotics should be used in patients having complaints of sinus or respiratory infections. Broad-spectrum antibi-

otics are also recommended in patients presenting with asplenia to fight off respiratory infections.
- Mucolytics and expectorants can be used to alleviate symptoms in patients presenting with primary ciliary dsykinesia in kartagener syndrome.
- Diuretics, ACE inhibitors, and certain ionotropic agents might be beneficial in certain cardiac anomalies patients might present with, in dextrocardia.

Surgical

In patients with associated cardiac anomalies such as transposition of great vessels (TGA), single ventricle (SV), ventral septal defect (VSD), and Tetrology of fallot (TOF) surgical intervention is required

- In surgical treatment primary goal is to treat the underlying defect. For this purpose, a fontan operation can be done or surgical exploration with anatomical correction can be performed.
- Patients having vascular anomalies and consequently heart blocks or defects in conduction of cardiac system can be evaluated for pacemakers.
- Dextrocardia patients with cardiac anomalies may require definitive treatment in the form of heart transplantation [44–48].

Complications

Depending on the type and associated anomalies untreated dextrocardia can progress to various systematic complications including:

Growth problems	Growth restriction, failure to thrive
Respiratory problem	Recurrent sinusitis, pneumonia, infections
Cardiac problems	Congestive cardiac failure
Intestinal problems	Intestinal malrotation and obstruction, asplenia
Genital problems	Infertility in males

Prognosis

Life expectancy and progress of patients with dextrocardia depend mainly on how the anomaly presents itself and what other congenital defects accompany it.

In isolated dextrocardia, mostly a disease-free life is expected without any complications relative to the location of the heart.

In newborns and younger children, complications like recurrent infections due to anomalies accompanying dextrocardia like asplenia can alter a patient's prognosis and prove to be fatal. Such conditions should be treated efficiently by using prophylactic antibiotics [47, 48].

Counseling and Educating Parents

If dextrocardia is identified at the time of birth timely counseling regarding its manifestation and presentation can be very helpful for the patient.

Parents must be informed regarding the heart's position, how it may affect their children's life, anomalies associated with it, and how it may lead to certain complications in them including infections, breathing problems, intestinal problems, and even infertility. They should also be informed how certain procedures like cardiac catheterization and surgical intervention might be a little more difficult in such patients.

Educating and communicating with the patients and their families regarding the disease is a very essential step in managing it [47].

Differential Diagnosis

There is a certain condition in which the heart can be located on the right side, it is important to identify them from dextrocardia so it can be timely managed.

These include kartageners syndrome, cardiac dextroposition, dextroversion, and heterotaxy [6].

Multiple Choice Questions

1. Which of the following period is critical for heart development and individuals with laterality defects like dextrocardia?
   A. Days 16–18.
   B. 20–24.
   C. 24–32.
   D. 32–36.
2. Congenital heart disease most frequently results from.
   A. Maternal medications.
   B. Rubella virus.
   C. Mutant genes.
   D. Fetal distress.
   E. Genetic and environmental factors.
3. When dextrocardia is associated with a normal position of other thoracoabdominal structures, it is called.
   A. Situs solitus.
   B. Situs inversus.
   C. Kartegner syndrome.
   D. Digeorge syndrome.
4. A 25-year-old primigravida visited the sonologist for routine US at 6 weeks. The sonologist told the mother that the heart tube has not yet differentiated into different chambers of heart. From the arterial to the venous end, the heart tube differentiates into which of the following chambers:
   A. Bulbuscordis, the ventricle, the atrium, sinus venosus.
   B. Bulbuscordis,, the atrium, the ventricle, sinus venosus.
   C. The ventricle, bulbuscordis, the atrium, sinus venosus.
   D. Bulbuscordis, the ventricle, sinus venosus, the atrium.
   E. The atrium, bulbuscordis, the ventricle, sinus venosus.
5. A female baby was born to a primigravida. After delivery the baby developed cyanosis. On US a defect was present between atrium and ventricles. This defect is known as which of the following:
   A. Foramen primum.
   B. Foraman ovale.
   C. Fossa ovalis.
   D. Foraman secundum.
   E. Crista terminalis.
6. Which of the following congenital defects is the direct outcome of malformation of the spiral partitioning of the conuscordis and truncusarteriosus?
   A. Double aortic arch.
   B. Transposition of the great vessels.
   C. Patent foramen ovale.
   D. Ventricular septal defect (VSD).
   E. Ectopiacordis.
7. A newborn baby is diagnosed with Fallotstetrology. The echocardiographic view shows the associated defects: pulmnory stenosis, ventricular septal defect, and hypertrophied left ventricle. The ventricular septal defect reflects a developmental failure of which of the following structures?
   A. Septum secundum.
   B. Bulbuscordis.
   C. Endocardial cushions.
   D. Truncusarteriosus.
   E. Sinus venosus.
8. Which of the following is important for establishing laterality during gastrulation for patterning the right and left sides of the heart:
   A. Serotonin (5-HT].
   B. TWISTI.
   C. MSX2.
   D. EFNB1 encodes ephrin-BI.
9. All the following are true with respect to heart development except.
   A. During weeks 2–3 the single heart tube is divided into four chambers.
   B. The right and left sides of the heart are separated from each other by the endocardial cushions.
   C. The endocardial cushions appear on the dorsal and ventral walls of the heart tube in the midline, grow toward one another, and fuse.
   D. Fusion of the endocardial cushions result in the right and left atrioventricular canals.
   E. Fusion of the endocardial cushions initiates the separation of the atria and ventricles of the heart.

10. All the following are true with respect to heart development except.

A. As the bulboventricular loop forms, the primitive atrium is carried behind (dorsal to) the primitive ventricle.

B. The sinus venosus attached to the primitive atrium has a left and right horn with three vessels entering each horn.

C. The vessels entering each horn of the sinus venosus are the supracardinal, subcardinal, and posterior cardinal veins.

D. As the two atria form, the right horn of the sinus venosus which has enlarged is incorporated into the wall of the right atrium.

E. The embryonic atrium persists as the right auricle, the rough-walled appendage of the atrium.

Answers

1. A.
2. E.
3. A.
4. A.
5. B.
6. B.
7. C.
8. A.
9. A.
10. C.

References

1. Perloff JK. The cardiac malpositions. Am J Cardiol. 2011;108(9):1352–61.
2. Mendelson M. Dextrocardia. In: ECG in emergency medicine and acute care. Philadelphia, PA: Elsevier; 2005. p. 227–9.
3. Grey DP, Cooley DA. Dextrocardia with situs inversus totalis: Cardiovascular surgery in three patients with concomitant coronary artery disease. Cardiovasc Dis. 1981;8(4):527–30.
4. Lev M, Liberthson RR, Eckner FA, Arcilla RA. Pathologic anatomy of dextrocardia and its clinical implications. Circulation. 1968;37(6):979–99.
5. Evans WN, Acherman RJ, Collazos JC, Castillo WJ, Rollins RC, Kip KT, et al. Dextrocardia: practical clinical points and comments on terminology. Pediatr Cardiol. 2010;31(1):1–6.
6. Rao PS. Dextrocardia: systematic approach to differential diagnosis. Am Heart J. 1981;102(3 Pt 1):389–403.
7. Rogel S, Schwartz A, Rakower J. The differentiation of dextroversion from dextroposition of the heart and their relation to pulmonary abnormalities. Dis Chest. 1963;44(2):186–92.
8. Bohun CM, Potts JE, Casey BM, Sandor GGS. A population-based study of cardiac malformations and outcomes associated with dextrocardia. Am J Cardiol. 2007;100(2):305–9.
9. Kennedy MP, Omran H, Leigh MW, Dell S, Morgan L, Molina PL, et al. Congenital heart disease and other heterotaxic defects in a large cohort of patients with primary ciliary dyskinesia. Circulation. 2007;115(22):2814–21.
10. Mitchell SC, Korones SB, Berendes HW. Congenital heart disease in 56,109 births. Incidence and natural history. Circulation. 1971;43(3):323–32.
11. Samánek M, Slavík Z, Zborilová B, Hrobonová V, Vorísková M, Skovránek J. Prevalence, treatment, and outcome of heart disease in live-born children: a prospective analysis of 91,823 live-born children. Pediatr Cardiol. 1989;10(4):205–11.
12. Hoffman JI. Incidence of congenital heart disease: I. Postnatal incidence. Pediatr Cardiol. 1995;16(3):103–13.
13. Gupta S, Handa KK, Kasliwal RR, Bajpai P. A case of Kartagener's syndrome: Importance of early diagnosis and treatment. Indian J Hum Genet. 2012;18(2):263–7.
14. Hanson JS, Tabakin BS. Primary and secondary dextrocardia. Their differentiation and the role of cineangiocardiography in diagnosing associated congenital cardiac defects. Am J Cardiol. 1961;8(2):275–81.
15. Wolla CD, Hlavacek AM, Schoepf UJ, Bucher AM, Chowdhury S. Cardiovascular manifestations of heterotaxy and related situs abnormalities assessed with CT angiography. J Cardiovasc Comput Tomogr. 2013;7(6):408–16.
16. Jacobs JP, Anderson RH, Weinberg PM, Walters HL 3rd, Tchervenkov CI, Del Duca D, et al. The nomenclature, definition and classification of cardiac structures in the setting of heterotaxy. Cardiol Young. 2007;17 Suppl 2(S2):1–28.
17. Lints TJ, Parsons LM, Hartley L, et al. Nkx-2.5: a novel murine homeobox gene expressed in early heart progenitor cells and their myogenic descendants. Development. 1993;119:419–31.
18. de la Cruz MV, Sanchez-Gómez C, Cayre R. The developmental components of ventricles: their significance in congenital malformations. Cardiol Young. 1991;1:123–8.
19. Black BL, Olson EN. Control of cardiac development by the MEF2 family of transcription factors. In: Harvey RP, Rosenthal N, editors. Heart development. London: Academic Press; 1999. p. 131–42.
20. Knauth A, McCarthy KP, Webb S, et al. Interatrial communication through the mouth of the coronary sinus defect. Cardiol Young. 2002;12:364–72.
21. Webb S, Kanani M, Anderson RH, et al. Development of the human pulmonary vein and its incorporation in the morphologically left atrium. Cardiol Young. 2001;11:632–42.
22. Queiroz RM, Filho FB. Kartagener's syndrome. Pan Afr Med J. 2018;29(160):160.
23. Arunabha DC, Sumit RT, Sourin B, Sabyasachi C, Subhasis M. Kartagener's syndrome: a classical case. Ethiop J Health Sci. 2014;24(4):363–8.
24. Dilorenzo M, Weinstein S, Shenoy R. Tetralogy of fallot with dextrocardia and situs inversus in a 7-year-old boy. Tex Heart Inst J. 2013;40(4):481–3.
25. Ortiz RO, Ali MJ, Lopez FA. CLINICAL CASE OF THE MONTH: a review of situs inversus and dextrocardia. J La State Med Soc. 2015;167(2):102–4.
26. Rubbo B, Lucas JS. Clinical care for primary ciliary dyskinesia: current challenges and future directions. Eur Respir Rev. 2017;26(145):170023.
27. Xie L, Zhao J, Shen J. Clinical diagnostic approach to congenital agenesis of right lung with dextrocardia: a case report with review of literature: lung agenesis. Clin Respir J. 2016;10(6):805–8.
28. Badui E, Lepe L, Solorio S, Sánchez H, Enciso R, García P. Heart block in dextrocardia with situs inversus. A case report. Angiology. 1995;46(6):537–40.
29. Fraser FC, Teebi AS, Walsh S, Pinsky L. Poland sequence with dextrocardia: which comes first? Am J Med Genet. 1997;73(2):194–6.
30. Fox CJ 3rd, Keflemariam Y, Cornett EM, Urman RD, Rapoport Y, Shah B, et al. Structural heart issues in dextrocardia: Situs type matters. Ochsner J. 2021;21(1):111–4.

31. Rapoport Y, Fox CJ, Khade P, Fox ME, Urman RD, Kaye AD. Perioperative implications and management of dextrocardia. J Anesth. 2015;29(5):769–85.

32. Fulcher AS, Turner MA. Abdominal manifestations of situs anomalies in adults. Radiographics. 2002;22(6):1439–56.

33. Yeo L, Luewan S, Markush D, Gill N, Romero R. Prenatal diagnosis of dextrocardia with complex congenital heart disease using fetal intelligent navigation echocardiography (FINE) and a literature review. Fetal Diagn Ther. 2018;43(4):304–16.

34. Walmsley R, Hishitani T, Sandor GGS, Lim K, Duncan W, Tessier F, et al. Diagnosis and outcome of dextrocardia diagnosed in the fetus. Am J Cardiol. 2004;94(1):141–3.

35. Offen S, Jackson D, Canniffe C, Choudhary P, Celermajer DS. Dextrocardia in adults with congenital heart disease. Heart Lung Circ. 2016;25(4):352–7.

36. Sharma P, Nagarajan V, Underwood DA. Heart on the right may sometimes be "right". Cleve Clin J Med. 2015;82(4):206–8.

37. Abd Elrazek AE, Shehab A, Elnour AA, Al Nuaimi SK, Baghdady S. Colon in the chest: An incidental dextrocardia A case report study. Medicine (Baltimore). 2015;94(6):e507.

38. Yusuf SW, Durand JB, Lenihan DJ, Swafford J. Dextrocardia: an incidental finding. Tex Heart Inst J. 2009;36(4):358–9.

39. Ogunlade O, Ayoka AO, Akomolafe RO, Akinsomisoye OS, Irinoye AI, Ajao A, et al. The role of electrocardiogram in the diagnosis of dextrocardia with mirror image atrial arrangement and ventricular position in a young adult Nigerian in Ile-Ife: a case report. J Med Case Rep. 2015;9(1):222.

40. Garg N, Agarwal BL, Modi N, Radhakrishnan S, Sinha N. Dextrocardia: an analysis of cardiac structures in 125 patients. Int J Cardiol. 2003;88(2–3):143–55. discussion 155-6

41. Huhta JC, Hagler DJ, Seward JB, Tajik AJ, Julsrud PR, Ritter DG. Two-dimensional echocardiographic assessment of dextrocardia: a segmental approach. Am J Cardiol. 1982;50(6):1351–60.

42. Ji Y-Q, Sun P-W, Hu J-X. Diagnosis and surgical treatment of congenital dextrocardia. Di Yi Jun Yi Da Xue Xue Bao. 2002;22(6):536–8.

43. Duong SQ, Godown J, Soslow JH, Thurm C, Hall M, Sainathan S, et al. Increased mortality, morbidities, and costs after heart transplantation in heterotaxy syndrome and other complex situs arrangements. J Thorac Cardiovasc Surg. 2019;157(2):730–740.e11.

44. Chang YL, Wei J, Chang C-Y, Chuang Y-C, Sue S-H. Cardiac transplantation in situs inversus: two cases reports. Transplant Proc. 2008;40(8):2848–51.

45. Guo G, Yang L, Wu J, Sun L. Implantation of VVI pacemaker in a patient with dextrocardia, persistent left superior vena cava, and sick sinus syndrome: A case report: A case report. Medicine (Baltimore). 2017;96(5):e6028.

46. Karigyo CJT, Batalini F, Murakami AN, Teruya RT, Gregori JF. Off-pump triple coronary artery bypass grafting in a patient with situs inversus totalis: Case presentation and a brief review of the Brazilian and the international experiences. Braz J Cardiovasc Surg. 2016;31(2):198–202.

47. Maldjian PD, Saric M. Approach to dextrocardia in adults: review. AJR Am J Roentgenol. 2007;188(6 Suppl):S39–49. quiz S35-8

48. Nesta M, Mazza A, Perri G, Bruno P, Massetti M. Repair of posterior infarct ventricular septal defect in a patient with dextrocardia and situs inversus: Repair of septal defect in dextrocardia. J Card Surg. 2016;31(3):147–9.

Double Inlet Left Ventricle

Ahmed Dheyaa Al-Obaidi, Abeer Mundher Ali,
Sara Shihab Ahmad, Abbas Kamil sh. Khalaf,
Ali Talib Hashim, and Mohammed Qasim Mohammed

Abstract

The double inlet left ventricle is a congenital cardiac abnormality, which means it exists from birth. The heart's top collecting chambers, the right and the left atria (plural to atrium), are attached to similar bottom ventricle or, pumping chamber, under this scenario. One of the ventricles of the heart's in some situations might be unusually small. Because neonates with common-inlet LV are extremely rare, those two concepts might be related to the development of the human heart and considered to be separate from septation of the atrioventricular canal apparently. The common-inlet right ventricle is a rare occurrence that usually arises in the context of heterotaxia syndrome. Benoit Bruneau, a developmental biologist, and his equals discovered molecular foundation related to the ventricular septum creation by an exclusive series of experiments. The presence of T-box Tbx5 (transcription factor) is connected to the creation of ventricular septum in mammals and humans (low in the right ventricle and high in the left one, and exactly in the location of the septum formation there is a sharp boundary of expression). The homozygous Tbx5 null mouse was found to be dead at 10.5 embryonic days with an LV that has severe hypoplasia and a slew of other abnormalities, highlighting the protein's importance in so many facets of embryonic development.

Keywords

Double inlet left ventricle · Single ventricle · Interstage remissions · Heterotaxy syndrome · Primary ciliary dyskinesia

Introduction

The double inlet left ventricle is a congenital cardiac abnormality, which means it exists from birth. The heart's top collecting chambers, the right and left atria (plural to atrium), are attached to similar bottom ventricle, or pumping chamber, under this scenario. One of the heart's ventricles may be unusually tiny in some situations. The right and left atriums (plural: atria) are located just at the upper area of the human heart, and the right and left ventricles are located at the bottom. The ventricle and atria transport blood into and at the same time from the body parts by arteries (which transfer the blood from the heart) and veins (which bring the blood into the heart). Blood that requires oxygen pass into the right atrium through huge veins known as the vena cava, then it passes to the right ventricle, which drives the blood via the pulmonary artery into lungs, where it is oxygenated. After that it returns back to the left atrium in the heart, as it will be collected and then transported to the left ventricle, which then drains the blood fully oxygenated to the whole-body parts through the aorta, a big artery. A left ventricle that functions normally (the chamber that pumps the blood into the body) and the presence of tiny right ventricle are common in babies with a left ventricle with double inlet (the chamber that pumps the blood into the lungs). The left ventricle receives the blood from the two atria. Therefore, the two types of blood one rich in oxygen and the other oxygen depleted are mixed together. The baby's lungs and body receive this blend of blood. The two inlets left ventricle is sometimes known as the single ventricle or common ventricle [1].

A. D. Al-Obaidi · A. K. s. Khalaf · M. Q. Mohammed
College of Medicine, University of Baghdad, Baghdad, Iraq
e-mail: abbas.kamel1700b@comed.uobaghdad.edu.iq;
Mohammed.Qasem1700d@comed.uobaghdad.edu.iq

A. M. Ali · S. S. Ahmad
M.B.Ch.B, Baghdad, Iraq

A. T. Hashim (✉)
Golestan University of Medical Sciences, Gorgan, Iran

Term "single ventricle" is used to refer to the double-inlet ventricle or common inlet ventricle, 2 (or more, if an atrium with double outlet is also present), a common AV orifice or AV orifices, that opens into single ventricular chamber, correspondingly. Early embryonic development in humans, a high-resolution analysis from Carnegie stages 13–23 (30–56 embryonic days) had confirmed that two processes at least must go wrong in order to develop a left ventricle (LV) with double inlet: loss of common (unseptated) AV canal to shift from its original into rightward forming an arrangement over the ultimate LV at day 30 and concomitant failure of the common (unseptated) atrioventricular canal to rightward movement.

Because neonates with common-inlet LV are extremely rare, these two processes might be linked in heart development of the human and to be free apparently of septation of the AV canal. The common-inlet right ventricle is a rare occurrence that usually arises in the context of heterotaxia syndrome [2].

Benoit Bruneau, a developmental biologist, and his equals discovered molecular foundation related to the ventricular septum creation by an exclusive series of experiments. The presence of T-box Tbx5 (transcription factor) is connected to the creation of ventricular septum in mammals and humans (low in the right ventricle and high in the left one, and exactly in the location of the septum formation there is a sharp boundary of expression). The homozygous Tbx5 null mouse was found to be dead at 10.5 embryonic days with an LV that has severe hypoplasia and a slew of other abnormalities, highlighting the protein's importance in so many facets of embryonic development. Tbx5 is expressed throughout the lone ventricular chamber during early development in an animal with only one ventricle as the turtle. Bruneau's lab genetically modified mice in order to express at a moderate level Tbx5 throughout the heart of the embryo, like in turtles, rather than the normal gradient steep left-right, to illustrate that the amount of the Tbx5 is considered to be causal rather than correlative of the formation of the ventricular septum. Despite the left-right differences in the expression in ventricular of other genes like atrial natriuretic peptide (Nppa) maintained, the offspring of these mice had no ventricular septum formation. A circulation of Fontan-type is characterized by biliary having and hepatic failure with cirrhosis probability, a low ejection efficiency paired with a high afterload, and protein-losing enteropathy. Short stature, atrial tachyarrhythmias, venous collaterals from systemic venous to pulmonary ones, thromboembolism, collaterals from systemic artery to pulmonary artery, esophageal varices, and plastic bronchitis are some of the most serious complications. Further information regarding the technical compo-

nents of the operation of modified Fontan can be found in other places.

DILV is associated with other congenital heart malformations:

- Coarctation of the aorta.
- Pulmonary stenosis.
- Pulmonary atresia.

Causes

In humans, the reason of a solitary ventricle is unremarkable. Till now, minimally ten targeted single-gene defects have resulted in mice in RV hypoplasia, which is similar to a single left ventricle (LV). Global nulls in Nkx2.5, Isl1, dHand (also known as Hand2), Mef2c, Fog-2, Fgf8 hypomorph, Foxh1, TGF 2, Bop, and Has2 are along the disruptions. A shared atrioventricular orifice is also seen in the Fog-2 null, which is virtually fully across the future LV (i.e., common-inlet ventricle). It has to be seen whether hypomorphic alleles of similar mutations in humans cause a single ventricle phenotype to develop but do not lead to mortality in embryonic life [3].

Tbx5 misexpression in the ventricles (as explained in the introduction section) and GATA4 inactivation in the myocardium cause a single ventricle.

Pathophysiology

Because the pulmonary and systemic circulations are normally parallel and connected at two levels: atrial and ductal, no circulatory abnormality is observed throughout fetal development. Postnatal cyanosis is caused by an inability of the systemic and pulmonary circulations to separate, with severity determined by the concurrent pulmonary outflow tract obstruction extent. Patients with an aortic arch obstruction and single ventricle are considered to be the least patients to develop cyanosis because pulmonary stenosis is never developed, but their lower body circulation is compromised due to the narrowing of the ductus arteriosus.

Prognosis

The great majority of patients should have a minimum of 20 years of life. Severe AV valve regurgitation is associated with a much worse prognosis. Unlike hypoplastic left heart syndrome, where completing only the first stage (Norwood procedure) is clearly superior, the vast majority of patients who have a single ventricle have a single (LV) left ventricle, so extremis is not present, and remain stable fairly for years after palliation initially, which includes a completed systemic to pulmonary connection [4].

Between 2000 and 2011, a retrospective analysis of 368 children with a single ventricle who received a procedure as Norwood and 118 children who received an aortopulmonary shunt indicated that both groups had comparable interstage mortality. In comparison to the surviving newborns, at surgery reduced weight and the occurrence of arrhythmias were considered as risk factors for interstage death in infants treated with shunt. Interstage remissions were common (75%) in another retrospective analysis (2012–2016) of 57 infants who had received hybrid surgical palliation stage 1, with 17% due to substantial side effects. Between phases, the mortality rate was found to be 7%. It's still unclear if the cavopulmonary circulation can duplicate or even outperform this level of life quality over a period of 30 years. In the pediatric population, the long-term effects of a mean systemic venous pressure greater than 10 mm Hg are unknown. The level of coexisting pulmonary outflow tract stenosis (or, alternatively, aortic blockage) as well as the ductus arteriosus reduction in the caliber establish the severity and timing of presentation. Before discharge to home screening could help identify those infants who have symptoms before they develop using newborn pulse oximetry [5].

Patients who have single ventricles and in the same time have extracardiac abnormalities have more risk factors more likely (e.g., low weight, prematurity), require a longer period of recovery following first-stage palliation, and have a higher interstage mortality and hospital rate.

Complications

Following the Fontan operation, patients may experience pleural effusions, pericardial effusions, and ascites. Thoracic and abdominal effusions, long regarded as the most agonizing postoperative early complication following Fontan completion, typically persisted for weeks and usually caused cardiac output impairment. Prior to early 1990s, those issues had a threat to exclude Fontan's principle application in the majority of patients who have a single ventricle. Despite there is a fact stating that the molecular and cellular basis of this situation is unknown, surgeons have begun to use several less-than-complete Fontan surgeries as a last resort.

Since higher than 80% of the patients acquired collaterals for intrahepatic venuses, that results in increased shunts from right to left, Lecompte's followed by Norwood's partial hepatic vein exclusion technique was widely abandoned. As a result, the fenestrated Fontan procedure proposed by Laks has been the most extensively used complete Fontan operation since the late 1990s. After the fenestrated Fontan (extracardiac conduit or lateral tunnel), early postoperative exuberant problems are minimized considerably, mostly because of a lower central venous pressure. However, rather than the mid-1990s found following nonpenetrated Fontan, saturation of arterial oxygen is frequently in low-1990s or in the upper 1980s [6].

Atrial Tachyarrhythmias

Are one type of tachyarrhythmia that affects the heart:

- This is considered the most common of the multiple late complications that can occur after various Fontan alterations, and it can be a symptom of hemodynamic deterioration. Due to the common comorbidity of dysfunction of sinus node, the reason for this problem is likely complicated, and treatment could be difficult. Surgical treatment looks to be more effective than medicinal treatment. Trauma during surgery to the sinus node or its concomitant blood supply is one of the current explanations for the origin of sinus node dysfunction. Also known as bidirectional Glenn surgery, subsequently extracardiac conduit (instead of the lateral tunnel) installation, was not successful in lowering the prevalence of sinus node dysfunction as a substitute to hemi-Fontan operation. This could be due to the fact that the sinus node region is considered not well defined by microscope, making measures to keep away from it (such as the bidirectional Glenn) ineffective.

Thromboembolism

Nearly 10% of those who survive the fenestrated Fontan procedure have venous thrombosis, but not arterial thrombosis. This complication's source is unknown. The pulmonary arteries and cerebral veins are examples of possible sites. Normal cardiac output, normal intracardiac blood flow pulsatility, and altered hepatic synthesis of thrombolytic pathway components endogenously had all been presented as plausible causes. The rule is hepatic dysfunction, as concluded by galactose elimination half-life and prothrombin time.

Malformations of the Pulmonary Arteriovenous System

This consequence of the hemi-Fontan surgery and its variants can occasionally be addressed following Fontan procedure lower than complete (of the lateral tunnel, hepatic vein exclusion varieties, or extracardiac conduit). When performed directly into the pulmonary arteries during cardiac catheterization, contrast echocardiography was found to be a method for the identification of pulmonary arteriovenous malformations with high sensitivity.

Plastic Bronchitis

The formation of mucinous bronchial casts is a symptom of this condition. Palliation has been described via atrial pacing, fenestration, or heart transplantation.

Systemic-to-Pulmonary Arterial Collaterals Are Formed

Collaterals from the systemic artery can transport the whole ventricular output and to the pulmonary artery which can take up to 40% of the total ventricular output. It is unknown whether it is due to the previous bidirectional Glenn or hemi-Fontan or the fenestration that was created surgically that results in arterial desaturation. While MRI is an efficient and non-invasive diagnostic tool for hemodynamic evaluation and screening, intervention and visualization by an angiography is usually required.

Clinical Features

History

Cyanosis occurs in newborns with a substantial pulmonary outflow tract obstruction and single ventricle, however additional symptoms are usually not found. Rapid breathing, lethargy, and poor feeding may occur in neonates who had a single ventricle and an aortic arch or systemic outflow tract obstruction.

Physical Examination

Keep the following in mind:

- Patients with significant pulmonary outflow tract stenosis have cyanosis.
- Patients having a single ventricle and at the same time having an aortic obstruction or significant systemic outflow tract have poor peripheral perfusion.
- Unless the right subclavian artery is abnormal, a blood pressure difference is noted between the lower extremity and right arm if interrupted or coarctation is involved with aortic obstruction.
- The first heartbeat is typical.
- The second heart sound is usually a single sound.
- Patients with pulmonary or systemic outflow tract stenosis have a systolic ejection murmur.
- Breathing problems.
- Poor feeding.
- Sweating may occur.
- Heart failure and heart murmur also.

Differential Diagnosis

The symptoms and signs of coexisting aortic arch blockage must be recognized. Inadequately alleviated the aortic stenosis, subaortic stenosis, or both should be recognized by clinicians. Children with single-ventricle cardiac physiology frequently require airway examination and intervention, and those who have undergone high-risk cardiac procedures are more likely to experience recurrent laryngeal nerve injury. Presence of subglottic stenosis appears to be the strongest predictor of the necessity for a tracheostomy in these patients [7].

When examining patients with a single ventricle, keep the following things in mind:

- Complicated malformation of the heart with arch blockage or aortic stenosis.
- Arch obstruction, or a component pulmonary stenosis or both of them as a complex heart malformation,
- Sepsis in newborns.

DD of Double Inlet Left Ventricle

1. The Double Outlet RV Surgery.
2. Heterotaxy, Polysplenia.
3. Heterotaxy Syndrome and Primary Ciliary Dyskinesia.
4. The Neonatal Sepsis.
5. A Pediatric Valvar Aortic Stenosis.
6. A Pediatric Hypoplastic Left Heart Syndrome.
7. Corrected Great Arteries Transposition by a Surgical Procedure.
8. A Protein-Losing Enteropathy.
9. The Valvar Pulmonary Stenosis.
10. The Surgical Treatment of Pediatric Hypoplastic Left Heart Syndrome.

Classification DILV (Fig. 1)

1. *DILV associated with leftward aorta and anterior (left-handed ventricular topology l-looped ventricles).*
   - Commonest variant.
   - Right-sided morphological left ventricle.
   - A left-sided subaortic with hypoplastic RV/incomplete cavity.
   - Straddling and severe overriding of the left-sided atrioventricular valve which results in its relation to the left ventricle,

   - The ventricular septal defect gives connection to a hypoplastic left side right ventricle.
   - The morphological size of the cavity of the RV might be different from being very hypoplastic to 75% only.
   - A restrictive VSD could be associated with obstruction of the subaortic area.

2. *DILV associated with rightward aorta and an anterior (right-handed/D-looped ventricular topology).*
   - Right-sided hypoplasia of the subaortic area incomplete/hypoplastic right ventricular cavity.
   - Ventricular septal defect offers connection to a hypoplastic RV.
   - Morphologic left ventricle which is left-sided.
   - The aorta is located rightward and anterior.
   - A restrictive VSD could be associated with obstruction of the subaortic area.

3. *DILV associated with normal great arteries (right-handed/D-looped ventricular topology).*
   - Known also as Holmes Heart.
   - Morphologic left ventricle on the left side.
   - Right-sided hypoplasia of the subaortic area incomplete/hypoplastic right ventricular cavity.
   - The VSD might function as a substitute for the obstruction of the pulmonary outflow tract which might be favorable to certain degree and will result in a stable circulation.
   - The ventricular septal defect gives connection into a hypoplastic RV.

Fig. 1 The classification of DILV

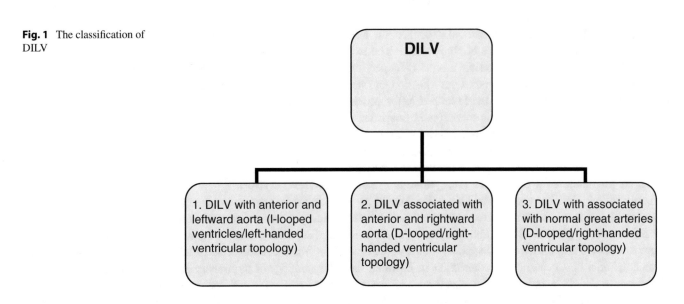

Diagnosis

Laboratory Investigations

In the preoperative investigations for the single ventricle, no special laboratory blood testing is required, though entire genome inexpensive sequencing will likely be helpful in the near future. Differentiating in between the conditions of single ventricle with arch blockage and the same conditions with severe pulmonary stenosis, aortic stenosis, or both of them can often be done with pulse oximetry or a measurement of arterial blood gas. When prostaglandin E1 is not given, a partial pressure of oxygen greater than 50 mm Hg reduces the chance of substantial pulmonary stenosis in a newborn with a single ventricle. The detection of fecal alpha1-antitrypsin after a Fontan operation is critical in monitoring for the complication of protein-losing. The reason behind that is the liver being the source of albumin endogenously, a low level of serum albumin suggests that the liver is unable to provide compensation for protein excessive loss or insufficient intake of protein [8].

Imaging

Two-Dimensional Echocardiography and Doppler Analysis

The single ventricle is diagnosed via two-dimensional echocardiography. It's simple to distinguish between pulmonary outflow tract stenosis, aortic stenosis, and an aortic arch obstruction. The specific atrioventricular connection also with the alignment ventricles are easily revealed. The two most famous kinds of single ventricle are the L-looped left ventricle associated with great arteries transposition and stenosis of the subpulmonary and the D-looped left ventricle associated with the same previous conditions. L-looped single left ventricle associated with great arteries transposition and hypoplasia of the aortic arch is considered as third mostly prevalent kind. D-looped single left ventricle that has regular alignment of great arteries (i.e., pulmonary artery from outflow chamber aorta from LV), often known as a Holmes heart, is the fourth most frequent type. The subaortic stenosis usually presents at the same time in single LVs with great arteries transposition and obstruction of the aortic arch because of a narrowing at the connection in between the rudimentary right ventricle (outlet chamber) and the LV. Bulboventricular foramen or exit foramen are common names for this opening.

Chest X-Ray

The results of chest radiography can differ. The cardiac silhouette could be normal to moderately enlarged in patients who have pulmonary stenosis. Vascularity of the lungs is not increased. The profile of the cardiac is usually modestly expanded in cases of arch blockage.

ECG

A septal q waves are found in precordial leads on the right side (in conditions with a single LV the L-looped type) and there is common findings like the presence of R/S pattern found monotonously over the anterior side of the precordium.

Holter Placement

It is particularly beneficial following the Fontan procedure done for surveillance to check the presence of sick sinus syndrome, supraventricular arrhythmias, and conduction blockage following a hemi-Fontan procedure (or a bidirectional Glenn procedure).

MRI

It is used to assess the following:

- The Physiology: cines of the systemic venous rout, Cines of the pulmonary arteries and cines of the short axis of the ventricle (to study ventricular performance).
- The inferior vena cava, superior vena cava, aorta, and branches of pulmonary arteries were all mapped for velocity.
- Viability imaging, three-dimensional reconstruction, and post-gadolinium injection.
- Anatomy: Bright blood images that are SSFP, which stands for steady-state free precession. Static images of dark blood shown as double inversion; and HASTE (half of Fourier acquisition single-shot turbo spin-echo sequences).

Catheterization

Cardiac catheterization is used to assess Fontan surgery candidacy, characterize post-Fontan hemodynamics, and manage supraventricular arrhythmic problems. In most patients, interventional correction (balloon angioplasty or endovascular stenting) of pulmonary artery stenosis, aortic recoarctation, and collateral vessel embolization has become the therapy of choice. Catheterization hazards include vascular disruption during balloon dilation, hemorrhage, nausea, vomiting, and pain, as well as arterial or venous blockage due to spasm or thrombosis.

Blood vessel rupture, bradyarrhythmias, tachyarrhythmias, and vascular blockage are all possible complications [9].

Treatment

Patients with a single ventricle should be admitted for tests and surgery. Patients with a single ventricle are supposed to be evaluated as an inpatient in an intensive care unit. Patients with severe pulmonary outflow tract or aortic arch obstruction should receive intravenous prostaglandin E1 immediately after birth. The initial arterial blood gas test is the best indicator of the requirement for an arterial line and assisted ventilation. Prior to the Fontan operation, patients' resting cardiac index ranges from 70 to 80 percent normally. Additionally, ability to raise cardiac output is limited and usually leads to a reduction in exercise capacity.

Surgical Procedures

There are three main procedures used to treat DILV which are:

1. *Blalock-Taussig shunt*: This is the initial surgery that is normally performed within the first weeks of the life of the baby, and it involves the use of a tiny tube to guide blood flow to the lungs.
2. *The Glenn treatment* is done within the first 6 months of the baby's life, and surgeons direct blood flow from the upper body to the pulmonary artery, allowing the blood to collect oxygen from the lungs without passing through the heart.
3. *Fontan procedure*: This is the third surgery, which is normally performed when the child is between the ages of two and three. The doctors will now separate the circulation so that blood does not mingle. The workload on the solitary ventricle is likewise reduced. Although this surgery does not restore the normal circulation of the blood to the body, it only improves it.

Complications of the Fontan Procedure Include

- Intolerance of heavy exercise.
- Protein-losing enteropathy.
- Poor ventricular function.
- Mortality.
- Heart blocks or dysrhythmias.

- Hepatomegaly and/or cardiomegaly.
- Ascites also might develop or edema of the limbs.
- Thrombosis of systemic veins.

Additionally, other operations may be necessary while the infant waits for the Fontan surgery, and the kid may require anticoagulants digitalis, diuretics, and ACE inhibitors for the remainder of his or her life or before and after surgery. In extreme circumstances, as the patient reaches maturity, a heart transplant may be necessary. It is critical to recognize that the Fontan method is constantly changing. Over extended follow-up periods, patients treated in this manner continue to be at risk for an increased incidence of heart failure, cardiac arrhythmias such as supraventricular arrhythmias, predominantly due to right atrial dilatation, and pulmonary hypertension.

Aortic Arch Blockage or Stenosis of the Pulmonary Outflow Tract

If pulmonary stenosis exists, the severity of the condition determines if a systemic-to-pulmonary artery shunt is required following the ductal closure. In the presence of an obstruction to the aortic arch, the commonest treatment is mainly done to restore the flow of the unobstructed aortic arch while restricting the pulmonary blood continue to flow. The reason is that most of the patients with arch obstruction have a bulboventricular foramen that is tiny, banding the pulmonary artery has given place to other means of reducing pulmonary blood flow. Bulboventricular foramen diameter has the tendency to shrink in overtime and might suddenly shrink in caliber after unloading treatment for the volume by pulmonary artery banding, even if it is not initially restricted (also the Fontan operations and hemi-Fontan) [10].

Reconstruction by a Norwood type (the anastomosis between the proximal pulmonary artery to the aorta) is now preferred to eliminate the potential of hemodynamically substantial systemic outflow tract stenosis. The reason is the proximity between conduction system and the occurrence of atrioventricular valve connection into the rim frequently, making the bulboventricular foramen larger by muscle resection is dangerous.

The Physiologic Sensitivity of Infants Treated with a Norwood-Type Operation Was Reduced

Although this is not always the case in single ventricle patients, physiology of palliation of newborn after treatment by Norwood-type had been generally noted to be frail relatively. This was found to be attributable to tiny aorta. Because the coronary artery flowing is primarily or could be completely dependent on retrograde aortic perfusion in the case of aortic valve atresia, the coexisting customized Blalock-

Taussig shunt creates "diastolic steal" incident that is considered extremely susceptible to pulmonary vascular resistance changes. Actually, the mortality during the transition from the first stage to the second stage had found to be high for decades, also in some facilities, patients are kept in the hospital for the whole interstate period.

Creating a Cavopulmonary Circulatory System

Due to the acute volume unloading there is an association with an acute upsurge in ventricular thickness of the wall, it is safer to create a cavopulmonary circulation in phases over 1–2 years. The diastolic performance of the single ventricle is significantly altered by this increase in wall thickness, which might decrease cardiac output. The hemi-Fontan procedure improves systemic blood flow (cardiac output) compared to the nonpenetrated "full Fontan" procedure since the cardiac output reduces by a smaller amount. The less-than-complete Fontan is now thought to offer the best blend of near-normal arterial oxygen saturation and low exuberant complication rates. As a result, even the "ultimate" step frequently leads to the formation of a fenestrated Fontan, where nearly all the vena cava flow is directed to the pulmonary arteries. Whatever the structure dividing the pulmonary venous pathway from the systemic venous pathway, a single 4 mm diameter hole in or numerous 2–3 mm in diameter holes are drilled. Although the latter form is characterized by final spontaneous closure, some patients develop protein-losing enteropathy and require placement of a catheter or surgery in order to establish a stable fenestration. Partial hepatic vein exclusion is a less-than-complete Fontan option. When the baffle is inserted, left anterior hepatic vein, one hepatic vein usually, could be expelled from the venous systemic stream. Hepatic vein drains into the pulmonary venous system were ruled out. Unfortunately, most patients who have had their hepatic veins partially removed eventually develop collaterals from the right hepatic vein to the left hepatic vein.

Transplantation of the Heart

Those who have had the Fontan operation and have experienced major problems, as well as the patients who has hemodynamics make them poor candidates for the Fontan procedure, may be candidates for cardiac transplantation.

Prevention

Due to the fact that the etiology of double inlet left ventricle is unknown, there is no method to prevent it entirely. However, you can begin preparing for a healthy pregnancy even before you get pregnant by taking care of yourself. Consider the following:

- Eat healthy types of foods and try to exercise regularly to keep or to get a healthy weight.
- Visit your healthcare professional before getting pregnant to find out how healthy you are and to share your family's health issues and history.
- Stop smoking if you are a smoker. As well as the same goes for drinking and/or using prescription or street drugs. As those things could harm your baby.
- Take a 400-mcg of folic acid supplement in order to prevent brain and spine defects.

Difference in Between the Double Outlet RV and the Double Inlet LV

Both (DORV) and (DILV) are congenital anomalies that result in single ventricle formation. This concludes that the heart, that ordinarily consists of 2 different chambers for pumping (left and right ventricles), now consists of a single functioning chamber.

DORV and DILV are both single ventricle abnormalities that are related to hypoplastic left heart syndrome and tricuspid atresia. Additionally, pulmonary atresia and some types of atrioventricular canal abnormalities may contribute to the development of the diseases associated with a heart with a single ventricular [11].

Generally, the RV which is the heart's chamber lying on the lower right, gets oxygen-depleted blood from the right atrium on its way to other parts of the body. The RV delivers blood to the lungs by the pulmonary artery. The left ventricle is the heart's chamber lying to the lower left which gets blood rich in oxygen from the lungs given by the atrium on the left. Left ventricle then pumps this blood under pressure which is high and distributes it to the other parts of the body through the aorta.

Great arteries (aorta and pulmonary artery) both of them find their exit through the right ventricle in DORV, and the patients are often found to have associated (VSD) ventricular septal defect. On the other hand, in people with DILV, the great arteries are inverted and both atria drain to an abnormal left ventricle as it is enlarged in its size.

The RV is typically reported in DILV to be small, and both atrial septal defects (ASDs) and VSDs may be present [12].

Multiple Choice Questions

1. The gene defect that mostly associated with single ventricle.
   A. Tbx5 misexpression in the ventricles.
   B. GATA4 inactivation.
   C. GATA3 inactivation.
   D. Both A and B.
2. Patients who are LEAST cyanotic, are those with aortic arch obstruction and a single ventricle because.
   A. Pulmonary stenosis does not develop.
   B. They usually develop pulmonary stenosis.
   C. They never develop aortic stenosis.
   D. Both A and C.
3. Most single-ventricle patients live.
   A. For at least 10 years.
   B. For at least 20 years.
   C. 10–15 years.
   D. 5 years only.
4. The most common of the multiple late complications that can occur after various Fontan alterations.
   A. Atrial tachyarrhythmias.
   B. Thromboembolism.
   C. Plastic bronchitis.
   D. Malformations of pulmonary AV system.
5. Which of the following is FALSE according to thromboembolic complications in DILV?
   A. Nearly 10% of those who survive the fenestrated Fontan procedure have venous thrombosis,
   B. Arterial thrombosis is common,
   C. The pulmonary arteries and cerebral veins are examples of possible sites.
   D. Altered hepatic syntheses of endogenous thrombolytic pathway components have all been presented as plausible etiologies.
6. According to the "DILV" with leftward and anterior aorta (left-handed ventricular topology/ l-looped ventricles) which one is false.
   A. It's the least common variant.
   B. Severe overriding in addition to straddling of Lt-sided AV valve leads to commitment of it to the left ventricle.
   C. VSD ensures a route of communication to the hypoplastic Lt-sided Rt ventricle.
   D. Obstruction in the subaortic area can be associated with VSD that is restrictive in type.
7. "DILV" with rightward and anterior aorta (right-handed ventricular topology/D-looped) which one is true.
   A. Left side hypoplastic subaortic incomplete/hypoplastic RV cavity.
   B. Morphologic Lt ventricle which is right side.
   C. VSD ensures a route of communication to hypoplastic Rt-ventricle.

D. Obstruction in the subaortic area can be associated with VSD that is restrictive in type.
8. In monitoring of the complication of protein-losing enteropathy (PLE) after a Fontan operation we depend on.
   A. The detection of fecal alpha1-antitrypsin.
   B. Lipoproteins lipase level.
   C. Doppler analysis.
   D. Holter Placement.
9. Regarding Glenn treatment which one is false.
   A. Performed when the baby is roughly 6 months old.
   B. Surgeons route blood flow from the upper body to the pulmonary artery.
   C. Allowing the blood to collect oxygen from the lungs without passing through the heart.
   D. It's the initial surgery.
10. The false statement regarding Fontan procedure.
    A. Normally performed when the child is between the ages of two and three.
    B. Separate the circulation so that blood does not mingle.
    C. The workload on the solitary ventricle is likewise reduced.
    D. Although this surgery restores normal blood circulation to the body.

Answers

1. D.
2. A.
3. B.
4. A.
5. B.
6. A.
7. C.
8. A.
9. D.
10. D.

References

1. Sanders SP. Hearts with functionally one ventricle. In: Lai WW, Mertens LL, Cohen MS, Geva T, editors. Echocardiography in pediatric and congenital heart disease: from fetus to adult. 2nd ed. Boston, USA: Wiley Blackwell; 2016. p. 509–40.
2. Earing MG, Hagler DJ, Edwards WD. Univentricular atrioventricular connection. In: Allen HD, Shaddy RE, Penny DJ, Feltes TF, Cetta F, editors. Moss & Adams' heart disease in infants, children, and adolescents, including the fetus and young adult. 9th ed. Lippincott Williams & Wilkins; 2016.
3. Penny DJ, Anderson RH. Other forms of functionally univentricular hearts. In: Anderson RH, Baker EJ, Penny DJ, Redington AN, Rigby ML, Wernovsky G, editors. Paediatric cardiology. 3rd ed. London: Churchill Livingston; 2010.

4. von Both I, Silvestri C, Erdemir T, et al. Foxh1 is essential for development of the anterior heart field. Dev Cell. 2004;7(3):331–45.

5. Sanford LP, Ormsby I, Gittenberger-de Groot AC, et al. TGFbeta2 knockout mice have multiple developmental defects that are non-overlapping with other TGFbeta knockout phenotypes. Development. 1997;124(13):2659–70.

6. Gottlieb PD, Pierce SA, Sims RJ, et al. Bop encodes a muscle-restricted protein containing MYND and SET domains and is essential for cardiac differentiation and morphogenesis. Nat Genet. 2002;31(1):25–32.

7. Camenisch TD, Spicer AP, Brehm-Gibson T, et al. Disruption of hyaluronan synthase-2 abrogates normal cardiac morphogenesis and hyaluronan-mediated transformation of epithelium to mesenchyme. J Clin Invest. 2000;106(3):349–60.

8. Zeisberg EM, Ma Q, Juraszek AL, Moses K, Schwartz RJ, Izumo S, et al. Morphogenesis of the right ventricle requires myocardial expression of Gata4. J Clin Invest. 2005;115(6):1522–31.

9. Pizzuto M, Patel M, Romano J, et al. Similar interstage outcomes for single ventricle infants palliated with an aortopulmonary shunt compared to the Norwood procedure. World J Pediatr Congenit Heart Surg. 2018;9(4):407–11.

10. Simsic JM, Phelps C, Kirchner K, et al. Interstage outcomes in single ventricle patients undergoing hybrid stage 1 palliation. Congenit Heart Dis. 2018;13(5):757–63.

11. Rydberg A, Teien DE, Krus P. Computer simulation of circulation in patient with total cavo-pulmonary connection: inter-relationship of cardiac and vascular pressure, flow, resistance and capacitance. Med Biol Eng Comput. 1997;35(6):722–8.

12. Poterucha JT, Anavekar NS, Egbe AC, et al. Survival and outcomes of patients with unoperated single ventricle. Heart. 2016;102(3):216–22.

Double Outlet Right Ventricle

Mays Sufyan Ahmad

Abstract

Dual outlet right ventricle (DORV) is a cardiac abnormality involving the outflow of the right ventricular system, the great arteries both originate from the right ventricle. Categorization of the group of abnormalities is based on the location of the VSD in relation to the aortic and pulmonary arteries. The location of the VSD has a significant impact on the physiologic symptoms of DORV as well as surgical concerns (subpulmonary, subaortic, committed, and non-committed VSD types). A comprehensive history of the patient's illness and physical examination to assess the precordium and respiratory system should be used to identify clinically relevant heart abnormalities. Echocardiography typically gives enough information for a precise and appropriate diagnosis, as well as the information needed to design the surgical strategy. The pulmonary stenosis presence greatly influences the patient's symptom profile and age at the time of clinical manifestation. Most of the patients were present earlier, in neonatal period. ECG, x-ray, cardiac angiography, and MRI were used but not standard or well-established diagnostic technique for this disease. CT scanning may be beneficial in determining coronary artery architecture in infants with TOF type. Medical and surgical treatment depends on the types of DORV and the associated anomalies. Palliative surgery can be done until the definitive treatment is possible. The prognosis also depends on whether the patient did a surgery or not, the type of intervention, and the underlying anomaly.

Keywords

Double outlet · Right ventricle · Congenital heart
Pulmonary stenosis · Congestive heart failure
Taussig-Bing heart · Committed VSD · Non-committed
VSD · Bidirectional Glenn · Tetralogy of Fallot

Introduction

The term "dual outlet right ventricle" (DORV) refers to a diverse group of related cardiac abnormalities involving the outflow of the right ventricular system in which both great arteries originate from the right ventricle. This anatomic defect can range from tetralogy of Fallot (TOF) to full transposition of the great arteries (TGA).

The incidence of DORV is estimated to be 0.09 per 1000 live births in the United States. About 1–1.5% of all congenital cardiac disease is caused by DORV. There has been no identification of a single causative agent or predicted event.

The clinical picture might range from severe cyanosis to fulminant congestive heart failure. DORV definition has been a source of contention among congenital cardiac surgery specialists. In general, classifying the lesion as DORV is appropriate from a surgical standpoint when more than 50% of both major arteries emerge from the right ventricle. Typically, one artery and the majority of the other vessels emerge from the right ventricle. Others specify that if the fibrous continuity between the arterial and atrioventricular valves is absent, then that is a characteristic feature of DORV. Lev et al. (1972) revised this categorization by proposing that aortomitral fibrous discontinuity be needed. Furthermore, Lev et al. started to categorize the group of abnormalities based on the location of the VSD (its location regarding the great vessels) [1].

The following are the occurrence rates of related cardiovascular anomalies:

- Pulmonary stenosis: 20–45% (most common with VSD of subaortic type).
- Atrial septal defect: 20–25%.
- Patent ductus arteriosus: 15%.
- Atrioventricular canal: 9%.
- Subaortic stenosis: 5–33%.
- Aortic coarctation, hypoplasia, or interruption: 3–46%.

M. S. Ahmad (✉)
College of Medicine, University of Baghdad, Baghdad, Iraq

G. Tagarakis et al. (eds.), *Clinical and Surgical Aspects of Congenital Heart Diseases*,
https://doi.org/10.1007/978-3-031-23062-2_21

- Mitral valve anomalies: 32%.
- And other non-cardiac associations: aneuploidy (trisomy 13,18) and tracheoesophageal fistula.

Pathophysiology

A VSD is usually often linked with DORV. The location of the VSD has a significant impact on the physiologic symptoms of DORV as well as surgical concerns. Four major categories can be identified:

1. Double outlet right ventricle with subaortic VSD.
2. Double outlet right ventricle with subpulmonary VSD.
3. Double outlet right ventricle with doubly committed VSD.
4. Double outlet right ventricle with noncommitted VSD.

According to the position of the great vessels:

1. Side by side great vessels position.
2. Right-sided position of great vessels.
3. Left-sided position of great vessels.

Subaortic VSD Type

It is the most frequent type of DORV. The degree of pulmonary stenosis determines the pathophysiology resulting in cyanosis (TOF type). When there is no pulmonary stenosis, the flow of blood increases, resulting in heart failure.

Subpulmonary VSD Type

The pulmonary artery gets oxygenated blood from the left ventricle, whereas deoxygenated blood from the right ventricle flows to the aorta (TGA type). The Taussig-Bing anomaly is a classic case of a DORV with subpulmonary VSD. A common connection is aortic arch hypoplasia. Associated with reversed differential cyanosis.

Doubly Committed VSD Type

Both the aortic and pulmonary valves are connected to the VSD because of the infundibular missing. The pulmonary stenosis determines the clinical characteristics if present [2].

Noncommitted VSD Type

This type is located far away from the aortic and pulmonary valves. The majority of patients with noncommitted VSD are treated with single ventricular palliative methods.

Clinical Features

The clinical appearance and therapy of DORV are largely determined by its type and the existence of concomitant cardiac abnormalities.

A comprehensive history of the patient's illness and its evolution and detailed physical examination to assess the precordium should be used to identify clinically relevant heart abnormal. Furthermore, pulmonary auscultation, as well as peripheral cyanosis and capillary filling, should be examined also.

The pulmonary stenosis presence greatly influences the patient's symptom profile and age at the time of clinical manifestation. Most of the patients were present earlier, in the neonatal period. Cyanosis is evident in patients with significant pulmonary stenosis, while congestive heart failure is seen in patients with the massive pulmonary flow [3].

Diagnosis

Electrocardiographic (ECG) results are rarely diagnostic. Right ventricular hypertrophy, right axis deviation, and, on rare occasions, indications of left ventricular hypertrophy are common findings. Routine laboratory testing includes the following: complete blood count (CBC), electrolyte levels, renal profile, hepatic function, coagulation profile, and assessment of nutritional status [2, 3].

Echocardiography

In neonates, echocardiography typically gives enough information for a precise and appropriate diagnosis, as well as the information needed to design the surgical strategy. Sanders and colleagues found that in 109 of 113 babies, conventional transthoracic echocardiogram (TTE) was utilized to diagnose conotruncal malformation. The diagnosis of DORV was confirmed with angiography in 11 of the 12 babies who had previously received a diagnosis based on subxiphoid two-dimensional echocardiography [4].

Cardiac Angiography

Heart catheterization, which was previously the gold standard, is now seldom used in the evaluation or preoperative planning of this cardiac disease.

When warranted, angiography offers numerous advantages, including the following: Hemodynamic parameters can be evaluated directly in an older child with a long-standing illness. The real anatomic variance can be described in the context of probable aberrant coronary architecture. When a Rastelli-type repair is considered, this knowledge can influence surgical strategy. Angiography can assist in identifying the major pulmonary branches, the pulmonary vascular tree, and the collateral arteries to the lungs in the setting of pulmonary vascular abnormalities.

Magnetic Resonance Imaging (MRI)

MRI has been used before but, it is not currently a standard or well-established diagnostic technique for this disease. MRI can provide additional anatomic information, such as the connection of the two ventricles.

Chest Radiography

Anteroposterior and lateral chest radiography results are dependent on the degree of pulmonary (or subpulmonary) stenosis. The pulmonary parenchyma is largely oligemic in the situation of severe stenosis, but in the setting of mild pulmonary stenosis (particularly with a Taussig-Bing heart), results are likely to be consistent with congestive heart failure. In either case, the chest picture demonstrates cardiomegaly.

Computed Tomography (CT) Scanning

Preoperative CT scanning may be beneficial in determining coronary artery architecture in infants with TOF type. A study that looked at the incidence and diagnostic accuracy of preoperative cardiac CT scanning for identifying detailed coronary artery anatomy in 318 children with TOF type discovered a 95% concordance between cardiac CT scanning and surgical findings, as well as a 96.9% diagnostic accuracy for cardiac CT scanning [5].

Management

Medical therapy of DORV is based on the abnormalities and underlying physiology. Maintaining patent ductus arteriosus is critical in the situation of insufficient pulmonary blood flow. Prostaglandin E (alprostadil) infusions are the standard of treatment until healing may occur. Having congestive heart failure is contradictory; cautious diuresis, inotropic support digoxin usage, and pulmonary blood flow management through intubation and blood gas manipulation may be needed [5].

Indications for Surgery

Because (DORV) is a disease that does not resolve on its own, the diagnosis alone is sufficient to warrant surgery. Sakakibara et al. reported the first successful biventricular repair for this condition in 1967.

The clinical appearance and surgical technique required for correction are determined by the relative anatomic abnormalities discovered. The accompanying VSD is generally big and nonrestrictive.

Palliative procedures are often done solely in patients who need short-term therapy, whereas noncardiac illness (e.g., sepsis) is addressed when anatomic characteristics do not allow for final repair [6].

In an ideal world, DORV is a procedure that repairs both ventricles, with the left ventricle linked to the aorta and the right ventricle attached to the major pulmonary artery. Palliative procedures differ depending on the subtype's physiology. With excessive pulmonary flow, banding can be done until definitive treatment. In case of insufficient blood flow, commonly a Blalock-Taussig shunt (an aortopulmonary shunt) can relieve symptoms until definitive treatment can be done.

Bidirectional Glenn operation is used for univentricular hearts or complicated congenital heart illness one of the DORV. In a retrospective cohort (4 years) study including 115 patients who underwent this surgery, the doctors determined that this procedure can enhance gas exchange and volume overload. Poor nutrition and late presentation increase the morbidity post-operation.

Contraindications for the Surgery

Significant left ventricular hypoplasia and severe atrioventricular valve overriding or straddling are absolute contraindications to double outlet right ventricle biventricular surgery. Single ventricle palliation would be suggested in individuals who are not candidates for biventricular surgery [7].

Preoperative Assessment

Preoperative investigations should be used to correctly assess surgically important characteristics such as pulmonary and tricuspid valve separation and their diameter, the presence of aortic coarctation, and anatomy of heart coronaries. Significance of pulmonary valve stenosis, VSD location, pulmonary stenosis, and size of major vessels are veryimportant to be assessed prior to surgery.

Intraoperative Assessment

Repair of DORV with Subaortic VSD Subtype

It is repaired usually by making an intraventricular tunnel that shunts blood from the left ventricle through VSD to the aorta. A patch (like polytetrafluoroethylene) can be used.

Post cardiopulmonary bypass by cannulation and cardiac arrest, the anatomy is examined by a right atriotomy. Through the tricuspid valve, the VSD can be visualized and connection to the aorta is done. The VSD can be enlarged if needed. This can be done superiorly and anteriorly, leading to the excision of some pieces of the infundibular septum [8].

The VSD closure by interrupted or a continuous suture. If the intraventricular tunnel bulges into the right ventricular outflow tract, the right ventriculotomy should be sealed by a patch. Surgery of subaortic VSD and pulmonary stenosis subtypes of RVO is done by the same procedure used in TOF. Before pulmonary bypass, it is important to locate the coronaries and plan for right ventriculotomy if indicated.

Subpulmonary VSD Type Repair

This type can be associated with aortic coarctation, so coarctation repair with a pulmonary artery band is the preferred method; however, repairing both defects can be done in one stage operation. If the VSD is restricted, it should be expanded to allow the blood flow from the left ventricle to the pulmonary artery. Other defects can be done concurrently [9].

Doubly Committed VSD-Type Repair

This is a rare type; the repair is done in the same manner as the subaortic VSD type method. The VSD mostly does not block the left ventricular flow through an intraventricular tunnel to the aorta. There may be a need for a conduit from the right ventricle to the pulmonary artery if there is a right ventricular obstruction or pulmonary stenosis.

Noncommitted VSD Repairs

The most difficult to repair and carry a high risk for the patient. This abnormality is distinguished by a persistent subaortic conus and a double infundibulum. The subaortic conus is larger than the typical right ventricular structure leading to aortic displacement normal position of the pulmonary artery and both of them are placed nearby.

Pulmonary artery banding is required for severe subaortic blockage, restrictive VSD, or aortic arch obstruction. Types with pulmonary stenosis should be managed conservatively or by modified Blalock-Taussig shunt which is a systemic to pulmonary shunt. The hypoplastic left ventricle and severe overriding of the atrioventricular valve are the main limitations to doing a biventricular repair. The surgery of choice when using combined atrial and ventricular methods is an intraventricular tunnel that links the VSD to the aorta [10, 11].

Outcome and Prognosis

Brown et al. reported a 56% of 15-year survival rate in individuals with DORV from 1980 to 2000 (including those who undergo the surgery and the patients that don't do it). The majority of non-complicated cases (95%) had a 15-year survival rate after surgery, whereas the Taussig-Bing abnormality had an 89% survival rate.

individuals with a double outlet right ventricle and a noncommitted VSD were at a greater risk of reoperation and mortality [12].

Multiple Choice Questions
1. The most useful diagnostic method for dual outlet right ventricle is:
   A. ECG.
   B. X-ray.
   C. CT scan.
   D. MRI.
   E. Echocardiography.

2. Patent ductus arteriosus should be kept open in some cases with pulmonary stenosis by administration of:
   A. Indomethacin.
   B. Alprostadil.
   C. Mifepristone.
   D. Aspirin.
   E. Baclofen.
3. Contraindication for biventricular repair:
   A. Left ventricular hypoplasia.
   B. Coarctation of aorta.
   C. Having ventricular septal defect.
   D. Aneuploidy.
4. In noncommitted type of double outlet right ventricle, the VSD location is:
   A. Subaortic VSD.
   B. Subpulmonary VSD.
   C. VSD that located far away from major vessels.
   D. VSD that is connected to both major vessels.
5. The most common type of DORV you can see in patients is:
   A. Subaortic VSD.
   B. Subpulmonary VSD.
   C. Committed VSD.
   D. Noncommitted VSD.
6. Taussig-Bing anomaly is a type of:
   A. Subaortic VSD.
   B. Subpulmonary VSD.
   C. Committed VSD.
   D. Noncommitted VSD.
7. Reversed differential cyanosis seen in subpulmonary VSD type in:
   A. Toes of the feet more than hand fingers.
   B. Fingers of the hand mostly.
   C. Equally in toes and fingers.
   D. There is no differential cyanosis in the subpulmonary type.

Answers

1. E.

   Explanation: Echocardiography typically gives enough information for a precise and appropriate diagnosis, as well as the information needed to design the surgical strategy.

2. B.

   Explanation: Alprostadil is a prostaglandin agonist that is used to keep ductus arteriosus open.

   Mifepristone is antiprogesterone and the other drugs are non-steroidal anti-inflammatory drugs that close the duct.

3. A.

   Explanation: Significant left ventricular hypoplasia and severe atrioventricular valve overriding or straddling are absolute contraindications to double outlet right ventricle biventricular surgery. Single ventricle palliation would be suggested in individuals who are not candidates for biventricular surgery.

4. C.

   Explanation: Located far away from the aortic and pulmonary valves

5. A.

   Explanation: Subaortic VSD.

6. B.

   Explanation: Subpulmonary VSD.

7. B.

   Explanation: Differential cyanosis is mostly seen in hand fingers associated with clubbing usually.

References

1. Goo HW. Double outlet right ventricle: in-depth anatomic review using three-dimensional cardiac CT data. Korean J Radiol. 2021;22(11):1894.
2. Yoo S-J, van Arsdell GS. 3D printing in surgical management of double outlet right ventricle. Front Pediatr. 2018;5:289.
3. Kariya T, et al. Personalized perioperative multi-scale, multi-physics heart simulation of double outlet right ventricle. Ann Biomed Eng. 2020;48(6):1740–50.
4. Yim D, et al. Essential modifiers of double outlet right ventricle: revisit with endocardial surface images and 3-dimensional print models. Circ Cardiovasc Imaging. 2018;11(3):e006891.
5. Goo HW. Coronary artery anomalies on preoperative cardiac CT in children with tetralogy of Fallot or Fallot type of double outlet right ventricle: comparison with surgical findings. Int J Cardiovasc Imaging. 2018;34(12):1997–2009.
6. Wang Z, et al. A new ISL1 loss-of-function mutation predisposes to congenital double outlet right ventricle. Int Heart J. 2019;60(5):1113–22.
7. Pang K-J, et al. Echocardiographic classification and surgical approaches to double-outlet right ventricle for great arteries arising almost exclusively from the right ventricle. Tex Heart Inst J. 2017;44(4):245–51.
8. Lu C-X, et al. A novel MEF2C loss-of-function mutation associated with congenital double outlet right ventricle. Pediatr Cardiol. 2018;39(4):794–804.
9. Ebadi A, et al. Double-outlet right ventricle revisited. J Thorac Cardiovasc Surg. 2017;154(2):598–604.
10. Bhatla P, et al. Utility and scope of rapid prototyping in patients with complex muscular ventricular septal defects or double-outlet right ventricle: does it alter management decisions? Pediatr Cardiol. 2017;38(1):103–14.
11. Lo CW, et al. Reply to 'double-outlet right ventricle is not hypoplastic left heart syndrome'. Nat Genet. 2019;51(2):198–9.
12. Kumar P, Bhatia M. Role of computed tomography in pre-and post-operative evaluation of a double-outlet right ventricle. J Cardiovasc Imaging. 2021;29(3):205.

Ebstein's Anomaly

Ahmed Dheyaa Al-Obaidi, Sara Shihab Ahmad,
Abeer Mundher Ali, and Rawaa Fadhil Al-Tofakchi

Abstract

Ebstein's anomaly, which is described by Wilhelm Ebstein, is one of the congenital heart diseases that are seldom encountered with a 1 per 200,000 live birth prevalence. It entitles the presence of deformity in the right side of the heart and the tricuspid valve and more specifically it is a downward displacement of septal and posterior leaflet into the right ventricle leading to enlarged atrium and atrialized ventricle. Many heart abnormalities can be associated with EA like ASD, conduction system abnormalities, PFO, pulmonary stenosis or atresia, and VSD. This anomaly has a wide range of manifestation depending on the severity of the lesion and it can be diagnosed by echocardiogram which is considered to be the diagnostic test for this anomaly. Management could be by observation in asymptomatic patient, medical therapy in mild cases while surgical intervention may be required in severe cases as well as valve replacement and heart transplantation.

Keywords

Ebstein's anomaly · Lithium therapy · MYH gene
Tricuspid valve · Atrialized right ventricle · Elevated JVP
Cyanosis · Starnes procedure · Valve replacement
Milrinone

Introduction

Ebstein's abnormality (EA) is one of the congenital heart diseases that are seldom encountered. It affects 1 in every two hundred thousand living-births and accounts for approximately 1% of all congenital heart disease occurrences.

Wilhelm Ebstein first identified this condition in 1866 in his report "Concerning a very rare case of insufficiency of the tricuspid valve caused by a congenital malformation." EA is a type of CHD marked by Rt-side of the heart and tricuspid valve (TR) abnormality. The inability of the leaflets of the TR to delaminate from the underlying cardiac-endocardium causes distinct characteristics [1]. There are different levels of downward displacement of the tricuspid leaflets into the Rt ventricle with the septal leaflet being the most significantly affected, followed by the posterior one; as a result, the annular circumference is often quite large, and the Rt atrium is quite enlarged; there is myopathic changes in the RV and it is divided into two distinct areas, an "atrialized" area of poor function, situated between the hinge point of the septal leaflet that is displaced apically and the true annulus, and the functional area which is located below the hinge point. This functional RV volume might be fairly small, its volume mainly depends on how much the leaflet is displaced. ASD, persistent patency of foramen ovale, abnormalities in the conductive system of the heart, VSD and stenosis or atresia of the pulmonary valve are among the cardiac abnormalities linked to EA [2]. EA manifests clinically as a spectrum ranging from minor types that become apparent in adulthood to severe forms that result in significant newborn mortality. EA can cause hydrops fetalis in the uterus, and cyanosis and dyspnea in children and adults, but the disease can manifest in a variety of ways and can become clinically severe at any moment during life. The diagnostic technique of choice for definitively diagnosing Ebstein's abnormality is echocardiography, which can also be used to characterize the degree of valvular insufficiency and the quality of the leaflets [3]. Other modalities, including an electrocardiogram (ECG), radiography of the chest, or prenatal ultrasonography, are frequently used to detect heart abnormalities and it is the initial tests that lead to additional investigation. When possible, valve repair is obviously preferred and it is more likely to succeed if the anterior leaflet is broad, sail-like, and relatively thin while thicker, muscularized anterior leaflet is an

A. D. Al-Obaidi · S. S. Ahmad · A. M. Ali · R. F. Al-Tofakchi (✉)
College of Medicine, University of Baghdad, Baghdad, Iraq
e-mail: rawaafadhil24@gemail.com

© The Author(s), under exclusive license to Springer Nature Switzerland AG 2023
G. Tagarakis et al. (eds.), *Clinical and Surgical Aspects of Congenital Heart Diseases*,
https://doi.org/10.1007/978-3-031-23062-2_22

unsuitable repair substrate. However, in other circumstances, replacement is required. Transplantation or single-ventricle palliation (Starne's technique) may be required in the neonatal period [3].

Associated Defects with EA

Ebstein's anomaly can be associated with congenital heart defects in any part of the heart, with mitral valve prolapse and left ventricular noncompaction (LVNC) being the two most prevalent [2, 3].

Associated Defects

- *Prolapse* of one or both mitral leaflets, focal fibrous thickening of the mitral leaflets, cord anomalies, and papillary muscle anomalies are all examples of mitral valve issues [4].
- *Left ventricular noncompaction* (LVNC) was linked to a greater mortality risk when compared to cases with EA by itself.
- *Arrhythmias*: "Wolff-Parkinson-White (WPW)" and due to dilated Rt atrium, EA patients can encounter a variety of atrial-originating arrhythmias such as: "atrial flutter, atrial tachycardia, atrial fibrillation, intra-atrial reentrant tachycardia in addition to AV node reentrant tachycardia, and ventricular arrhythmias [4]."
- *Structural abnormalities*: ASD, patent foramen ovale (right-to-left shunting across these defects explains why certain individuals exhibit relative hypoxia), pulmonary stenosis or atresia (requiring surgical intervention), and ventricular septal defect [5].

Teratogens and the Role of Genetics in EA

EA has a quite heterogeneous etiology. In most cases (80%), EA is a non-syndromic and an isolated defect, while in about 20% of cases, it occurs in association with other anomalies that are extracardiac in origin as in cases where Mendelian or chromosomal defects are present. All patients have chromosomal abnormalities affecting genes involved in the early development of cardiac structures [6].

Non-syndromic EA is a sporadic abnormality that affects families. In familial situations, inheritance patterns were "autosomal recessive," with reappearance in siblings, and "autosomal dominant with reduced penetrance," with recurrence in nephews and uncles. This could be because the genes that are responsible for heart morphology formation are mutated, such as the NKX2.5 and MYH7 genes, have

been found in some EA patients. Nonetheless, EA is likely to be characterized by genetic variation as well as multifactorial inheritance, as screening of the"NKX2.5 and GATA4 genes" mutations in other EA-suffering individuals has come up negative [6, 7].

Syndromic EA Could Be Due To

Chromosomal abnormalities, such as deletions, may cause syndromic EA. Facial dysmorphisms, microcephaly, mental retardation, CHD, plus genital anomalies are characteristics of 8p23.1 deletion. CHD affects 40–65% of affected patients, with an AV canal defect, stenosis of the pulmonary valve, and Fallot tetralogy being the most frequent abnormalities. The GATA4 gene, which is expressed throughout the development of the heart and maps to the 8p23.1 crucial area, is frequently deleted in disease-suffering patients and is the main cause of CHD [8, 9].

Micro chromosomal Anomalies: One of the most prevalent is terminal deletion Ip36, which is characterized by epilepsy, poor cognition, and facial dysmorphisms. CHD, with anatomical anomalies and cardiac myopathy in addition to the specific hallmarks of Lt ventricular non-compaction, is identified in nearly half of these patients. Ebstein anomaly has been found in many cases, indicating that this genetic condition should be investigated in patients with syndromic EA and poor cognition, both with and without epilepsy [9].

Numerous chromosomal anomalies have been described, including: "duplication 9p, deletion and duplication 11q, duplication 15q, terminal deletion 18q, trisomy 18, trisomy 21, and the 5q35 microdeletion syndrome," as well as a wide range of Mendelian illnesses. Risks of recurrence and the inheritance patterns of chromosomal or Mendelian illnesses are followed in genetic counseling for syndromic EA. Factual risk statistics are implemented to evaluate the possibility of recurrence in ensuing pregnancies of those having a kid with EA in the case of non-syndromic Ebstein abnormality. If one sibling is affected, the probability of CHD recurrence in first-degree relatives of patients with EA is estimated to be around 1% [10]. When multiple relatives are affected, the danger is increased. When two siblings are impacted, the couple's recurrence risk is approximately 3%. If we look for teratogens that aid in the development of EA, lithium therapy (drug to treat bipolar disorder) during the initial three months of pregnancy was considered strongly linked to the development of EA in the fetus. However, newer epidemiological researches have not supported these observations, suggesting that the use of lithium medication during pregnancy is of minor consequence as a risk factor for illness development. Maternal exposure to benzodiazepines may contribute to developing the anomaly [11].

Pathophysiology of EA

Many distinct lesions have been identified and are relevant to surgical treatment:

- The delamination of the TV leaflets has failed.
- Appropriate level of attachment of the anterior leaflet; however, it is sail-like or large in appearance. Numerous attachments of the chordae to the wall of the ventricle are present, as well as aberrant fenestration [12].
- The RV is thin and dilated in the area above the functional annulus ("atrialized right ventricle"), with varying hypertrophy. The real annulus of the tricuspid valve is virtually always enlarging and descending apically [13].
- The effective RV's cavity is reduced.
- The excess anterior leaflet's tissue and its chordal attachments to the infundibulum frequently obstruct the RV's infundibulum.

These anomalies result in that blood flows backward from the tricuspid valve into the RA when the RV contracts. The RA enlarges as a result of this. The elevated pressure in the RA maintains opening of the PFO, if the tricuspid regurgitation is severe enough, this defective connection permits blood that is deoxygenated to pass from the RA to the LA, bypassing the lungs and directly reaching the body (right-to-left shunting) [14]. Lower oxygen levels in the blood will arise as a result of this. This is the reason behind the fact that patients with EA may seem "cyanotic," or bluish in color, have lower than normal oxygen saturations (arterial desaturation), paradoxical embolism, and pulmonary oligemia, congestive heart failure can also result [15].

The degree of apical displacement of the septal leaflet (≥ 8 mm/m^2 body surface area) is the critical distinguishing feature of EA from other congenital regurgitant lesions. Ebstein's anomaly can range from mild to severe, depending on the extent of valvular displacement and so EA can be classified into many types. The anatomic severity of Ebstein's abnormality can be described in two ways. The first method is based on the appearance of the anomaly on echocardiography, which is classified as "anatomically mild, moderate, or severe." The degree of right ventricular dilatation and the quantity of leaflet displacement and tethering are measured. This classification is a little imprecise, but it gets the job done. The second technique is to detail the actual architecture of each of the heart's relevant structures as seen during surgery. The features that surgeons consider crucial when deciding whether to repair or replace the tricuspid valve are highlighted in this nomenclature system. Celermajer et al. established an enhanced Glasgow Outcome Scale grading system depending on echocardiographic findings, with grades ranging from 1 to 4.19. The functioning right ventricle and left heart are compared to the total area of the RA and atrialized RV (ratio less than 0.5, grade 1; ratio 0.5–0.99, grade 2; ratio 1.0–1.49, grade 3; ratio more than 1.5, grade 4) [16].

In 1988, Carpentier et al. depending on the exact anatomy of lesion suggested a classification of EA as follows:

1. *Type A.*
   Mild apical leaflet displacement, mild FRV size reduction, and normal silhouette of the anterior leaflet.
2. *Type B.*
   The leaflets are moderately apical displaced, the FRV volume is moderately reduced but generally adequate, and the anterior leaflet could appear to have normal mobility but aberrant chordal attachments.
3. *Type C.*
   Leaflets with severe apical displacement and a small FRV. RVOT blockage due to anterior leaflet constriction caused by aberrant chordal attachments.
4. *Type D.*
   "Tricuspid Sac." The leaflets are completely nondelaminated, with only the infundibular section of the RV remaining.

Clinical Manifestation

EA manifest as a wide spectrum ranging from very mild to very severe cases with many clinical findings due to highly variable natural history, in many times severe cases are unable to reach birth and lead to fetal loss or hydrops fetalis while if severe cases reach the birth, they will be critically ill at birth with apparent cyanosis which is considered to be the cardinal sign. They usually depend on the ductus arteriosus and need prostaglandin E2 infusion to maintain the patency of the duct. Supraventricular tachycardia (rate > 300 beats per minute) and heart failure may also occur and require immediate intensive care [17].

The remainder of the spectrum of Ebstein anomaly can remain remarkably symptomless throughout childhood and tolerate the TR very well, growth and development are generally normal in patients suffering from EA. Some young patients have cyanosis, due to right to left shunt. Children may complain from palpitation which is usually described by children as "my heart beats in a funny way." They may become tired faster than their peers, especially on the playground. Symptoms may improve with age as the pulmonary vascular resistance falls allowing the blood to flow to the lungs and tricuspid valve regurgitation becomes less, as a result cyanosis and other symptoms become better. Some not presenting until adulthood. In patients of young age, the sensation of difficulty in breathing, palpitations, and feeling of chest pain can be the initial symptoms. Progressive cyanosis can be one of the manifestations and sudden cardiac death is also possible [18].

Diagnosis

In Ebstein's abnormality, the tricuspid valve does not develop in the appropriate way during the initial weeks of intrauterine life. A process known as delamination begins to create the AV valve leaflets from the tissues of the ventricular myocardium around week 7. The tricuspid valve is fully established by the end of week 12. Normal cardiac structure involves that the tricuspid valve has three leaflets: " anterior, posterior, and septal." That means the tricuspid valve and right ventricle are malformed in EA. Fetuses with EA can be diagnosed prenatally using fetal echocardiography, or heart sonography [19]. This is the diagnostic test of choice for Ebstein's anomaly because it can accurately assess the tricuspid valve leaflets as well as the size and function of the cardiac chambers. The main hallmark of Ebstein's abnormality is apical displacement of the septal leaflet of the tricuspid valve, which can be seen on sonography. There is also a significantly enlarged RA and the RV is atrialized. Tricuspid valve regurgitation is common as a result of the valve's abnormality, albeit the location and severity vary. Echocardiography can also be used to determine the viability of valve repair.

Postnatal diagnosis depends on physical examination and many imaging techniques.

Appearance and Physical Examination Show

Patients may have a blue-colored face depending on the degree of cyanosis and Rt-Lt shunting, cyanosis is usually found in patients younger than 1 year old [20].

1. Vitals.
   The pulse may be weak or impalpable due to right-sided heart failure.
2. Skin.
   No apparent skin findings are usually found in EA patients.
3. Neck.
   Elevated jugular venous pressure can be caused by tricuspid regurgitation and increased right atrial pressure. These patients have a prominent "a" wave in their dilated jugular veins. Because of the damping effect of the large atrium, the V wave of TR is rarely seen in the jugular pulse. However, in severe TR cases, a prominent "v" wave may be seen.
4. Heart.
   - *Inspection.*
     - Asymmetrical chest due to an enlarged right heart.
     - An apical impulse may be visible.
   - *Palpation.*
     - On the apex of the heart, a palpable impulse can be detected.

- A systolic thrill can be felt near the left side of the lower sternal border.
- The right ventricular heave is faint due to the right ventricle's small size.
- *Auscultation.*
  - Wide-splitting of the first and second heart sounds due to the RBBB (Rt bundle branch block) that is frequently encountered with this illness.
  - A loud first heart sound (S1) of tricuspid regurgitation.
  - It's possible to notice a noticeable S3 and S4.
  - A grade 3 pansystolic murmur caused by tricuspid regurgitation, loudest near the left-lower border of the sternum and increasing with inspiration (without radiation), in association with a "mid-diastolic murmur" caused by the elevated diastolic flow volume over the tricuspid valve.
  - A click sound may be heard if the anterior leaflet moves abnormally.

5. Lung.
   - Lung examination is usually normal in patients with Ebstein's anomaly but some patients may have tachypnea or dyspnea.
   - Abdomen.
   - Tricuspid regurgitation and a high right atrial pressure might cause hepatomegaly.
   - Back (no observed clinical findings).
   - Genitourinary (no observed clinical findings).
   - Neuromuscular (no observed clinical findings).
6. Extremities.
   - Clubbing.
   - Cyanosis.
   - Cool periphery.
   - No pedal edema.

While Imaging Techniques Include

Echocardiography of the heart is the principal diagnostic procedure for determining the definitive diagnosis of Ebstein's abnormality and identifying any concomitant cardiac abnormalities. It allowed the cardiologist to accurately estimate the level of valvular displacement, insufficiency or stenosis severity, heart chambers size, and whether foramen ovale has remained patent. This test also helps to diagnose patients whose clinical features were not pathognomonic. The presence of septal leaflet tissue and movement of the anterior leaflet with a "free leading edge" are both favorable echocardiographic markers for TV repair. Any delamination of the septal and inferior leaflet helps in completing circumferential reconstructive planning successfully. Leaflet anchoring to the endocardium with muscularization, on the other hand, indicates a more challenging repair. Severe annular dilatation, which can reach 8 cm or more in adults, is another factor that makes effective repair difficult. A chest x-ray, which is used to determine the heart size, may frequently reveal considerable right atrial enlargement and cardiomegaly, giving the appearance of a "wall-to-wall," "clock face," "box-shaped," "globe-shaped" heart that occupies most of the cavity of the chest. Due to the presence of an abnormally big heart that is easily seen on chest X-ray, Ebstein anomaly is frequently suspected. The pulmonary vasculature could be normal or abnormal [21].

Cross-sectional investigations from the "apical four chamber view" were particularly useful for measuring septal-leaflet displacement, which is invariably >15 mm in individuals with EA. If severe hypoplasia of the lungs is a danger, a CT scan may be beneficial. Cardiac MRI is very helpful for determining the function and size of the RV. RV volumes and tricuspid regurgitation can be measured using magnetic resonance imaging with gadolinium contrast, as well as the size and function of the left ventricle. The inclusion of the area of the RV that is atrialized in the quantification of its ejection fraction and volume calculations varies majorly, and this must be kept in mind when trying to interpret results. Velocity mapping perpendicular to the regurgitant jet is used to quantify tricuspid regurgitation, and a jet cross section of more than 6 mm × 6 mm is considered severe.

An electrocardiogram can help verify the imaging technique's findings or make a differential diagnosis of Ebstein abnormality if performed first. It generally consists of the following:

1. RA hypertrophy—seen as tall P wave of more than 3 mm.
2. First-degree heart block—seen as PR interval prolongation of duration >0–10 s.
3. Complete heart block.
4. Complete or incomplete RBBB with QRS duration >0–06 s.
5. Atrial tachycardia(arrhythmia) including atrial fibrillation, atrial flutter, ectopic beats, or atrioventricular nodal reentrant tachycardia.
6. Patients may have additional conducting pathways such as "Wolff-Parkinson-White syndrome" and this enhances the possibility of sudden cardiac death.

An electrocardiogram (ECG) is a test that records the beat of the heart. If the patient has complained of tachycardia and the test results are normal, the patient may be given a recorder to wear at home to try to capture the tachycardia episodes. An exercise stress test may be done on the patient to better measure cardiac function during exercise. Additional electrophysiologic testing may be required for some people with irregular heart rhythms in order to properly diagnose and perhaps treat their heart rhythm disorders. When a pre-excitation route is present, a preoperative electrophysiologic examination is recommended, and most patients can be treated percutaneously. Cardiac catheterization is an invasive diagnostic test which is not performed today as in the past. Catheterization was used previously to define the cardiac anatomy and function but by the development of imaging technique and the ability of echocardiograms and cross-sectional imaging to provide a necessary information about anatomy and function of the heart, catheterization become contraindicated due to its serious complication like arrhythmias and cardiac arrest.

Treatment

Asymptomatic patients can be treated medically and monitored for years. Arrhythmias, progressive RV widening, and worsening of RV systolic performance should all be constantly monitored. When patients develop symptoms like worsening exercise capacity, paradoxical embolism, progressive RV changes, cyanosis, and the appearance of new arrhythmias, and if repair of the tricuspid valve is applicable in a setting where morbidity and mortality are low, they should be considered for operative intervention.

Medical Management of Patients with EA

Medical therapy is mainly used in order to make surgery less of a necessity, especially when the patient is still a neonate, when the risk of death from any surgical procedure is highest. Medical care helps to gradually reduce pulmonary vascular resistance, allowing surgical repair to be undertaken if necessary. With low oxygen supplementation and prostaglandin infusions, relatively stable newborns can be observed. Maintaining ductal patency is critical, especially in infants with anatomical pulmonary atresia. To minimize pulmonary over circulation and heart volume overload, supplemented oxygen should not exceed 21% fractional inspired oxygen. During this time, keep blood oxygen saturation between 75 and 85%. Prostaglandin therapy can be stopped if pulmonary vascular resistance reduces. As the ductus closes, they allow for accurate measurement of the antegrade flowing pulmonary blood. If oxygen saturation falls below 80%, medications to lower the pulmonary vascular resistance, like supplementary oxygen and nitric oxide, can be used to enhance the antegrade flow passing through the right ventricle. In functional pulmonary atresia, however, a trial of prostaglandin removal may be required. Similarly, prostaglandins may worsen the symptoms of heart failure as a circular shunt is being established in the presence of pulmonary valve regurgitation. Blood pathway starting from the left ventricle to the aorta, then through the big ductus into the pulmonary artery, then the retrograde flow starts through the pulmonary valve into the RV to the RA by the tricuspid valve which is incompetent, and finally by the ASD it will be back again to the heart's left side. This process results in cardiac failure with a high output. In this instance, early prostaglandin removal may be necessary. A two-step procedure can be used to treat neonates with a circular shunt. The main pulmonary artery is ligated first, with or without branch PA bands, and then a Starnes surgery is performed once the patient is stabilized. Cardiogenic shock develops as hemodynamic instability worsens [21]. Mechanical ventilation and intubation with tidal volumes considerably large are essential in these cases to ensure sufficient breathing in case of patients having significant cardiomegaly. Paralysis and sedation might also be required to minimize oxygen demand. To help improve cardiac output, inotropic assistance such as milrinone combined with epinephrine or dopamine in low doses might also be required. Milrinone is a highly effective medication since it affects the right ventricle in both lusitropic and inotropic ways. It also lowers pulmonary vascular resistance, allowing for increased antegrade pulmonary blood flow. Because of the wide separation of tachyarrhythmias in this particular group of patients, there should be an imitation of catecholamine inotropes with caution.

Frequent echocardiograms are helpful in determining the antegrade flow via outflow tract of the RV and the extent of TV regurgitation during medical treatment. If the condition worsens, this assessment will be of help in guiding the weaning of prostaglandins and nitric oxide and inotropes initiation, or going ahead with the surgical surgery.

Some newborns may require extracorporeal membrane oxygenation (ECMO) support for stabilization prior to surgical surgery, and despite the minimal incidence of endocarditis in this abnormality, prophylaxis for endocarditis is indicated [19–22].

Indication for Surgical Repair

Because surgery for Ebstein's abnormality has an elevated risk of mortality, particularly in infants, it is rarely indicated unless the patient has severe symptoms. Surgery can be delayed until symptoms arise in asymptomatic or mildly symptomatic children, allowing them to enjoy a relatively normal life. If there is a good likelihood of a good repair in children between the ages of 2 and 5, operational intervention is indicated. This is critical in order to avoid additional cardiomegaly, particularly due to the dilatation of the atrialized right atrium. EA patients who have an anatomic pulmonary atresia, presence of circular shunt, a need for mechanical ventilation or prostaglandins, symptoms like fatigue and exercise intolerance, new onset of atrial and ventricular arrhythmias paradoxical embolism,, worsening cyanosis

(systemic oxygen saturation below 75%), or presence of heart failure associated with feeds intoleration as a result of mesenteric congestion, and severe forms in general like C/D type Carpentier, (G.O.S.E) score Great Ormond Street Echocardiography is more than three or if the patient has right heart failure, a surgical intervention will be required throughout neonatal period.

Surgical Procedures

Many surgical techniques for the treatment of newborn EA have been described so far. The goal of operative intervention is to repair the tricuspid valve. This typically involves reduction of RA, RV plication, and total or subtotal closure of the atrial septum. As the valve repair is considered as the preferred outcome, the outcomes of tricuspid replacement in the adult patients show that it is safe as well as successful. The two competing strategies for surgical treatment for neonatal EA are whether to perform a biventricular repair or a single ventricle palliative procedure (Starnes Procedure). Which repair method is appropriate for neonates with EA is considered as a controversial subject. Mizuno et al. experience with neonatal EA repair was shared at their center. The result shows that the biventricular repair group had a higher survival when compared to single ventricle palliation (Starnes Procedure) 0.60% vs. 25%, respectively. Kumar et al. analyzed median seven years Starnes operation follow-up in neonatal repairs for 27 cases in a recent study. Their total survival rate was 81% after follow-up for 5 years. The outcomes of neonatal biventricular repair for EA were described by Boston et al. In their study, early survival was 78.1%, but 15-year survival was 40 and 79% for EA whether anatomical pulmonary atresia is present or not respectively. As a result, in EA newborns who have anatomical pulmonary atresia the biventricular repairs is the method of choice which should be done with caution [22].

A tertiary care center should provide comprehensive care with a multidisciplinary team that includes a pediatric cardiologist, high-risk obstetrician, pediatric cardiothoracic surgeon, and intensivist for newborn. Medical care during the newborn period lowers mortality rates. The goal is to restore both atria and ventricles. If there is severe RV dilatation or dysfunction, a 1.5 repair for the ventricle (valvuloplasty + bidirectional Glenn -BDG-) might be required.

Biventricular Repair Procedures

Danielson at Mayo Clinic's was the first to define some of the fundamental concepts of biventricular repair for any age group having EA. This comprises: the atrialized section of

RV free wall is plicationed, posterior tricuspid annuloplasty is performed, ASD is closed, and right reduction atrioplasty is performed. Addition of papillary muscles anteriorly near to the septum of the ventricle using the "Sebening stitch" to enable coaptation of the leaflet with ventricular septum is one of the subsequent Danielson adjustments.

The following are the main processes in a biventricular repair:

1. Tricuspid valve leaflets are being mobilized. The degree of leaflet mobilization is determined by the valvuloplasty procedure utilized.
2. The right ventricle being atrialized is plicated also obliterated.
3. Real annulus is reduced.
4. Right atrioplasty reduction. This gives the lungs greater room to breathe.
5. The atrial septum is fenestrated or partially closed.
6. Where atresia of the pulmonary valve is encountered, establishment of the RV-PA continuity is a must.
7. VSD closure if present.

The upcoming are the 2 most popular biventricular repair procedures for neonates tricuspid valvuloplasty techniques:

Technique of Knott–Craig Monocusp

This procedure has changed EA neonatal therapy via providing the option of a biventricular repair in the EA group with a difficult-to-treat group category. The main focus of repair is appropriate anterior leaflet mobilization with a movable leading edge supported well in order to aid in achieving valvular competency by coapting with the ventricular septum. The leaflet of the ventricular septum is preserved because it is considered one of its structures. The important steps are as follows:

By placating the posterior leaflet from the coronary sinus to the anteroposterior commissure, the posterior leaflet is destroyed. The primary tricuspid orifice and a caudal orifice are formed as a result. The ARV is also eliminated by obliterating the caudal orifice with a vertical plication suture. During the plication, take care that right coronary artery is not to be included.

In circumstances when the ventricular wall is adherent to the anterior leaflet however, it is not big enough in extent to the ventricular septum, as a result a determination might be needed as its body could be augmented. It is considered vital to have free edge that's both mobile and well supported. By providing a more stable point to hinge a "Sebening stitch" that is modified as formed from the ventricular septum to the anterior leaflet even more strength will be present.

- Fenestrated patch closes the ASD.
- Atrioplasty is used to produce reduction in the right atrium size.
- Relying upon how well annuloplasty works, a monocusp-associated transannular patch or an RV-PA conduit is utilized to treat pulmonary atresia.

da Silva Cone Repair Procedure

Cone reconstruction is a new procedure that was first reported by da Silva in 2007 and has since been the treatment of choice for EA tricuspid valve repair. The technique of Carpentier has formed the basis for this technique in which the inferior and septal leaflet tissues are to be organized to utilize all three leaflets of the TV, and then its sides were rotated clockwise and reattached in a method to produce leaflet tissue that is 360 degrees in width and shares a central blood flow. After that, the genuine annulus was reattached again to the newly built "cone" resulting in nearly anatomic repair. There has been an increase in reports numbers of the Cone technique being used for EA in neonates.

The following are the important steps in this procedure:

- Mobilizing leaflets from functional annulus: from functional annulus all 3 leaflets are detached except for certain portions in the anterior leaflet (in between 10–12 clock—the points of anterior leaflet divergence from true annulus), a rim of valvular tissue 1–2 mm in size is left on the annulus in order for reattachment facilitation. The name given to this edge is "Cut edge."
- Delamination of the leaflets: By dividing fibromuscular adhesions, the leaflets' bodies are moved away from the ventricular wall and septum. From the annulus, this is performed for about two-thirds of the body of the valve. This stage provides great subvalvular apparatus exposure. Small fenestrations might occur throughout this process due to the leaflets thinning downwards, which if they found to be not a part of coapting surface should be fixed carefully.
- After mobilization of the leaflets body, the following step is ensuring that the leaflets "Leading edge," known also as the coapting edge, is subtended by existing from the primary chords or has an autologous neochord that had been derived from ventricular wall fibro-muscular tissue, typically being arisen from papillary muscle as a consequence of the process of delamination. Fibro-muscular tissue being extended from free edge (especially the posterior and septal leaflets) can be quite collinear at times, requiring longitudinal fenestrations to produce neo-chords that are separate to allow input into the ventricle without any restriction. For a successful repair, it's crucial to have an unattached and well-supported leading edge.

- The leaflet cut edge lying posteriorly is carried to the leaflet's septal cut edge by a rotation clockwise once all three leaflets have been mobilized, creating 360 degree "Cone" of tricuspid tissue. To avoid the presence of any distortion, it's best to utilize interrupted stitches. This symbolizes a "Cone," with the mobilized leaflet cut edges forming the base and the leading edge associated with subtending structures of the chords forming the apex. If it is considered very small, then the posterior leaflet's cut edge is carried to the septal edge anterior leaflet in order to for the cone generation.
- ARV reduction and plication of anatomic annulus: The ARV is plicated longitudinally from the tip to the bottom, as it keeps the geometry better than placating horizontally. The portion of the RV that is non-trabeculated is referred to as ARV. This reduces the genuine annular size to some amount as well. During this stage, be careful not to include or deform the right coronary artery. Furthermore, the annulus may be so dilated that simply plicating the ARV may not be enough to reduce it. By intermittently plicating it along the annulus's other half, particularly the anterior side, a more symmetric decrease of the real annulus can be achieved.
- Sutures are used to attach the "Cut edge" to plicated true annulus, which might be continuous or interrupted. An additional security is provided by the presence of second suture line.
- When there are concerns about right heart dysfunction, closing of the ASD is being done in valved or fenestrated form, functioning like a "pop-off" with right into left shunt.
- Before atrial closure, a superfluous piece of the enlarged right atrium is excised in a reduction atrioplasty.

Pulmonary hypertension, older ages (> 60 years), presence of biventricular dysfunction (30% ejection fraction for left ventricule), deficiency of leaflet septal tissue and anterior leaflet minimal delaminated tissue (50%), and severe enlargement of RV with corresponding right atrioventricular junction severe dilation are all potential contraindications to cone reconstruction.

The subsequents are the main steps in a univentricular repair technique:

- If the valve is inadequate, the major pulmonary artery and the PDA are ligated.
- Patch with fenestrated holes (modified Starnes procedure). To allow for RV decompression, the TV must be closed. Gortex patch with 4 mm fenestration, or a Sano RV exclusion treatment, is more expected to maintain the underlying structures of the valve for valvuloplasty in the future. The idea is to generate a functional tricuspid atresia that is more tolerated.

- An unobstructed atrial septum is created.
- A shunt known as Blalock-Taussig shunt is created.
- To allow lung development the atrioplasty on the right side was reduced.
- A bidirectional Glenn surgery and a Fontan technique are used to further channel the patients down the single ventricle palliation. Again, at each step, an assessment should be performed to consider the possibility of enlisting the RV as a subpulmonary ventricle that has a valvuloplasty/valve replacement, if this is feasible. As a result, either ventricle of 1.5 or a biventricular reparation is possible.

The following are the two most popular univentricular repair procedures:

- Starnes procedure
  It's a successful single ventricle palliation approach for neonates that helped increase survival in a group that was previously difficult to treat and had a high death rate. An autologous non-fenestrated pericardial patch that is treated by glutaraldehyde was employed in the original study. In order to avoid any harm to the system of conduction, this patch at the "anatomic" level of tricuspid valve is sutured and coronary sinus has been kept on the RV excluded side. Since then, the method has been changed to include 4 mm patch fenestration (patch of GORE-TEX, it is expected to provide protection for the leaflets more likely) and the coronary sinus which drains in the right atrium. With pulmonary atresia, fenestration is considered especially critical in preventing the excluded RV persistent expansion and compression of the LV subsequently. Coronary sinus is also inserted on the RA side in order to provide prevention of presence of any extra place of flowing blood. A septectomy of the atrial septum allows for optimal mixing. To create a regulated source of the pulmonary blood flowing, a modified shunt of Blalock-Taussig-Thomas is used. With bidirectional Glenn and Fontan surgeries, most newborns having RV Starnes exclusion technique then are directed toward a single ventricular conduit.
- Sano RV exclusion procedure
  Another single ventricle palliation approach is this one. Regardless of TV orifice closing by a Gortex patch fenestrated type, the right ventricular free wall is removed as it is redundant and thinned out; the resulting damage is corrected primarily. Thus, the volume of dilated RV is reduced and compression of the LV is also reduced by limitation of the late diastolic migration of ventricular septum to the left. It helps with the lungs' bulk effect also. Coronary sinus is kept in the right side of the atria (lower pressure chamber) and patch is lined in distance from the membranous septum to avoid heart block occurrence, as opposed to standard Starnes method. The Sano method,

on the other hand, has the disadvantage of being unable to transfer into a biventricular repair when the excluded right ventricle grows.

Heart transplantation is more effective in neonates who have coupled dysfunction of the LV or unusual associations like a hypoplastic syndrome of the left heart.

- Tricuspid valve replacement

A replacement of tricuspid valve is required when there is no possibility for a repair is or failure had occurred. Each effort for valve repair should be taken, particularly in patients who are younger, such as newborns and young children, who have limited valve replacement alternatives. On the other hand, for patients with older ages (more than sixty years old) who have a substantially enlarged RV or TV annular dilatation, replacement is considered more beneficial than a difficult and perilous reparation requiring more periods in the operating room. In the tricuspid position, mechanical valves have higher thrombogenicity, as a result bioprosthetic valves are preferred and usually in case of RV severe dysfunction they are avoided owing to the possibility of motion anomalies in the disc. The main fact is the avoidance of the septal surface conduction system of the implant's, as well as right coronary artery on the implant's inferior and anterior sides. It's possible that the suture line will be placed more atrially rather than via the annulus. It's possible that the coronary sinus will be kept on the RV side. Bioprosthetic valve Struts also should be directed so no occlusion of AV nodal site is present nor an obstruction to the RVOT. In valve replacement a percutaneous TV valve, usually with melody valve, is a future possibility that can be accomplished with low risk.

When LV function is severely low, heart transplantation should be considered. A diastolic and systolic dysfunction, non-compaction cardiomyopathy might be present on the left side. However, with the inclusion of a BDG, patients who have older ages associated LVEF that is as low as 30% could be saved with a TV replacement or repair. As the time passes, part of those individuals sees an enhancement in the function of their LV. In the RV there is an increased index of the end-diastole >200 mL/m^2 as well as 40%EF, and age is more than 50 years. There might be an advantage in quick intervention in EA therefore the need for a heart transplant might be avoided, according to the risk factors for RV failure postoperatively.

- Ablation using a catheter

In individuals with Ebstein's abnormality who develop tachyarrhythmias, electrophysiological assessment and ablation by radiofrequency to the accessory symptomatic pathway(s) when possible should be undertaken. Patients who have the abnormality had a poorer success rate with catheter ablation than patients with normal hearts struc-

turally, and higher recurrence risk is present. At the time of surgical correction, ablation of the supraventricular tachyarrhythmia present at the same time with an Ebstein's abnormality is possible to be done also.

Prognosis

EA of the tricuspid valve is a rare cardiac condition with poor prognosis. TR (tricuspid regurgitation) severity, extent of tricuspid valve displacement (TVD), cardiothoracic (CT) ratio, hepatomegaly, associated cardiac defects like VSD, requiring mechanical ventilation and medication, pulmonary valve defects, patent arterial duct, oxygen saturation (SaO$_2$) which is presented as cyanosis, and the time of presentation (young age a) can all affect the outcome in neonates. But yet no identifiable reliability regarding risk factors can predict the mortality in this population who have complex congenital heart disease. Prenatal illness diagnosis and fetal death are frequently associated with individuals on the severe end of the range. The echocardiographic appearance and existence of accompanying lesions can suggest fetal presentation, which is related to more severe outcomes. The history nature of more severe Ebstein anomaly variants is terrible without therapy. According to certain research, just half of the patients live to be 13 years old. Those with milder variants, on the other hand, have a life expectancy that is more usual, while drugs treated children have few problems and great outcomes, and the majority of the patients who survive till childhood have few symptoms or no symptoms at all and reasonably a heart with normal function. The existence of concomitant cardiac abnormalities and severe displacement of the tricuspid valve are potential predictors for surgical palliation needed in the period of newborn, and children who have surgery perform well. Ebstein's anomaly early mortality in the newborn has decreased considerably as a result of improved diagnostic procedures, contemporary neonatal care, and significant advancements in innovative surgical approaches during infancy and youth, all of which have helped to increase the survival rate of this age group. Incidental findings and arrhythmia are prevalent in older children and adults, and the long-term result is better.

Multiple Choice Questions

1. Which heart valve is affected in Ebstein's anomaly.
    A. Bicuspid valve.
    B. Pulmonary valve.
    C. Aortic valve.
    D. Tricuspid valve.
2. Which leaflet is the most affected in the valve?
    A. Septal leaflet.
    B. Anterior leaflet.

C. Posterior leaflet.

D. All of the above.

3. What is the diagnostic feature of Ebstein anomaly in PA X-ray.

A. Box-like shape.

B. Wall-to-wall shape.

C. Clock face.

D. All of the above.

4. Which of the following is considered to be the gold standard procedure to diagnose Ebstein's anomaly?

A. Echocardiogram.

B. Prenatal sonography.

C. X-ray.

D. ECG.

5. All of the following could be seen in the ECG of the patient with Ebstein's anomaly except.

A. PR interval prolongation.

B. Atrial arrhythmia.

C. features of Wolff-Parkinson-White syndrome.

D. Short P wave.

6. Ebstein's anomaly may be associated with which of the following.

A. Kidney problems.

B. Hematological disease.

C. Aortic valve atresia.

D. ASD.

7. Clinical examination of the patient with Ebstein's anomaly may reveal.

A. Elevated JVP.

B. Skin dehydration.

C. Altered sensation.

D. All of the above.

8. All of the following are considered to be contraindication to cone reconstruction except.

A. Old age group.

B. Large septal leaflet.

C. Pulmonary hypertension.

D. Severe enlargement of RV.

9. Which one of the following medications is effective in the case of Ebstein's anomaly?

A. Propranolol.

B. Milrinone.

C. Amoxicillin.

D. Salbutamol.

10. Which of the following is the distinguishing feature of EA?

A. Right-sided heart failure.

B. ASD.

C. VSD.

D. Apical displacement of septal leaflet.

Answers

1. D.

   Explanation: Ebstein's anomaly is a congenital heart disease characterized by deformity of the tricuspid valve and right side of the heart.

2. A.

   Explanation: Apical displacement of septal leaflet presents in all Ebstein' anomaly patients.

3. D.

   Explanation: Right atrial enlargement and cardiomegaly, giving the appearance of a globe-shape.

4. A.

   Explanation: This particular test provided the pediatric cardiologist the ability to determine valve insufficiency severity (leakage) or the valve stenosis (narrowing), degree of valve displacement, heart chambers size, and whether an open (patent) foramen ovale was present or not. This test also helps to diagnose patients whose clinical features were not pathognomonic.

5. D.

   Explanation: Because of the presence of right atrial hypertrophy, that means a tall P wave greater than 3 mm.

6. D.

   Explanation: Ebstein' anomaly may be associated with structural abnormalities like ASD, VSD, and PFO.

7. A.

   Explanation: Elevated jugular venous pressure can be caused by tricuspid regurgitation and increased right atrial pressure.

8. B.

   Explanation: Because the da silva-cone reconstruction procedure depends on mobilization of leaflets, a small leaflet states failure of procedure.

9. B.

   Explanation: Milrinone is a highly effective medication since it affects the right ventricle in both lusitropic and inotropic ways. It also allows for increased ante-grade pulmonary blood flowing by lowering pulmonary vascular resistance.

10. D.

Explanation: The degree of apical displacement of the septal leaflet (≥ 8 mm/m^2 body surface area) is the critical distinguishing feature of EA from other congenital regurgitant lesions.

References

1. Tudorache S (2018) Congenital anomalies: from the embryo to the neonate
2. Giamberti A, Chessa M (2014) The tricuspid valve in congenital heart disease
3. Digilio MC, Bernardini L, Lepri F, Giuffrida MG, Guida V, Baban A, Versacci P, Capolino R, Torres B, De Luca A, Novelli A, Marino B, Dallapiccola B. Ebstein anomaly: genetic heterogeneity and association with microdeletions 1p36 and 8p23.1. Am J Med Genet A. 2011;155(9):2196–202.
4. Yuan S-M. Ebstein's anomaly: genetics, clinical manifestations, and management. Pediatr Neonatol. 2017;58(3):211–5.
5. Cabin HS, Roberts WC. Ebstein's anomaly of the tricuspid valve and prolapse of the mitral valve. Am Heart J. 1981;101(2):177–80.
6. Gerlis LM, Ho SY, Sweeney AE. Mitral valve anomalies associated with Ebstein's malformation of the tricuspid valve. Am J Cardiovasc Pathol. 1993;4(4):294–301.
7. Holst KA, Connolly HM, Dearani JA. Ebstein's anomaly. Methodist DeBakey Cardiovasc J. 2019;15(2):138–44.
8. Cincinnatichildrens.org (2019) Ebstein's anomaly in children | symptoms, repair & treatment
9. Barron DJ. Core topics in congenital cardiac surgery. Google books. Cambridge University Press; 2018.
10. Cha M-Y, Won H-S, Lee M-Y, Woo K-H, Shim J-Y. An unusual ultrasonographic manifestation of a fetal Ebstein anomaly. Obstetr Gynecol Sci. 2014;57(6):530–3.
11. Augustin N, Schmidt-Habelmann P, Wottke M, Meisner H, Sebening F. Results after surgical repair of Ebstein's anomaly. Ann Thorac Surg. 1997;63(6):1650–6.
12. Radford DJ, Graff RF, Neilson GH. Diagnosis and natural history of Ebstein's anomaly. Br Heart J. 1985;54(5):517–22.
13. Root MC, Fisher KL. Prenatal sonographic detection of Ebstein's anomaly. J Diagn Med Sonogr. 2017;33(3):225–30.
14. Marcu CB, Donohue TJ. A young man with palpitations and Ebstein's anomaly of the tricuspid valve. Can Med Assoc J. 2005;172(12):1553–4.
15. Driscoll DJ, Mottram CD, Danielson GK. Spectrum of exercise intolerance in 45 patients with Ebstein's anomaly and observations on exercise tolerance in 11 patients after surgical repair. J Am Coll Cardiol. 1988;11(4):831–6.
16. Pflaumer A, Eicken A, Augustin N, Hess J. Symptomatic neonates with Ebstein anomaly. J Thorac Cardiovasc Surg. 2004;127(4):1208–9.
17. Sainathan, S., da Fonseca da Silva, L., and da Silva, J.P. (2020). Ebstein's anomaly: contemporary management strategies. J Thorac Dis, 12(3), pp.1161–1173
18. Attenhofer Jost CH, Connolly HM, Dearani JA, Edwards WD, Danielson GK. Ebstein's anomaly. Circulation. 2007;115(2):277–85.
19. Kaiser L, Kron IL, Spray TL. Mastery of cardiothoracic surgery. Google books. Lippincott Williams & Wilkins; 2013.
20. Lee LA, Kulik TJ, Sandhu SK, Goldberg CS, Mosca RS, Bove EL, Charpie JR. Prognostic stratification of neonatal Ebstein's anomaly. Pediatr Res. 1999;45(7):26–6.
21. Celermajer DS, Bull C, Till JA, Cullen S, Vassillikos VP, Sullivan ID, Allan L, Nihoyannopoulos P, Somerville J, Deanfield JE. Ebstein's anomaly: Presentation and outcome from fetus to adult. J Am Coll Cardiol. 1994;23(1):170–6.
22. Kapusta L, Eveleigh RM, Poulino SE, Rijlaarsdam ME, du Marchie Sarvaas GJ, Strengers JL, Delhaas T, de Korte CL, Feuth T, Helbing WA. Ebstein's anomaly: factors associated with death in childhood and adolescence: a multi-centre, long-term study. Eur Heart J. 2007;28(21):2661–6.

Hypoplastic Left Heart Syndrome

Mahnoor Sukaina and Irfan Ullah

Abstract

An embryonic heart and a fetal heart are different from the neonatal heart. The heart of the human embryo when 10 mm from crown to rump, it is symmetrical in the sense that the septa formation is in the middle of atria and ventricles. The plane of septa extends from the anterior part of the anterior interventricular sulcus to the posterior part of the atrial septum. In congenital heart defects (CHDs), the position of the heart has a different appearance when seen through ultrasonographic guidance. Such as when the right ventricle is underdeveloped, the cardiac apex has an anterior position, while in the hypoplasia of the left ventricle, the cardiac axis is found to be posterior. Moreover, anatomically and functionally, a left heart is different from the right. The tissues forming the left atrium are smoother, refined, and comprised of narrow and tubular appendages. Similarly, trabeculae carneae of the left ventricle is comprised of a thin and smoother layer, while the fibrous continuum exists in the bicuspid and aortic valves. In the fetal heart, the left atrium is in situ posterior chamber, while the pulmonary vein exists inferiorly and shifts cranially by the start of the 12th week of gestation. It affects 1–8% of all the CVMs. The disease is fatal without surgical intervention, and even in the case of survival, the data and research lack a definite answer on the life span and other associated comorbidities of these patients. Nonetheless, HLHS even after the surgical interventions the survival chances are only 65% until the age of 5 and 55% at the age of 10. This chapter provides a comprehensive overview regarding the anatomy, etiology, epidemiology, genealogy, morphology, pathogenesis, management, and surgical intervention of HLHS.

M. Sukaina (✉)
Karachi Medical and Dental College, Karachi, Pakistan

I. Ullah
Kabir Medical College, Gandhara University, Peshawar, Pakistan

Keywords

Epidemiology · Hypoplastic left heart syndrome
Congenital heart defects · Anatomy · Fetal heart
Genealogy · Diagnosis · Norwood procedure · Palliative
treatment · Pathogenesis · Morphology

Background

The chapter provides a comprehensive overview of hypoplastic left heart syndrome (HLHS), which is a rare congenital heart defect. The topics discussed in this chapter are:

- *Postnatal anatomy of a human heart*: a refresher is provided in terms of human heart anatomy, and functionality of the four chambers of the heart in the systemic and pulmonary circulation.
- *Anatomy of a fetal heart*: the formation of the embryonic heart and fetal heart is discussed. This anatomy provides an understanding of the discussion in the later sections when the influence of genes is discussed in the causality of the HLHS.
- *Heart of the newborn:* this section discusses the differences in the heart of a newborn, and the difference between the fetal and adult heart. Readers will find out that the pressure on the newborn heart is proportionately much higher than the adult heart. And in this scenario, the complications arising from the HLHS can be fatal. The subsections discuss the structure of the right heart and its abnormalities, and the structure of the left heart and its abnormalities.
- *What is HLHS*: the definition is given for the HLHS and its epidemiology.
- *Genecology and genealogy of the HLHS*: This section is divided into two subsections; the role of specific genes that play roles in the causality of the HLHS, and the hereditary influences and probands health conditions that pose risk to the children.

G. Tagarakis et al. (eds.), *Clinical and Surgical Aspects of Congenital Heart Diseases*,
https://doi.org/10.1007/978-3-031-23062-2_23

- *Morphology and pathogenesis of the HLHS*: this section discussed morphology and pathogenesis of the HLHS in light of the main hypothesis and other subvariants.
- *Management of the disease*: various management techniques and important research are discussed in this section, and how does HLHS can cause long-term comorbidities and health complications in the postnatal survivors.
- *Diagnosis of the HLHS*: diagnosis of the HLHS is discussed in light of three subsections: prenatal, at birth, and postnatal.
- *Surgical intervention*: different surgical interventions are discussed in this section, including prenatal surgical intervention, stage-1,2,3 palliative treatment, heart transplantation, and hybrid approach.

Postnatal Anatomy of a Human Heart

The inner cavity of the human heart has four chambers: left atrium, right atrium, left ventricle, and right ventricle. In between the left atrium and left ventricle lies the left atrioventricular valve, and similarly in between the right atrium and right ventricle lies the right atrioventricular valve. The left and right atria are separated by the interatrial septum, while the left and right ventricles are separated by the interventricular septum. The interatrial septum and interventricular septum are separated by the atrioventricular septum, which is a fibrous membranous septum. The left atrioventricular junction (AVJ) has a bicuspid or mitral valve, while the right AVJ has a tricuspid valve. The valves (mitral or tricuspid) are elongated by chordae tendineae that joins the papillary muscle. These muscles are attached to the innermost layer of the heart called the endocardium, followed by a relatively thicker middle layer called myocardium, then the two parts of the outermost layer epicardium: visceral pericardium and parietal pericardium separated in-between by pericardial space. The left and right ventricles also have ridge muscles called trabeculae carneae that is thin in the left ventricle and coarse in the right ventricle, and assist chordae tendineae in preventing the regurgitation of blood into the atrium.

Functionalities of the Four Heart Chambers

As for the functionalities of these chambers; the superior vena cava (SVC) carries deoxygenated blood from the upper body of a human: neck, brain, arms, and shoulder. It extends out from the brachiocephalic veins to enter the right atrium. Inferior vena cava (IVC) carries deoxygenated blood from the lower body of the human, which extends out from the iliac veins to enter the right atrium. The venous blood directs the flow from the right atrium to the right ventricle via the tricuspid valve. The right ventricle is involved in pulmonary circulation by pumping venous blood into the lungs through the pulmonic valve into pulmonary arteries. The oxygenated blood is pumped back into the left atrium through pulmonary veins from the lung. The left atrium fills the left ventricle with oxygenated blood through the bicuspid valve. The left ventricle supplies the oxygenated blood through the aortic valve to the aorta that pumps it to the rest of the body.

Anatomy of the Fetal Heart

The heart of the human embryo when 10 mm from crown to rump, it is symmetrical in the sense that the septa formation is in the middle of atria and ventricles. The plane of septa extends from the anterior part of the anterior interventricular sulcus to the posterior part of the atrial septum [1]. Soon after that, the rotation occurs when the apical part of the anterior interventricular sulcus moves to the left, and the posterior part of the atrial septum moves to the right. In the second trimester, when the fetus is about 100 mm [1], the plane of the atrial and ventricular septa is at 45° to the sagittal and coronal plane of the body [2]. This angulation of the septa plays an imperative role in revealing the fetal heart with the postnatal heart. The details of the development are omitted from this section, as it is out of the scope of the chapter, but the readers are encouraged to refer to the article by Walmsley and Monkhouse [1] that discusses the development in detail.

The length of the fetal heart at the 12 weeks of gestation is 8 mm, which becomes 16 mm between the 12th and 17th week, and 24 mm at the end of the 21st week of gestation [2]. Readers are also encouraged to refer to an article by Moorman et al. [3] that discusses in detail the formation of heart tubes, through the process called gastrulation, which happens in the third week of embryonic development. The formation of three germ layers: ectoderm, mesoderm, and endoderm occurs at this stage. Heart tissues are formed by the mesodermal layer, which forms the crescent; later extending to the neural plate, which is formed by the ectodermal layer. At this point of development, the plate of promyocardial cells is intertwined with the plexus of endothelial cells. The endocardial cells form the tube, which is partially wrapped around by the myocardial cells, and maintain modularity with the splanchnic mesoderm and developing mediastinum at the dorsal mesocardium [3].

In congenital heart defects, the position of the heart has a different appearance from the ultrasonographic scan. When the right ventricle is underdeveloped, the cardiac apex has an anterior position; while in the hypoplasia of the left ventricle, the cardiac axis is found to be posterior. This discussion is delayed for the further sections when hypoplastic left heart syndrome is elaborated.

Heart of a Newborn

A child born in a normal term that is eight and a half to 9 months, weighs around seven pounds, while a premature child that is 7 months weighs around three pounds. The cardiac output in a newborn is 550 ml per minute as compared to an adult that is 3 L per minute. However, the difference is the heart of a newborn is proportionally exerting more pressure in context to the size of the body as compared to an adult. This is why, the pulse rate of an embryo in a fetus is 65 per minute at the end of the third week, which near the term of the birth reaches up to 150 per minute, and 180 per minute at the time of birth, 170 per minute after 10 min of the birth, 120–140 per minute 15 min to an hour after birth, and 113–127 per minute 6 months to a year after birth [4 p. 40]. This transition in the pulse rates indicates that at the time of birth, a newborn's baby is pumping and circulating rapidly; one prime reason is that the circulation system of a fetus is dependent on the placenta and umbilical cord. However, at birth, when the umbilical cord is cut off, a newborn's heart starts the circulation on its own.

The weight of a heart of a newborn is about 20 gm at the time of birth, 100 gm at about 6 years of age, 200 gm at about 14–15 years of age, and slightly less than 300gm at adulthood. In a normal newborn, the weight of the ventricle in comparison to the atrium is 4–5:1 at the time of birth, and later in adulthood is slightly more than 6:1. It is the left ventricle versus the right ventricle that weighs a quarter proportion more (1.25:1); however, the growth of the left ventricle is about twice that of the right ventricle at the end of 2 years after the birth [4 p. 41]. The size of the left and right ventricles is not the only difference; the thickness of the lateral walls also differs between the left and the right ventricle. At birth, the thickness of both the left and right ventricles is approximately equal, which is about 5 mm. However, the lateral wall of the left ventricle is twice thicker than the right ventricle nearly at the end of 24 months after the birth, and three times thicker when the child reaches puberty [4 p. 42].

Right Heart

It is out of the scope of this chapter to discuss the structure and abnormalities of the right heart, and any reader interested in it is referred to the article by Cook et al. [2], which elaborates this section with minute details. Briefly, the morphological appearance of the right atrium possesses its properties by the tenth week of gestation, where the appendage is more triangular as compared to the left atrium, which is tubular and bendy. The pectinate muscles of the right atrium elongate from the tip of the atrial appendage around AVJ to the crux of the heart. However, in the left appendage, the pectinate muscles are confined to the tubular situs, hence exhibiting a smooth posterior AVJ. During the development of the normal fetal heart, superior and inferior caval veins in the right atrium extend to the cranial and caudal ends. By the mid-trimester of the pregnancy, the inferior caval vein is parted from the right atrium by the Eustachian valve. The coronary sinus also enters the right atrium as the systemic venous tributaries. The right ventricle has coarse trabeculation in its apex, as compared to the left ventricle whose trabeculae carneae is thin and smoother as compared to the right ventricle. Tricuspid inlet valve in the right ventricle closes in trifoliate modularity. The inlet and outlet of the right ventricle are segregated by the part of subpulmonary infundibulum known as conus; crista supraventricularis [2].

In the fetal heart, before the 12th week of gestation, the tricuspid valve is not fully developed. The developing leaflet of the tricuspid valve from the inferior AV cushion is in the process of bending and delaminating from the right ventricle septum, whose failure can result in Ebstein's malformation, resulting in tricuspid valvar incompetence and cardiomegaly. Another anomaly is the absence of the connection of the right atrium and the right ventricle resulting in tricuspid atresia.

Left Heart

The tissues forming the left atrium are smoother, refined, and comprised of narrow and tubular appendages. Similarly, trabeculae carneae of the left ventricle is comprised of a thin and smoother layer, while the fibrous continuum exists in the bicuspid and aortic valves. In the fetal heart, the left atrium is in situ posterior chamber, while the pulmonary vein exists inferiorly and shifts cranially by the start of the 12th week of gestation. Therefore, a solitary pulmonary venous channel branches out to four solely pulmonary veins and enters the top left of the left atrium. As stated above in the opening section of the chapter the left side of the heart has a mitral or bicuspid valve. It consists of two uneven and nonsymmetric leaflets, the anterior side referred to as the aortic or arterial leaflet is evident at the crux of the heart. It consists of one-third of the mitral annulus ring and approximately two-thirds of the valvular orifice [5]. The parasternal short-axis view, also known as ring or doughnut view, reveals the orientation of the valvar orifice to be oblique to the ventricular septum. The arterial leaflet of the bicuspid valve pivots from the apex of the transverse sinus. The second leaflet of the mitral valve is the posterior leaflet, also referred to as a mural or ventricular leaflet, and comprises two-thirds of the mitral annulus. The prime functionality of the mitral valve leaflets is during diastolic filling blood from the left atrium to the left ventricle, and during systolic preventing blood to reverse from the left ventricle to the left atrium [5].

Likewise tricuspid valve abnormality, the mitral valve may have a similar problem, when the leaflets do not close properly, it may result in mitral valve regurgitation. Similarly, there can be a complete absence of the connection between the left atrium and left ventricle, called mitral atresia, or there can be partial mitral stenosis. One of the major abnormalities of the left heart is hypoplastic left heart syndrome (HLHS), and until now the chapter wanted its readers to understand the importance of the anatomical structure of the heart, whether fetal or newborn. The obstructions in the left ventricular outflow tract (LVOT) are the leading and most severe form of congenital heart defects, which includes coarctation of the aorta (CoA), bicuspid aortic valve (BAV), aortic valve stenosis (AVS), and hypoplastic left heart syndrome (HLHS) [6]. The subsequent section will highlight the discussion around the various aspect of the HLHS, its epidemiology and etiology, and its management, diagnosis, and treatment.

What Is HLHS?

The underdevelopment of left heart chambers together with malformations of ascending aorta and aortic arch was discussed by Lev in 1952. However, it was in 1958 when Noonan and Nadas highlighted the mitral and aortic atresia, hence opening the field of discussion on hypoplastic left heart syndrome.

Definition

Hinton et al. define HLHS as "atresia or stenosis of the aortic and mitral valves and hypoplasia of the left ventricle and ascending aorta" [7]. Öhman et al. [8] exclude the stenosis of the aortic valves from the definition. The signs and symptoms according to the ICD 10 code 2021 edition (Q23.4) include tachypnea, cyanosis, dyspnea, and lethargy. It is to be noted that the ventricular septum remains intact, and so do the great arteries in the HLSH [9].

The disease is fatal without surgical intervention, and even in the case of survival, the data and research lack a definite answer on the life span and other associated comorbidities of these patients. Nonetheless, HLHS even after the surgical interventions the survival chances are only 65% until the age of 5 and 55% at the age of 10 [9, 10]. However, Barron et al. [10] emphasized that the gravity of HLHS is so austere that if not treated then 25–40% of neonatal death within a few weeks will be due to this defect, which affects 95% of the cases.

Epidemiology of the HLHS

Hypoplastic left heart syndrome is a rare and severe congenital heart defect (CHD) that results in cardiovascular malformation (CVM) [7]. It affects 1–8% of all the CVMs [8–10]. It is the leading cause of infant mortality and morbidity in children [7], by affecting 1 in 5–10,000 neonates each year and causing 1 in 4 deaths in an infant due to CHD [11]. In the absence of selection in the pregnancy, HLHS may affect from 8 to 25 per 10,000 live births in neonates [8]. Barron estimates that 200–260 neonates are born annually with the HLHS in the UK. In the USA, there is about 2000 annual incidence of the HLHS [9]. Complications in terms of delayed motor development and severe impairment in cognitive functioning are found across all the phenotypes in HLHS. The prevalence of HLHS is higher in the male population, and increased maternal age is another factor [6].

Genecology and Genealogy of HLHS

Genecology

The MIM# for HLHS is 241,550, this number will be useful for further and future readers, who would be interested in dwelling further into the gene-causality of this defect. In a periodically and rapidly evolving field of genetics, various reasons are hypothesized to be associated with the malformation in cardiac. At the embryogenesis stage the Drosophila tinman NK-homeobox genes Nkx2–5, Nkx2–3, and Nkx2–6 result in the malformation of the heart [12, 13]. Nkx2–5-Cre and Mef2c-AHF-Cre lineage cells have a major contribution to aortic and mitral valves [13]. Serum response factors (SRF) and myocardin transcription factors (MTF) play a vital role in the formation of mesoderm, which forms the heart tissues [12]. Other external gene factors involve bone morphogenetic protein (BMP), fibroblast growth factor (FGF), and the WNT family of protein that influences cardiac development and its abnormalities. Wnt1-Cre plays a major contribution only to the aortic valve [13]. The genetic depletion of T-box transcription factor Tbx5 results in the atria and left ventricle [12]. It is found that ablation of the histone deacetylase-dependent transcriptional Bop protein results in the hypoplastic right ventricle, its association with the HLHS is not exploited. Similarly, the Irx4 homeodomain transcription impacts the fate of the ventricle chamber. The presence of Fgf10 mRNA is observed in the development of secondary heart field in the mesoderm, and at this point of development Tbx1, transcription factor Tbx1 may play a role in the 22q11 deletion syndrome [12]. Mef2c-AHF-Cre has also a significant dedicated role in secondary heart field cells [13].

Chromosomal anomalies such as trisomy 18 (Edwards syndrome), 22q11.21–2 deletion (DiGeorge syndrome), monosomy X (Turner syndrome) in 5–13% of HLHS cases, 11q deletion (Jacobsen syndrome) in 10% of the HLHS cases,10 1q21.1 microduplication (tetralogy of Fallot), have also been found to be associated with the HLHS [9]. Other limited studies have found an association of other genes as the cause of HLHS; however, further studies including a wide array of subjects and cohort studies are required for confirmation. This group of genes defects includes connexin43 gene mutation, in which arginine codons at positions 362 and 376 are replaced by glutamines codons [14, 15], or reduction in connexin43 and N-cadherin [15]. Other studies of gene mutations are NOTCH116 that affects the left ventricular outflow tract, and HAND1 and GATA4 are not the cause of HLHS [16, 17].

Genealogy

It is found in the studying of the probands of the HLHS that the malformation of the left- and right-sided valve dysplasia, or the presence of bicuspid aortic valve (BAV) in the lineage or family members; 18.3% first-degree relative [9]. Hinton et al. [7] found a strong hereditary association in probands and the neonate born with HLHS. In his study, 55% of the families had greater than one affected individual with heart defects. All the subjects in his HLHS probands had either hypoplasia or dysplasia. 94% of his subjects had mitral dysplasia, 56% had tricuspid dysplasia, and 11% had pulmonary dysplasia [7]. Limited research has been conducted that found the causality of the HLHS by the non-chromosomal genetic conditions, including Smith-Lemli-Opitz syndrome, Rubinstein-Taybi syndrome, Holt-Oram syndrome, vertebral defects, anal atresia, cardiac defects, tracheoesophageal fistula, renal anomalies, and limb abnormalities (VACTERL) association, and Noonan syndrome. The detailed association is omitted from the discussion as it is out of the scope of this chapter; therefore, only a reference is made for the readers interested in exploring further reasons.

By using whole-genome sequencing, Theis [18] found the HLHS to be heritable by discovering the presence of pathogenic MYBPC3 nonsense variant in the first proband who had the transplantation due to diastolic heart failure. Another proband was identified with the presence of a pathogenic RYR2 variant. The hereditary risk factors that may contribute toward the outcome of HLHS in the offspring include dilated or hypertrophic cardiomyopathy, left ventricular noncompaction (LVNC), bicuspid aortic valve (BAV), and the rare presence of MHY6 variants [18]. Helle et al. [19], in a cohort study in Finland, could not find any association of MHY6 in probands as the pathogenic factor to cause HLHS.

Morphology and Pathogenesis of HLHS

The generally adopted hypothesis in terms of the pathogenesis of HLHS is the variations in the blood circulation at the embryonic development, including premature narrowing of the foramen ovale, or obstruction in the aortic valve [9]. The BMP and transforming growth factor-beta (TGF-β) molecules send signals from the myocardium of the atrioventricular canal. TGF-β molecules induce epithelial to the mesenchymal transformation that forms the valves via endocardial cushions. Improper secretion of the TGF-β2 from the myocardium to endocardial cushion may result in the deletion of BMP receptor gene ALK3, thus, resulting in the absence of valve formation [12].

Barron et al. [9] discuss that neonate with HLHS has patent ductus arteriosus at birth, which affects the systemic circulation. The deoxygenated (venous) blood from SVC and IVC empties into the right atrium, which is filtered to oxygenated blood via patent foramen ovale to enter the tricuspid valve. At this stage of the circulation, the pulmonary venous can enter the systemic circulation through the foramen ovale to reach the atrial septum. In HLHS due to mitral atresia or stenosis, the oxygenated and deoxygenated blood is mixed to create cyanosis. If no external intervention is done in the neonates with HLHS, the duct naturally closes failing the systemic circulation.

The left heart components including the aortic arch, the ascending aorta, the aortic valve, the mitral valve, the outflow tract, and the LV cavity are simultaneously involved in the circulation process rather than in isolation. In the aortic atresia or mitral stenosis, there is an inflow but not the outflow into the LV cavity. Further complications in about 7.5% of the HLHS cases may arise from the transposition of the great vessels, atrial isomerism, and total anomalous pulmonary venous drainage (TAPVR); in which the four pulmonary veins fail to connect to the left atrium [9].

Crucean et al. [13] identified three subtypes of the HLHS in their study based on the valve patency; a slit-like left ventricle was found in 24% of their subjects, in which aortic atresia and mitral atresia were evident in all. Miniaturized left ventricle found in 6% exhibited the presence of small aortic and mitral valves. While 70% had thickened left ventricle with endocardial fibroelastosis that showed various aortic valve malformation with different thicknesses of the left ventricle.

Management of the Disease

The advancement in biotechnology and the advent of different branches of medicines and educational programs have provided several inputs on the management of various congenital heart defects. These start with the prenatal diagnosis [20],; which includes fetal ultrasonography, echocardiography, or in selected cases a magnetic resonance imaging can be also used, and so does a positron emission tomography by using lower dosages of specific markers [21, 22]. A magnetic perfusion imaging scan can also be performed in pediatric cardiology to diagnose several cardiac defects in children [22, 23]. Four decades back the m-mode 2D-Doppler was the best option in terms of safety and accuracy was available for cardiac sonography [22, 24]. Although, in many countries, it is still a widely used method for cardiac imaging, especially in the many developing countries with densely rural populations. A comparative study from 1990–2010 in Sweden estimated that due to prenatal diagnosis the incidence of live birth decreased from 15.4 to 8.4 per 10,000 [8]. This includes prenatal diagnosis increasing from 27% to 63%, and termination of pregnancies increasing from 19% to 56% [8].

Other management methods include counseling, disseminating knowledge, and promoting awareness by obstetricians and gynecologists. The advancement in fetal medicine and the opening of fetal medicine centers also contribute toward the management protocols. A maternal-fetal medicine doctor specializes in the treatment and surveillance of fetal complications in pregnancy. Similarly, pediatric cardiologists and heart centers have neonatal intensive care units that manage to eliminate or mitigate the risks pose to neonates. Finally, life-long surveillance is observed in patients with cardiac abnormalities, and efforts are made to intervene in a timely fashion including surgical interventions at the later stages. A study found central nervous malformations and acquired brain anomalies in 29% of the child with HLHS [25]; similarly, brain abnormalities are associated with other congenital heart defects [26].

Diagnosis of the HLHS

Prenatal Diagnosis

A prenatal diagnosis can be made by the OB/GYN or the sonographer by observing the abnormality of the four-chamber view of the fetal echocardiography between the 18–24-week duration of gestation. Barron et al. [9] discuss the two ultrasounds practice; the first in the first trimester, in that nuchal translucency measurement of more than 95th percentile for crown-rump length can predict the presence of congenital heart defect at birth. Statistically, 46% of the prediction of the CVM at this stage of screening is related to either inflow or outflow obstruction, which is a precursor of the HLHS. It is beneficial to conduct the first screening at the 14th week of gestation, and repeat the screening in the second trimester if any chance of CVM is suspected. The second-trimester screening can be conducted between the

18–24 weeks of gestation, ideally the 20th week. Statistically, the screening at this stage can identify up to 70% of the CVM by visualizing the evident defects.

There are several advantages of prenatal screening and diagnosis. First, it can provide an option for the parents to terminate the pregnancy. Second, it can provide sufficient time for the parents to decide on the surgical intervention. Parents need to be both mentally and financially prepared for the outcomes. Third, timely education and awareness can be disseminated to the parents. Fourth, parents can plan for the postnatal care and management of their neonates. In a cohort study in the UK [9], the termination of the pregnancy fell from 71% to 44% (1994–2000) to 25% (2000–04). On the contrary, the cohort study in Sweden found an increase in the termination due to prenatal diagnosis resulting in a decrease in a child born with HLHS per 10,000 [8].

At Birth Diagnosis

At the time of delivery, the child is seen normal as it is attached to the umbilical cord. However, the condition of the child starts deteriorating at a rapid pace due to cyanosis. Symptoms that may suggest the presence of a large patent duct include continuous heart murmur and wide pulse pressure. Additional symptoms may manifest that of cardiomegaly, pulmonary plethora, and hepatomegaly with increasing tachypnoea. Without surgical intervention, the situation may quickly lead to respiratory distress, increasing acidosis, and circulatory collapse [9].

In some cases, femoral pulses can be weak or absent, which may suggest the presence of a moderate obstruction in the patent ductus arteriosus. These children may exhibit the symptoms of mild to moderate congestive heart failure, due to the presence of high pulmonary blood flow and high systemic overload. A neonate will become symptomatic a few days after the birth as the duct starts constricting. Some of the symptoms might overlap with other LVOT-caused abnormalities, including CoA, AVS, and interrupted aortic arch. Chest X-ray and BNP test may expose the cardiomegaly, such as edema or pulmonary plethora, or increase in the B-type natriuretic peptide (BNP).

The acute case of HLHS in neonates at birth is seen in the form of restrictive patent foramen ovale, or intact atrial septum. In this scenario, a child may have pulmonary venous edema and atrial hypoxemia, therefore this child will have tachypnoea and cyanosis since birth.

Postnatal Diagnosis

The prime objective of a child born with any of the above-stated symptoms at birth is to save the child. The foremost strategy adopted in this situation is to secure the patency of the duct, for that, an intravenous infusion is done with prostaglandin E1 (PGE1). Different imaging and blood tests are conducted to rule out the diagnosis. Once the diagnosis is narrowed or identified, then respective treatment is followed. Diuretics are the first-in-line option for congestive heart failure to drain the pulmonary edema. However, if the symptoms get worsened with acute exacerbation, tachypnoea, and acidosis with peripheral constriction then inotropic support commonly with dobutamine 5–10 µg/kg/min is provided to reduce the volume load on the right ventricle. The child is kept in the cardiac care intensive unit and is kept on intubation and ventilation to achieve respiratory and hemodynamic stabilization. In rare acute cases, hypercapnia and the addition of nitrogen to the ventilator circuit have been opted [9].

Surgical Intervention

Prenatal Surgeries

Fetal interventional surgeries are also an option including balloon septostomy in the restrictive atrial septum or balloon valve surgery in acute aortic stenosis [27]. One has to be very cautious in carrying out this precarious procedure, as there is the probability of one in five loss of the fetus [27].

Postnatal Surgeries

Once the CHD is identified based on the symptoms of the neonate, the decision is made for the operative response. The surgical intervention has subdued the risk posed by HLHS. The prognosis of the disease has improved due to several operative interventions in the past few decades. This section discusses these techniques. Among these techniques, Barron et al. [9] segregate these techniques into three broader categories. Conventional procedures where the right heart overlooks the functionalities of the left heart, neonatal heart transplantation, and the hybrid techniques. Before the 1980s, there was no known treatment for the HLHS, it was then in the UK when a thesis was proposed and suggestions were carried out in the early 1990s. This treatment included the utilization of the right ventricle to support the circulation system in the body of those affected. Among the most adapted surgical technique is the 3-staged palliative treatment. The stage-1 is the Norwood operation, which is done typically to 2–7 days after birth. The stage-2 is the Hemi-Fontan or the Glenn procedure, which is done between 4–6 months after the birth. Finally, stage-3 is the Fontan procedure, which is done between 18–24 months after the birth.

Stage-1: Palliative Treatment: Norwood Operation

We discussed above that in the case of HLHS, there is a right ventricular overload, but the right heart is not blocked in the systemic circulation process. The purpose of this surgery is to protect the right ventricle concerning the systemic circulation, however, providing the stable input flow from the right ventricle through the pulmonary artery to maintain the pulmonary circulation. The first step in this procedure is atrial septectomy, which is removing the atrial septum. Then reconstruction of the aortic arch is done to eliminate any hypoplasia or coarctation. Then the pulmonary artery is connected to the newly reconstructed arch. This reconstructed loop restores the systemic circulation. The second part of the procedure to provide stability in the pulmonary circulation is achieved by inserting a small Gore-tex shunt connecting the systemic and pulmonary circulatory network. There are two methods to place this; either conventionally through the Blalock-Taussig (BT) shunt, or the Sano shunt that involves placing a conduit between the right ventricle and the pulmonary artery (RV-PA).

There are few indications to perform the Norwood procedure. Size of reconstruction to preserve the blood flow toward the lungs and restriction of residual pressure gradient after completion of surgical correction of aortic arch reconstruction [28]. Norwood procedure carries a risk of increase in mortality if conducted after 14 days of birth [28, 29]. Premature infants are more vulnerable to mortality associated with the Norwood procedure. Furthermore, it extends its risk to postoperative morbidity and ICU stay [29].

Blalock Taussig Fistula

This procedure was first demonstrated in 1945 by Alfred Blalock and Halen Taussig. The main notion of this procedure is to create a fistula that acts as a shunt to divert the systemic circulation from the subclavian artery into the pulmonary artery. A 4 mm shunt is created that links the subclavian artery or right innominate artery to right pulmonary artery through a polytetrafluoroethylene tube [30]. A complication of coronary steal arises with the BT Fistula procedure. Due to the differences in the pressure gradient of pulmonary arterial pressure and pulmonary vascular resistance than systemic vascular resistance, this leads to low diastolic pressure due and reduced coronary perfusion if the increased amount of blood is directed to the pulmonary circulation. This can result in malignant arrhythmias, myocardial dysfunction, or in extreme lethal cases can lead to sudden cardiac death. Furthermore, a hypoxic condition may arise with acute obstruction of pulmonary blood flow (PBF) due to stenosis or thrombosis of shunt created by BT Fistula [30, 31].

Right Ventricle to Pulmonary Artery Conduit

The RV-PV conduit started to be considered for HPLS as stage 1 palliation to improve the pulmonary blood circulation. However, an optimal result in comparison to BT fistula is still not established [32]. There is still a debate over RV-PV conduit over BT-fistula due to complications of systemic hypoxia and the risk of early-age mortality associated with both procedures [32]. The conventional RV-PA conduit maintains the diastolic pressure of the aorta and restricts the systolic pulmonary blood flow. Some studies suggest that RV-PV conduit reduces the hospital mortality rate [31]. However, a concerning drawback is the regurgitation of blood flow that perhaps leads to ventricular dysfunction and arrhythmias due to right ventricle infundibulotomy in addition to that, direct right ventriculotomy could result in injury to the myocardium [27, 31, 32]. A decrease in volume load of the ventricle could result in the early onset of post-surgical cyanosis [33].

Reconstruction of the Aortic Arch

One of the postoperative complications due to the Norwood procedure is the compression of the pulmonary artery caused by the tightening of the aortopulmonary space [34]. This may occur due to bronchial and pulmonary artery stenosis or neoaorta coarctation [35]. One of the ways to treat or avoid having this condition is by creating arch-angle augmentation with glutaraldehyde-treated autologous pericardium [35]. Multidetector computed tomography angiography can be used to create the arch images, and their geometric parameters to minimize the complications during or after the Norwood operation. Aortopexy is another option that can be used to open the aortopulmonary space; however, it is not a feasible option in those with total cavopulmonary connection repair that requires two sternotomies [36]. In such a complex situation, neoaortic extension is a useful option as proposed by Baker et al. However, the novel approach by Asada et al. [34] is seen as a useful alternative in the complex situation as it does not compress the left pulmonary artery. Also, this may be a useful technique to avoid the complication of developing tricuspid regurgitation in these patients. The material to construct a patch for the aortic arch could be autologous, homologous, or xenologous [29]. Reconstruction starts from the descending part to the arch, to the ascending aorta, using a continuous polypropylene suture. The successful strategy is to make a patch as tailored as possible.

Tricuspid Regurgitation and Right Ventricular Dysfunction

Tricuspid regurgitation to some degree is a common problem among patients with HLHS, while one in four patients is noted to have moderate to severe tricuspid valve dysfunction [29]. This prevents the completion of the single ventricle pathway, therefore requires repair of the right ventricle, oth-

erwise increasing the risk of mortality and morbidity. The primary hypothesis for the tricuspid regurgitation is the annular dilation caused by the stroke volume overload. Other reasons may include the structural abnormalities of the leaflets and the subvalvular apparatus. Post-stage-1 palliation myocardial ischemia can be another reason to cause this anomaly. Echocardiogram (transthoracic, m-mode, Doppler, 2D or 3D) is often used to evaluate the occurrence of regurgitation or dysfunction. MRI can also be done in the suspected patients or to rule out the suspicion. Surgeons can identify the structural abnormalities, whereas prolapse can be identified by the sonographers.

Stage-2 Palliative Treatment: Glenn Procedure/ Hemi-Fontan

There are two options available at the stage-2 palliative treatment: either the Hemi-Fontan procedure or the bidirectional Glenn anastomosis. The objective of stage 2 palliative treatment is the conversion of the high-pressure right ventricle or aorta arterial source of PBF to the venous source [31]. This is achieved through the anastomosis of the superior vena cava to the pulmonary arteries [31]. The ideal age to perform this procedure is when a child is between 4–6 months of age; however, if desired then it can be performed on a child aged 3 months or less.

In the bidirectional Glenn procedure or cavopulmonary shunt, the shunt placed during stage-1 is removed, disconnecting the superior vena cava from the heart and connecting it to the cranial part of the right pulmonary artery [10, 31]. The azygous vein is tied off to prevent the venous flow to the lower body region, and although seems a complicated procedure, the survival rate is between 96–99% in this procedure [10].

In the Hemi-Fontan operation, a slight modification is done to the functional work of the Glenn procedure in which the need for disconnecting superior vena cava from the heart is felt unnecessary. This is achieved by creating a patch at the central pulmonary arteries, then joining the right atrial-to-superior vena cava junction and pulmonary arteries, after this closing the right atrial-to-superior vena cava junction patch [30].

Stage-3: Modified Fontan Procedure

The final stage of palliation for the surgical treatment of HLHS is named after Dr. Francois Fontan, who was the first to create the pulmonary and the systemic circulations in series, by utilizing only one ventricle [31]. As the name suggests, there is a modification to the original procedure done by Fontan. In this procedure, the right ventricle is bypassed by creating a circuit, in which the inferior vena cava return is redirected through the pulmonary vasculature [28]. By doing so, all the systemic venous blood runs passively into the lungs. It can be done by creating either the intra-atrial lateral tunnel or the extracardiac conduit that connects the inferior vena cava to the pulmonary artery [28, 30, 31]. The extracardiac conduit reduces the outcome complications associated with the lateral tunnel; including atrial clot formation, atrial arrhythmias, and left atrial dilation [28]. The communication between the Fontan circuit and atrium is called Fontan fenestration, which could be improved by providing adequate oxygen saturation. Thus, improving the systemic ventricular filling and ensuring the baby is not cyanosed [28].

Heart Transplant

A heart transplant is another viable option as compared to going through three-stage palliative care. However, there are a few considerable risks associated with this procedure, but the benefits outweigh the risk. The limitations are lack of desired organ donors, ABO-incompatibility, immunosuppression, and the greater risk of organ unacceptance by the body [27]. Since the first human heart transplantation (HHT) in 1967 by Dr. Christiaan Barnard in South Africa, the field of HHT is making considerable progress. Thanks to the advancement in immunosuppressive regimens, gene expression profiling, and microarray technology; acute cellular rejection and antibody-mediated rejection have declined [37].

Endomyocardial biopsies (EMB) is the first and optimum protocol to evaluate the criteria of rejection. The use of gene profiling test (AlloMap®), serum biomarkers donor-derived cell-free DNA (ddcfDNA), and the Molecular Microscope MMDX® system are three important advanced techniques that can assist in curbing the rejection rates by the organ donor [37–40]. Besides the formerly stated techniques, other techniques, such as organ engineering, stem cell therapy, mechanical circulatory assist device, and xenotransplantation are available, and readers are referred to the article by Kobashigawa [40], who discussed these techniques in detail. A study found an increase in the life span of the infants ($n = 322$) who received the HT due to CHD in their infancy [41]. 59% of the infants were able to live 25 years after the HT, while 35% died due to allograft vasculopathy nearly 25 years after HT, 20% had post-transplant lymphoma, chronic kidney disease stage-3 was noted in 31% of the survivors [41]. The quality of life between the ones who get HT is better versus those neonates who get staged palliative surgery [27].

Hybrid Procedure

The hybrid approach imitates the functional purpose of the Norwood procedure with an added advantage of minimizing the cardiopulmonary bypass, hence waning the risk of circulatory collapse. The aim is to go the least invasive by combining the surgical technique by cardiac surgeon, with the interventional cardiology technique, by the interventional cardiologist, under the imaging guidance in an operation theater [42]. The surgeon places the branch pulmonary artery banding bilaterally [30], with a small median sternotomy, while the cardiopulmonary bypass is avoided [31]. This increases the pressure in the main pulmonary artery, and prevents pulmonary hypertension, therefore decreasing vascular resistance while securing appropriate systemic circulation. The interventional cardiologist places a metal transcatheter stent to adjust the patency of ductal arteriosus in the main pulmonary artery above the pulmonary valve [29]. Afterward, either atrial septectomy or balloon atrial septostomy is done to ensure sufficient systemic and pulmonary venous mixing return at the atrial level.

The risk of circulatory arrest can be mitigated by using the hybrid approach over the Norwood procedure. Also, the major open-heart surgery in the infants can be deferred to an older age of their lives in this approach. The probability of survival as found during a cohort study between 2002–2007 found an 82.5% success ratio [42]. However, the higher success ratio in the hybrid stage-1 procedure is associated with its limitation, which Galantowicz et al. [42] did was in their inclusion/exclusion criteria. Any higher-risk candidate was not included as their subject to carry out the procedure. Based upon their criteria, it is noted that classic cases of HLHS were included; aortic atresia/stenosis with mitral atresia/stenosis. Hybrid is also a viable and preferable procedure over the Norwood in high-risk frail neonates, such as prematurely born, or are susceptible to life-threatening diseases such as necrotizing enterocolitis and neonatal sepsis [30]. It is a time-sensitive procedure, and one of the critical success factors is this should be done within 2–5 days after being born, and is deemed to diminish in success if it is done after 14 days [29].

The physiological conditions of the neonates who have undergone hybrid procedure versus Norwood operation are similar [30]. However, the cerebral and coronary perfusions are remarkably different between them. There is an anterograde blood flow through the aorta into coronary and cerebral vascular beds after the Norwood operation. However, there is a retrograde blood flow into coronary and cerebral vascular beds through the native aortic arch, due to blood being ejected into the pulmonary artery that transverse the ductus arteriosus. There is a chance of having stenosis at the junction that connects ductus arteriosus with the native aorta. This complication is termed retrograde aortic arch obstruction and may affect 10–24% of the neonates, with higher mortality in the subjects with this complication [30].

Hybrid Interstage 1 Monitoring and Pharmacology

The hybrid procedure improves the survival chances and increases the life expectancy in patients with HLHS. As discussed above that the major open-heart surgery is delayed until a later age. During this period known as interstage, the surveillance and routine check-up is deemed as important. Parents need to observe home monitoring as this increases the chance of survival in these neonates. Moreover, the pediatric cardiologists may start the neonates onto medications. The interstage medication regimen includes the use of any or in a combination of diuretics with and without digoxin, HR-oriented b1-receptor blockers combined with spironolactone (cardiac fibrosis influencing dosage), and angiotensin-converting enzyme (ACE) inhibitors if there is persistently increased systemic vascular resistance [29].

Further Reading for Surgical Intervention

In light of the scope of the chapter and exhaustiveness of the readers, advanced and detailed discussion about the surgical intervention is omitted from this comprehensive overview of the HLHS. Readers interested in attaining the knowledge about these three-staged palliative treatments and other techniques are highly recommended to read articles (especially by) Alphonso et al. [29] and Feinstein et al. [31].

Multiple Choice Questions

1. Hypoplastic left heart syndrome is characterized by underdevelopment of left heart chamber along with:
   A. Mitral stenosis.
   B. Mitral regurgitation.
   C. Malformation of ascending aorta.
   D. Malformation of Pulmonary arteries.
2. Nkx2–5-Cre and Mef2c-AHF-Cre lineage cells are involved with congenital defect of.
   A. Aortic and mitral valve.
   B. Tricuspid valve.
   C. Myocardium of left ventricle.
   D. Foramen ovale.
3. Ablation of histone deacetylase-dependent transcriptional Bop protein results in.
   A. Hypoplastic left heart syndrome.
   B. Hypoplastic right heart syndrome.
   C. Overriding of aorta.
   D. Outflow tract alignment.
4. Improper secretions of the TGF-β2 from the myocardium to endocardial cushion may result in the deletion of BMP receptor gene ALK3 may contribute towards.
   A. Boot-shaped heart.
   B. Valve stenosis.

C. Valve atresia.
D. Absence of valve formation.
5. A prenatal diagnosis can be made by the OB/GYN or the sonographer by observing the abnormality of the four-chamber view of the fetal echocardiography between the gestation of.
   A. 5–6-week
   B. 18–24-week
   C. After viability.
   D. None of the above.
6. Cardiomegaly such as edema or pulmonary plethora in neonates can be diagnosed initially by.
   A. Chest X-ray.
   B. ECG.
   C. Electrocardiography.
   D. Cardiac catheterization.
7. A complication of coronary steal arises with the BT Fistula procedure because.
   A. Differences of pressure gradient pulmonary artery and systemic vascular resistance.
   B. Thrombus formation leading to diastolic insufficiency.
   C. Blood directed from pulmonary circulation to systemic circulation.
   D. None of above.
8. Most common problem among patients with HLHS.
   A. Tricuspid stenosis.
   B. Mitral atresia.
   C. Patent ductus arteriosus at birth.
   D. Tricuspid regurgitation.
9. Risks of circulatory arrest can be mitigated in HLHS by using.
   A. Hybrid procedure.
   B. Norwood procedure.
   C. Heart Transplant.
   D. Blalock Fistula.
10. HLHS can be improved with chances of survival greatly by.
   A. Stage 1 palliative.
   B. Blalock fistula.
   C. Hybrid procedure.
   D. Norwood procedure.

Answers
1. C.
2. A.
3. B.
4. D.
5. B.
6. C.
7. A.
8. C.
9. A.
10. C.

References

1. Walmsley R, Monkhouse WS. The heart of the newborn child: an anatomical study based upon transverse serial sections. J Anat. 1988;159:93–111.

2. Cook AC, Yates RW, Anderson RH. Normal and abnormal fetal cardiac anatomy. Prenat Diagn. 2004;24(13):1032–48.

3. Moorman A, Webb S, Brown NA, Lamers W, Anderson RH. Development of the heart: (1)~formation of the cardiac chambers and arterial trunks. Heart. 2003;89(7):806–14.

4. Crelin ES. Functional anatomy of the newborn. New Haven, CT: Yale University Press; 2005.

5. Sanchez Vaca F, Bordoni B. Anatomy, thorax, mitral valve. In: Stat Pearls. Treasure Island, FL: StatPearls Publishing; 2021.

6. McBride KL, Marengo L, Canfield M, Langlois P, Fixler D, Belmont JW. Epidemiology of noncomplex left ventricular outflow tract obstruction malformations (aortic valve stenosis, coarctation of the aorta, hypoplastic left heart syndrome) in Texas, 1999–2001. Birth Defects Res A Clin Mol Teratol. 2005;73(8):555–61.

7. Hinton RB Jr, Martin LJ, Tabangin ME, Mazwi ML, Cripe LH, Benson DW. Hypoplastic left heart syndrome is heritable. J Am Coll Cardiol. 2007;50(16):1590–5.

8. Öhman A, El-Segaier M, Bergman G, Hanséus K, Malm T, Nilsson B, et al. Changing epidemiology of hypoplastic left heart syndrome: results of a national Swedish cohort study. J Am Heart Assoc. 2019;8(2):e010893.

9. Benson DW, Martin LJ, Lo CW. Genetics of hypoplastic left heart syndrome. J Pediatr. 2016;173:25–31.

10. Barron DJ, Kilby MD, Davies B, Wright JGC, Jones TJ, Brawn WJ. Hypoplastic left heart syndrome. Lancet. 2009;374(9689):551–64.

11. Cole CR, Eghtesady P. The myocardial and coronary histopathology and pathogenesis of hypoplastic left heart syndrome. Cardiol Young. 2016;26(1):19–29.

12. Bruneau B. The developing heart and congenital heart defects: a make or break situation. Clin Genet. 2003;63(4):252–61.

13. Crucean A, Alqahtani A, Barron DJ, Brawn WJ, Richardson RV, O'Sullivan J, et al. Re-evaluation of hypoplastic left heart syndrome from a developmental and morphological perspective. Orphanet J Rare Dis. 2017;12(1):138.

14. Dasgupta C, Martinez A-M, Zuppan CW, Shah MM, Bailey LL, Fletcher WH. Identification of connexin43 (α1) gap junction gene mutations in patients with hypoplastic left heart syndrome by denaturing gradient gel electrophoresis (DGGE). Mutat Res. 2001;479(1–2):173–86.

15. Mahtab EAF, Gittenberger-de Groot AC, Vicente-Steijn R, Lie-Venema H, Rijlaarsdam MEB, Hazekamp MG, et al. Disturbed myocardial connexin 43 and N-cadherin expressions in hypoplastic left heart syndrome and borderline left ventricle. J Thorac Cardiovasc Surg. 2012;144(6):1315–22.

16. Esposito G, Butler TL, Blue GM, Cole AD, Sholler GF, Kirk EP, et al. Somatic mutations inNKX2-5,GATA4, andHAND1are not a common cause of tetralogy of Fallot or hypoplastic left heart. Am J Med Genet A. 2011;155(10):2416–21.

17. Firulli BA, Toolan KP, Harkin J, Millar H, Pineda S, Firulli AB. The HAND1 frameshift A126FS mutation does not cause hypoplastic left heart syndrome in mice. Cardiovasc Res. 2017;113(14):1732–42.

18. Theis JL, Hu JJ, Sundsbak RS, Evans JM, Bamlet WR, Qureshi MY, et al. Genetic association between hypoplastic left heart syndrome and cardiomyopathies. Circ Genom Precis Med. 2021;14(1):e003126.

19. Helle E, Pihkala J, Turunen R, Ruotsalainen H, Tuupanen S, Koskenvuo J, et al. Rare variants in genes associated with cardiomyopathy are not common in hypoplastic left heart syndrome patients with myocardial dysfunction. Front Pediatr. 2020;8:596840.

20. American College of Obstetricians and Gynecologists' Committee on Practice Bulletins-Obstetrics, Committee on Genetics, Society for Maternal-Fetal Medicine. Practice Bulletin No. 162: Prenatal diagnostic testing for genetic disorders. Obstet Gynecol. 2016;127(5):e108–22.

21. Donnelly JP, Raffel DM, Shulkin BL, Corbett JR, Bove EL, Mosca RS, et al. Resting coronary flow and coronary flow reserve in human infants after repair or palliation of congenital heart defects as measured by positron emission tomography. J Thorac Cardiovasc Surg. 1998;115(1):103–10.

22. Wiles HB. Imaging congenital heart disease. Pediatr Clin N Am. 1990;37(1):115–36.

23. Kondo C. Myocardial perfusion imaging in pediatric cardiology. Ann Nucl Med. 2004;18(7):551–61.

24. Nelson TR, Pretorius DH, Sklansky M, Hagen-Ansert S. Three-dimensional echocardiographic evaluation of fetal heart anatomy and function: acquisition, analysis, and display. J Ultrasound Med 1996;15(1):1–9 quiz 11

25. Glauser TA, Rorke LB, Weinberg PM, Clancy RR. Acquired neuropathologic lesions associated with the hypoplastic left heart syndrome. Pediatrics. 1990;85(6):991–1000.

26. Licht DJ, Wang J, Silvestre DW, Nicolson SC, Montenegro LM, Wernovsky G, et al. Preoperative cerebral blood flow is diminished in neonates with severe congenital heart defects. J Thorac Cardiovasc Surg. 2004;128(6):841–9.

27. Rai V, Gładki M, Dudyńska M, Skalski J. Hypoplastic left heart syndrome [HLHS]: treatment options in present era. Indian J Thorac Cardiovasc Surg. 2019;35(2):196–202.

28. Shillingford M, Ceithaml E, Bleiweis M. Surgical considerations in the management of hypoplastic left heart syndrome. Semin Cardiothorac Vasc Anesth. 2013;17(2):128–36.

29. Alphonso N, Angelini A, Barron DJ, Bellsham-Revell H, Blom NA, Brown K, et al. Guidelines for the management of neonates and infants with hypoplastic left heart syndrome: the European Association for Cardio-Thoracic Surgery (EACTS) and the Association for European Paediatric and Congenital Cardiology (AEPC) Hypoplastic Left Heart Syndrome Guidelines Task Force. Eur J Cardiothorac Surg. 2020;58(3):416–99.

30. Yabrodi M, Mastropietro CW. Hypoplastic left heart syndrome: from comfort care to long-term survival. Pediatr Res 2017;81(1–2):142–9

31. Feinstein JA, Benson DW, Dubin AM, Cohen MS, Maxey DM, Mahle WT, et al. Hypoplastic left heart syndrome. J Am Coll Cardiol. 2012;59(1):S1–42.

32. Ghanayem NS, Jaquiss RDB, Cava JR, Frommelt PC, Mussatto KA, Hoffman GM, et al. Right ventricle-to-pulmonary artery conduit versus Blalock-Taussig shunt: a hemodynamic comparison. Ann Thorac Surg. 2006;82(5):1603–9. discussion 1609-10

33. Reinhartz O, Reddy VM, Petrossian E, MacDonald M, Lamberti JJ, Roth SJ, et al. Homograft valved right ventricle to pulmonary artery conduit as a modification of the Norwood procedure. Circulation. 2006;114(1 Suppl):I594–9.

34. Asada S, Yamagishi M, Itatani K, Yaku H. Chimney reconstruction of the aortic arch in the Norwood procedure. J Thorac Cardiovasc Surg. 2017;154(3):e51–4.

35. Hasegawa T, Oshima Y, Maruo A, Matsuhisa H, Tanaka A, Noda R, et al. Aortic arch geometry after the Norwood procedure: the value of arch angle augmentation. J Thorac Cardiovasc Surg. 2015;150(2):358–66.

36. Baker CJ, Wells WJ, Derby CA, Rizi S, Starnes VA. Ascending aortic extension for enlargement of the aortopulmonary space in children with pulmonary artery stenosis. Ann Thorac Surg. 2005;80(5):1647–51.

37. Benck L, Sato T, Kobashigawa J. Molecular diagnosis of rejection in heart transplantation. Circ J [Internet]. 2021; https://doi.org/10.1253/circj.CJ-21-0591.

38. Shah KS, Kittleson MM, Kobashigawa JA. Updates on heart transplantation. Curr Heart Fail Rep. 2019;16(5):150–6.
39. Gordon PMK, Khan A, Sajid U, Chang N, Suresh V, Dimnik L, et al. An algorithm measuring donor cell-free DNA in plasma of cellular and solid organ transplant recipients that does not require donor or recipient genotyping. Front Cardiovasc Med. 2016;3:33.
40. Kobashigawa JA. The future of heart transplantation: the future of heart transplant. Am J Transplant. 2012;12(11):2875–91.
41. Chinnock RE, Bailey LL. Heart transplantation for congenital heart disease in the first year of life. Curr Cardiol Rev. 2011;7(2):72–84.
42. Galantowicz M, Cheatham JP, Phillips A, Cua CL, Hoffman TM, Hill SL, et al. Hybrid approach for hypoplastic left heart syndrome: intermediate results after the learning curve. Ann Thorac Surg. 2008;85(6):2063–70. discussion 2070-1

Hypoplastic Right Heart Syndrome

Lolita Matiashova, Aparajeya Shanker,
Dimitrios V. Moysidis, Andreas S. Papazoglou,
and Christos Tsagkaris

Abstract

"Hypoplastic right heart syndrome is a rare collection of congenital heart defects characterized by the hypoplasia of right heart structures and subsequent cyanosis in neonates." Its etiology is still unknown but certain genetic factors, related to heart development are thought to be implicated. The failure of pulmonary circulation is responsible for circulatory collapse and mortality with timely surgical management aiming to restore pulmonary circulation. A three-stage reconstructive palliation surgery involving Blalock-Taussig Shunt, Glenn's Shunt, and Fontan Procedure with modern variations remains the definitive method of treatment and all these aspects are discussed in this chapter.

Keywords

Hypoplastic right heart syndrome · Neonate's cyanosis
Hypoplasia of right heart · Congenital heart defects
Genetic factors · Blalock-Taussig Shunt · HRHS
Cyanotic congenital heart defect · Palliation surgery
Fontan procedure

Introduction

"Hypoplastic right heart syndrome (HRHS) is a collection of congenital heart defects characterized by the underdevelopment of right-sided heart structures, with cyanotic presenta-

L. Matiashova (✉)
L.T.Mala NIT NAMSU, Kharkiv, Ukraine

A. Shanker
Medical University Pleven, Pleven, Bulgaria

D. V. Moysidis · A. S. Papazoglou
Aristotle University of Thessaloniki, Thessaloniki, Greece

C. Tsagkaris
University of Crete, Heraklion, Greece

tion at birth" [1]. The involved underdeveloped structures are: hypoplastic ventricles, tricuspid and pulmonary valves, pulmonary vein, and artery. HRHS may present with a concomitant atrial-septal defect of the ostium secundum type [1]. HRHS is a very rare congenital anomaly accounting for fewer than 1 in 60,000 births in the United States [1].

Etiology

The etiology of HRHS is yet not well understood. Research on several potential environmental and genetic causes has identified some relevant etiological factors which might contribute to the development of HRHS. The occurrence of HRHS in siblings in some studies conducted in the 1960s and 1970s suggests a familial component to the genetics of HRHS [2]. A population study conducted in 2017, which examined live births between 1998-225, found copy number variations (CNVs) in genes responsible for right ventricular and valve development [2]. The study discovered a case where the LBH gene, responsible for limb and heart development, had a 27Mb duplication at 2p23.2–2p16.2. This mutation was part of a partial trisomy 2p chromosomal mutation [2]. A further study of CNVs discovered existing mutations in the ERBB4 gene [3]. ERBB4 is responsible for cardiomyocyte regulation and differentiation and although the study sample was restricted, other cases involved showed duplications in 16q11-12. Mutations in this region have been previously implicated in other congenital heart anomalies [3]. Further suspected genes behind the HRHS are the RPGRIP1L, RBL2, SALL1, and MYLK3 genes. Nonetheless, all these studies did not identify any demographic risk factors related to the age of the mother, race, ethnicity, or sex of the fetus as significant for the HRHS etiology; yet further studies are still warranted to investigate any potential etiopathological correlation of drug or alcohol consumption during pregnancy and maternal diabetes with the occurrence of HRHS.

Pathogenesis

Hypoplastic right heart syndrome results in the lack of biventricular circulation, and in the loss of adequate hemodynamic balance between pulmonary and systemic circulation. In HRHS, the right-sided blood flow, responsible for pulmonary circulation is compromised and this leads to hypoxia. The severity of the subsequent hypoxia and cyanosis depends on the phenotype of the HRHS. Hemodynamic correction is achieved by bypassing the ventricle in reconstructive procedures, as discussed later in this chapter. So far, five phenotypes have been identified and they may exist either independently or in combination with each other. These phenotypes of HRHS are:

1. *Tricuspid Stenosis*: Which is defined as an abnormal narrowing of the tricuspid foramen resulting in a diastolic pressure difference between the right atrium and foramen. This diastolic pressure difference causes venous congestion and reduced cardiac output [4].
2. *Tricuspid Atresia*: Which is defined as the absence of the tricuspid valve, often comorbid with hypoplastic right ventricle, tricuspid stenosis, and ventricular septal defect (VSD). The combination of these pathological variations leads to a decrease in pulmonary blood flow and a subsequent increase in right ventricular pressure. Sometimes, tricuspid atresia is also combined with hypoplastic pulmonary arteries which may worsen the occurring hypoxia and cyanosis [5].
3. *Pulmonary stenosis*: Which is defined as the narrowing of the pulmonary valve or the pulmonary arteries. It is classified into valvular, subvalvular, and supravalvular type, based on the location of the obstruction. The most common type of pulmonary stenosis is the valvular stenosis. The valves can be bicuspid, tricuspid (normal), or quadricuspid. The pathophysiology is the same irrespective of the location of the obstruction; blood pressure increases before the obstruction and an overload of an often hypoplastic right ventricle leads to progressive right heart failure [6].
4. *Pulmonary Atresia*: Which is defined as the underdevelopment of the pulmonary valve, leading to pulmonary hypertension. This occurs in combination with a hypoplastic right ventricle and, therefore, there is not enough force generated to pump blood into pulmonary circulation [7].
5. *Right Ventricle Hypoplasia*: Which is defined as the underdevelopment of the right ventricle characterized by a small-sized right ventricle and a decrease in pumping function [8].

The exact HRHS phenotype as well as its combination with one or more of the above abnormalities determine the severity of the HRHS clinical presentation. The spectrum of HRHS ranges from one abnormality listed above to a combination of two or more abnormalities occurring together. The occurrence of multiple comorbid abnormalities explains the high mortality rates encountered in neonatal patients with HRHS.

Clinical Manifestation

Hypoplastic right heart syndrome manifests in neonates as a cyanotic congenital heart defect with one or more of the following features:

1. Cyanosis.
2. Dyspnea.
3. Tachycardia.
4. Difficulty in feeding.
5. Lethargy.
6. Poor weight gain and growth.
7. Fatigue.
8. Cold and grey skin.
9. Circulatory collapse.

Physical Examination

Upon physical examination, neonates are in clear distress, with cyanotic lips, and heart murmurs can be heard. General appearance should be noted for lethargic babies with poor responses, rapid, strained breathing, and difficulties with feeding. Low cardiac output is most frequently apparent, and pulse oximetry disorders may present just 24–48 h after birth. This pattern of clinical presentation resembles the hypoplastic left heart syndrome [9].

Diagnosis

The diagnosis of HRHS is primarily made prenatally using fetal echocardiograms and ultrasounds. Ultrasound will demonstrate absent or decreased flow through the tricuspid and pulmonary valves. The ultrasound may also demonstrate an absent or small pulmonary artery. Furthermore, the right ventricle may be small and hypertrophic (Fig. 1) [10].

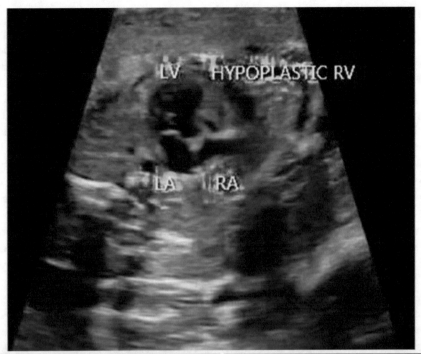

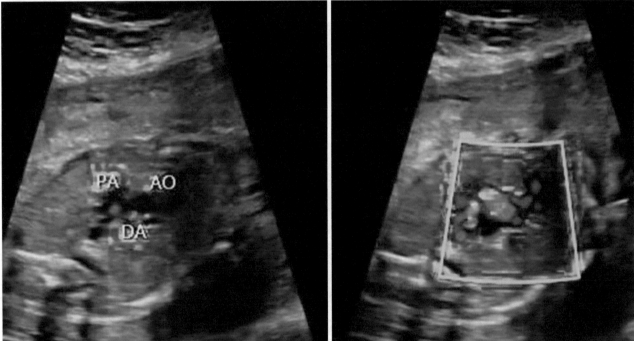

Fig. 1 Prenatal echocardiographic images of a case with hypoplastic right heart syndrome

Management

The management of HRHS is based on the timely identification of the hypoplastic structures and on the surgical interventions that aim to restore pulmonary blood flow and hemodynamics in the patient. The management of HRHS is tailor-made for each patient due to its rarity and variation in underlying etiology. The first line of management in neonatal patients is to alleviate the respiratory distress and to achieve adequate oxygenation and hemodynamic stabilization. The gold standard approach for the severe spectrum of HRHS requires extensive cardiac surgery, which is discussed in the next section.

Surgical Management

Surgical management remains the best, and in most cases, the only option for comprehensively managing HRHS. The surgical management consists of a three-stage reconstruction procedure where the aim is to balance systemic and pulmonary circulation. The main principle of surgical management is based on the creation of a shunt, on maintaining its patency and viability and thereby completely bypassing the absent or hypoplastic ventricle. The first line approach in the surgical management of all cyanotic congenital heart defects is the Blalock-Taussig Shunt. It is a form of palliation surgery, where the first aim is to relieve distress in the neonate and improve circulation to the pulmonary system. This procedure is performed within the first week of birth in the interest of time and for the best results.

However, there are also two other surgical procedures, performed after the Blalock-Taussig Shunt, which are known as the Glenn procedure and the Fontan procedure. The Glenn procedure is performed between 4–6 months of age and aims to connect the pulmonary artery with the superior vena cava. The Fontan Procedure, which is the final procedure, is usually performed between 2 and 4 years of age and is used to bypass the ventricle by creating a direct connection between the pulmonary artery and the inferior vena cava. Each procedure is discussed below.

Blalock-Taussig Shunt

The Blalock-Taussig Shunt is the first stage of palliation in the three-step palliation strategy for HRHS. The classic Blalock-Taussig Shunt is a shunt performed between the subclavian and pulmonary artery using part of the opposing subclavian artery graft as a shunt. A thoracotomy is performed for access. However, the classic Blalock-Taussig Shunt has been replaced by the Modified Blalock-Taussig Shunt, where a polytetrafluoroethylene (PTFE) shunt is used instead of a graft. The length of the shunt is important as it determines the hemodynamics of flow into the pulmonary circulation. The ductus arteriosus is also closed and the oxygen saturation is monitored. If the saturation is above 85%, the shunt is oversized, and if the oxygen saturation is below 75%, the shunt is too small. In both cases, the shunt needs to be revised. The main advantage of the Modified Blalock-Taussig Shunt over the Classical approach is that the shunt can be revised as needed, while the risk of nerve injury and Horner's syndrome is significantly lower [11].

Nevertheless, there have been also reported some complication associated with the Blalock-Taussig Shunt [11]:

1. Thrombosis.
2. Leaking of serous fluid from shunt into mediastinum.
3. Pseudoaneurysm, with consequential fatal hemoptysis.

Glenn Procedure

The Glenn Procedure, also known as the Glenn's shunt, is the second stage in the palliation of HRHS. It is performed in patients under 2 years of age and is a form of cavopulmonary shunting [12]. There are two forms of the Glenn Shunt: the Classic Shunt (also known as the Unidirectional Glenn Shunt), and the more modern, bidirectional Glenn Shunt (also referred to as a hemi-Fontan). In the Classic Glenn Shunt, the superior vena cava is directly attached to the right pulmonary artery. The left pulmonary artery is sutured shut after being dissected. The right atrium is then connected to the right pulmonary artery.

The bidirectional Glenn Shunt is an emerging modern variation, where the superior vena cava is connected to the right branch of the pulmonary artery and only the right atrium is bypassed. The right atrium is sutured shut and the continuity of the pulmonary trunk is completely maintained. This procedure is physiologically equivalent to half a Fontan procedure and is therefore referred to as a hemi-Fontan procedure by some authors [12].

Two main complications of the Glenn's procedure are [12]:

1. Progressive cyanosis due to venous collaterals.
2. Formation of diffuse arteriovenous shunts.

Fontan Procedure

The Fontan Procedure refers to any procedure in which systemic blood reaches the pulmonary circulation without entering a ventricle [13]. In the context of HRHS, the Fontan procedure is the third stage of the palliation procedure which aims to bypass the right ventricle. Currently, modern approaches of the Fontan procedure aim toward bypassing both the right atrium and the right ventricle by creating two direct anastomoses, one between the inferior vena cava and the right pulmonary artery, and another between the superior vena cava and the right pulmonary artery [13].

The modern approach of the Fontan procedure involves the formation of an intra-atrial tunnel. This intra-atrial tunnel is grafted from a homograft constructed from parts of the right atrium. It connects the inferior vena cava to the right pulmonary artery and is placed inside the right atrium. In some cases, an extracardiac circuit is created where the anastomosis is placed completely outside the heart. The extracardiac circuit method utilizes PTFE graft material to create a tube that can be attached to the inferior vena cava. The limitation of the extracardiac method is that it can be only used in patients older than 3 years old and in selected patients where the hemodynamics of an adult inferior vena cava can be tolerated [13].

The main complications reported after the Fontan procedure are [13]:

1. Dilatation with poor turbulent flow.
2. Thrombosis.
3. Pulmonary arteriovenous malformation.

Conclusion

Hypoplastic right heart syndrome is a very rare collection of congenital heart defects caused by the underdevelopment of right heart structures. These abnormalities usually present with hypoplastic right ventricle, pulmonary atresia, and pulmonary stenosis, and may occur either alone or in combination. The usual clinical manifestation of HRHS is cyanosis and hypoxia, with a significant risk for circulatory collapse and mortality in neonates. The primary step in HRHS management is to stabilize the critically ill patient and to prepare them for cardiac surgery, which follows a three-stage palliation plan. The ultimate aim of the surgeries is to achieve a total bypass of the right ventricle, a sustainable pulmonary flow, and stable hemodynamics, which is achieved by creating multiple shunts at various stages to ensure their patency.

Multiple Choice Questions

1. What is the incidence of hypoplastic right heart syndrome?
   A. In every second newborn.
   B. Commonly in adults.
   C. 1 in 60,000.
   D. 5 in 100,000.
2. What is the most commonly accepted theory of the etiology of HRHS?
   A. Genetic factors.
   B. Entirely environmental factors.
   C. Combination of genes and environment.
   D. Not clearly understood.
3. Why is prenatal diagnosis of HRHS important?
   A. Because mother should take special medication.
   B. Because prompt surgical management after birth is the only way to increase survival.
   C. Because child should have prenatal surgery.
   D. Because the pregnancy must be terminated.
4. HRHS characterized by
   A. Tricuspid stenosis/atresia.
   B. Pulmonary stenosis/atresia.
   C. Right ventricle hypoplasia.
   D. All of the above.
5. Why does HRHS present with cyanosis?
   A. Decreased pulmonary blood flow.

B. Overload of the left ventricle.
C. Right-to-left bleeding,
D. All above.

6. What is the principle of management of HRHS?
   A. Restoring cardiac function.
   B. Restoring pre-cyanotic status.
   C. Restoring pulmonary blood flow.
   D. All of the above.
7. What is the distinguishing factor of the Modern Blalock-Taussig Shunt?
   A. It is a aortopulmonary bypass.
   B. It is a grafting shunt that utilizes the superior vena cava.
   C. It utilizes the subclavian artery as a shunt.
   D. It utilizes a PTFE shunt.
8. Which of the following statements refers to the Hemi-Fontan procedure?
   A. It is a bidirectional flow procedure where the shunt is created between the superior vena cava and the right branch of the pulmonary artery.
   B. It is a bidirectional flow procedure where the shunt is created between the superior vena cava and the right atrium.
   C. It is a bidirectional flow procedure where the shunt is created between the right branch of the pulmonary artery and the superior vena cava.
   D. None of the options are correct.
9. What is the aim of the Fontan Procedure?
   A. Ventricular repair.
   B. Bypassing the atria only.
   C. Creating atrioventricular connections.
   D. Bypassing a ventricle.
10. Which of the following statements best describes the management of a patient with hypoplastic right heart syndrome?
    A. Restoring pulmonary circulation and hemodynamics with palliation surgery.
    B. Restoring systemic circulation through extensive repair of the atrial septal defects only.
    C. Restoring both pulmonary and systemic blood flow.
    D. None of the above.

Answers
1. C.
2. A.

   Explanation: Genetic factors are theorized to be the most probable cause behind the development of HRHS. Although the exact mechanisms have not been identified, limited studies suggest that duplications in genes responsible for cardiomyocyte development may be responsible.

3. B.

   Explanation: Prompt surgical management to improve hemodynamics is the only way to improve the odds of survival. Increasing pulmonary blood flow and increasing oxygen saturation is the aim of the Blalock-Taussig Shunt, which is the first step in the surgical management of HRHS.

4. D.

   Explanation: HRHS is characterized by hypoplastic congenital changes in right heart structures such as tricuspid stenosis/atresia, pulmonary stenosis/atresia, and right ventricle hypoplasia.

5. A.

6. C.

   Explanation: Hypoplastic right heart structures compromise pulmonary blood flow. This compromised pulmonary blood flow results in cyanosis and respiratory distress in neonates.

7. D.

   Explanation: PTFE stands for polytetrafluoroethylene, a material commonly used in surgery. The modern Blalock-Taussig Shunt utilizes a PTFE shunt to create a connection between the subclavian artery and the pulmonary artery. This is different from the classic Blalock-Taussig Shunt, where the opposing subclavian artery is grafted and used as a shunt.

8. A.

   Explanation: The Hemi-Fontan procedure is another name for the bidirectional Glenn procedure.

9. D.

   Explanation: Any procedure which aims to bypass a ventricle (right or left) is called a Fontan procedure.

10. A.

References

1. Dib C, et al. Hypoplastic right-heart syndrome presenting as multiple miscarriages. Tex Heart Inst J. 2012;39(2):249.
2. Dimopoulos A, Sicko RJ, Kay DM, et al. Rare copy number variants in a population-based investigation of hypoplastic right heart syndrome. Birth Defects Res. 2017;109(1):8–15.
3. Giannakou A, Sicko RJ, Kay DM, Zhang W, Romitti PA, Caggana M, Shaw GM, Jelliffe-Pawlowski LL, Mills JL. Copy number variants in hypoplastic right heart syndrome. Am J Med Genet A. 2018;176(12):2760–7.
4. Baumgartner H, De Bonis M, Lancellotti P. Tricuspid stenosis. In: ESC CardioMed. Oxford: Oxford University Press; 2018–2012.
5. Minocha PK, Phoon C. Tricuspid atresia. [Updated 2021 Aug 9]. In: StatPearls [Internet]. Treasure Island, FL: StatPearls Publishing; 2021.
6. Heaton J, Kyriakopoulos C. Pulmonic stenosis. [Updated 2021 Aug 11]. In: StatPearls [Internet]. Treasure Island, FL: StatPearls Publishing; 2021.
7. Sana MK, Ahmed Z. Pulmonary atresia with ventricular septal defect. [Updated 2020 Dec 12]. In: StatPearls [Internet]. Treasure Island, FL: StatPearls Publishing; 2021.
8. https://rarediseases.info.nih.gov/diseases/4721/right-ventricle-hypoplasia
9. Kritzmire SM, Cossu AE. Hypoplastic left heart syndrome. [Updated 2021 Jun 9]. In: StatPearls [Internet]. Treasure Island, FL: StatPearls Publishing; 2021.
10. Rajiah P, Mak C, Dubinksy TJ, Dighe M. Ultrasound of fetal cardiac anomalies. Am J Roentgenol. 2011;197:W747–60. https://doi.org/10.2214/AJR.10.7287.
11. Kiran U, Aggarwal S, Choudhary A, Uma B, Kapoor PM. The Blalock and taussig shunt revisited. Ann Card Anaesth. 2017;20(3):323–30.
12. Jacobstein MD, et al. Magnetic resonance imaging in patients with hypoplastic right heart syndrome. Am Heart J. 1985;110(1):155–8.
13. Fredenburg TB, Johnson TR, Cohen MD. The Fontan procedure: anatomy, complications, and manifestations of failure. Radiographics. 2011;31(2):453–63.

Mitral Stenosis

Abdallah Reda, Ahmed Dheyaa Al-Obaidi,
Sara Shihab Ahmad, and Abeer Mundher Ali

Abstract

Mitral valve stenosis, or mitral stenosis, "is a part of valvulopathies and represents the narrowing of the mitral orifice, blocking the blood flow from the left atrium to the left ventricle." Rheumatic fever is the most prevalent cause of mitral stenosis, although it can also be caused by immunological illnesses such as RA (rheumatoid arthritis) or SLE (systemic lupus erythematosus). Thus, mitral stenosis has been classified into 4 grades based on the Wilkins score, which takes into consideration the aspects of the valve, like its mobility, thickening, and calcification, and these classifications make the approach less complicated. To confirm the diagnosis, there are too many steps that should be done, from the physical examination to the EKG, echocardiography, chest X-ray, and many other ways to confirm the diagnosis. The mitral stenosis treatment plan includes 3 stages, starting with the pharmacological treatment and medical treatment until we get to the surgical interventions.

Keywords

Mitral valve stenosis · Mitral stenosis · Rheumatic fever
Lautenbacher syndrome · Rheumatoid arthritis
Pulmonary hypertension · Pulmonary congestion
Pulmonary edema · Atrial fibrillation

A. Reda (✉)
Carol Davila University of Medicine-Faculty of General Medicine,
Bucharest, Romania
e-mail: abdallah.reda@stud.umfcd.ro

A. D. Al-Obaidi
College of Medicine, University of Baghdad, Baghdad, Iraq

S. S. Ahmad · A. M. Ali
M.B.Ch.B, Baghdad, Iraq

Introduction

The human heart has four chambers, two atria, and two ventricles, and it contains four valves [1, 2]:

- The tricuspid valve.
- The mitral valve.
- The pulmonary valve.
- The aortic valve.

The mitral valve connects the left atrium with the left ventricle [3].

And before talking about mitral stenosis, we should talk a little bit about its structures and anatomy. It has six structures [4]:

1. The left wall of the atria.
2. Annulus.
3. Leaflets.
4. Chordae tendineae.
5. Papillary muscles.
6. The left wall of the ventricle.

Mitral stenosis is the inability of the mitral valve to open completely in the diastole phase due to the narrowing of the mitral orifice [5].

The normal mitral orifice diameter is 4–6 cm^2.

The most common cause is represented by the shuffle of the mitral valve and the subvalvular mitral structure caused by the AAR.

Epidemiology

Already, we have said that the mitral stenosis commonest cause is represented by the AAR (rheumatic fever). That is caused by a specific bacterium. We have also observed that the frequency related to this cause has decreased in recent years, especially in advanced countries, due to many things and many changes that have appeared in their lifestyle or their mentality that concern their health. For example, people become more interested in visiting their doctors from time to time. Their access to medical centers and facilities has become easier, and their medical culture has become richer, especially in the way they use antibiotics. Another etiology could be a congenital defect, especially for kids. Rheumatic mitral stenosis could be associated with an atrial septal defect (Lautenbacher syndrome).

Also, we can list other causes:

1. Some autoimmune diseases include systemic lupus erythematosus and rheumatoid arthritis [6].
2. Left atrial myxoma may mimic mitral stenosis.

Pathological Anatomy

As we said before, the normal mitral valve orifice is 4–6 cm^2. The apparition of the valve-related syndrome is related to the level of stenosis and the aria of the valve, such that the patients will experience it when the valve area reaches 1 cm^2.

When the aria decreases, the pressure of the left atria increases. As a result, we get passive pulmonary hypertension followed by pulmonary arterial vasoconstriction. It leads to the migration of the fluid into the pulmonary interstitium, causing dyspnea. Rheumatic mitral stenosis affects the endocardium, leading to inflammation and the formation of fibrous scars with thickening and calcification of the valves.

Pathophysiology

The narrowing of the mitral valve leads to various consequences which can or by making other sites suffer and causing radical changes in their roles. The normal mitral orifice area = 4–6 cm^2, and under normal physiologic conditions, during diastole, blood flows freely out of the left atria into left ventricle, and between the two chambers, the pressure is equal. The flowing of blood from left atrium is difficult in individuals with mitral stenosis, and the gradient of pressure throughout mitral valve appears as early as an area of 2 cm^2. The diastolic pressure of the left ventricle is normally 5 mmHg. The atrioventricular gradient is 20 mmHg when the mitral valve area is reduced by approximately 1 cm^2, so the left atrial pressure is approximately 25 mmHg. The increasing pressure in left atria will be transmitted to the pulmonary veins and the pulmonary capillaries. Also, as a result of the increased pressure in the left atria and the fact that this pressure level remained high, atria size on the left will grow, increasing the risk of atrial fibrillation appearing during this

period. Thus, that a big role in pulmonary hypertension: in the first place, the transmission of the left atria's pressure to the pulmonary veins (reversible), and then the pulmonary arteriolar vasoconstriction (reversible) leads to obstructive changes in the pulmonary vascular circulation (most likely irreversible) that can lead to pulmonary edema in advanced stages.

Also, in advanced stages, shunts may occur between the pulmonary and bronchial veins. Pulmonary hypertension causes the left ventricle to expand owing to prolonged stasis induced by lung injury, which can result in left ventricular hypertrophy and secondary tricuspid insufficiency [7–10].

Clinical Features

Patients with mitral stenosis progress over many years from being asymptomatic to having symptoms of heart failure. Many patients remain asymptomatic for a long time despite increased left atrial pressure, but reduce their physical effort depending on tolerance. The symptoms are diverse and differ in severity and risk of threatening the patient's life:

- Dyspnea, fatigue, and low tolerance are the most common symptoms observed in mitral stenosis patients.
  Dyspnea is often associated with hemoptysis, and nocturnal cough or effort.
- Hemoptysis is caused by the rupture of brachial veins after a sudden increase in left atrial pressure.
- Dysphagia.
- Palpitation represents a frequently encountered syndrome, and supraventricular arrhythmias are common in mitral stenosis patients due to the modifications in the left atrial structure [11].
  Atrial fibrillation appears in 50% of these patients.
- Thromboembolism occurs when the left atrium increases in volume.
  As a result, nearly 15% of patients experience embolic episodes associated with atrial fibrillation. Also, when the left atria or the pulmonary artery develops compression over the recurrent laryngeal nerve, it may lead to dysphonia.

And in later stages, the patient may suffer from right heart failure symptoms (such as jugular venous distention, hepatomegaly, parasternal heave, or ascites) associated with pulmonary hypertension, orthopnea, hemoptysis, and paroxysmal nocturnal dyspnea. The presence of mitral facies (pinkish-purple patches on the cheeks) indicates chronic severe mitral stenosis. [12–14].

Mitral Valve Classification of the Stenosis Severity [15]

1. Mild stenosis.
   - The mean gradient (mmHg) below 5.
   - Systolic pressure (mmHg) of the pulmonary artery is below 30.
   - Valve area (cm²) of less than 1.5.
2. Moderate stenosis.
   - Mean gradient (mmHg): 5–10.
   - Systolic pressure (mmHg) of the pulmonary artery is 30–50.
   - The area of the valve (cm²) 1.0–1.5.
3. Severe stenosis.
   - The mean gradient (mmHg) greater than 10.
   - Systolic pressure (mmHg) of the pulmonary artery greater than 50.
   - The area of the valve (cm²) is below 1.0.

Using the Wilkins score accordingly [15, 16]:

Grade 1 [15]
- The mobility: The valve mobility is high, with restriction of the leaflet tips only.
- The thickness of leaflet: Leaflet thickness is close to normal (4–5 mm).
- Calcification: A single area of increased echo brightness.
- Thickening: Just below the mitral leaflets, there is a minimal thickening.

Grade 2
- The mobility: Normal mobility of the leaflets' mid to base parts.
- Normal mid leaflets: Margins are considerably thickened (5–8 mm).
- At the leaflet margins, there are confirmed scattered areas of brightness,
- Subvalvular thickening: Chordal structures are thickened reaching to one of the lengths of the chord ai.

Grade 3 [17]
- The mobility: In diastole, the valve continues to move forwardly, from the base mainly.
- Thickening: Thickening reaching throughout the whole leaflet (5–8 mm).
- Calcification: The brightness extending to the middle part of the leaflets.
- Subvalvular thickening: Thickening reaching to the distal third of the chords.

Grade 4 [18]
- The mobility: In diastole, forward movement of the leaflets is no or minimal.
- All leaflet tissue has a considerable thickening (greater than 8 –10 mm).
- Calcification: Much of the leaflet tissue has a brightness found extensively [15].
- Subvalvular thickening: Thickening is extensive and shortening of all chordal structures reaching along to papillary muscles. [15].

Physical Examination

General Inspection

Presence of mitral facies with patches of pink and purple on the cheeks.

There may be a malar flush (plum-red discoloration on the high cheeks) due to the CO_2 retention and its vasodilatory effects.

Also, jugular venous distention is present.

In advanced stages, when right heart failure occurs, ankle and sacral edema are present.

Auscultation

S1: The initial sound is emphasized because of the increased force of the mitral valve shutting. If pulmonary hypertension is severe, the pulmonic element of the second auscultation will be loud. And when pulmonary hypertension develops, the Graham-Steell murmur (murmur of pulmonary regurgitation), tricuspid regurgitation, and a right-sided S3 will be heard [19, 20].

S3: It would be heard in certain pathological conditions where there is coexisting aortic or mitral regurgitation. A fourth heart sound may be produced if we have right ventricle hypertrophy with sinus rhythm. A mid-diastolic murmur is detected following the opening snap is present, and this type of murmur is best heard in the apical region. To make the murmur more accentuated, it is recommended to roll the patient toward the left.

To see the severity of the mitral stenosis, we should look at the duration of the murmur and not at its intensity.

In the presence of pulmonary hypertension, a pulmonary eject sound is detected, which reduces with inspiration. [21, 22].

A high-pitched decrescendo diastolic murmur (Graham-Steell murmur) induced by pulmonary regurgitation might be audible at the sternal border upper side.

Diagnosis

ECG: The electrocardiogram detects suggestive left atrial enlargement, pulmonary hypertension, right ventricular hypertrophy, and atrial fibrillation. [23].

Left atrial enlargement: It produces a bifid P wave (P mitral) in lead II, with a total P wave duration of >110 ms, and the negative portion of the p wave will be wide in V1 [24]. Right ventricular hypertrophy: the presence of its signs depends on the pulmonary hypertrophy grade [24]. That could include:

Right axis deviation of +80° or more.
*R/S ratio > 1 in V1 [25].
*S/R ratio > 1 in V6 [25].
RV1 + SV5 or SV6 > 10 mm.
*P pulmonated or right atrial enlargement or P congenital.
*Inverted *T* wave in the anterior precordial leads [26].
*The *R* wave is bigger than the *S* wave in V1 [26].

Atrial fibrillation: irregular rhythm with absent P waves. Also, we can obtain ECG signs suggestive of left ventricular hypertrophy that could appear in some associated valvular lesions (aortic or mitral regurgitation).

In mitral stenosis patients, the physical exam, ECG, and radiography of the chest, in the majority of cases to the correct diagnosis. Thus, we need some other investigations to reveal the severity of the mitral stenosis so we can avoid the consequences and find the best treatment options. Echocardiography plays a major role in detecting the severity of mitral stenosis and choosing the best medical intervention. It also helps to control the consequences that could appear after a medical or surgical intervention. [27].

Transthoracic 2D Echocardiography

It confirms the diagnosis by visualizing the thickened, calcified mitral valve with limited opening force. Stenosis of the mitral valve can be seen using different views including subcostal, apical, and parasternal views with the latest being the preferred view among the rest. In rheumatic mitral stenosis, in the parasternal long axis, we can visualize that the anterior mitral leaflet is in a "hockey-stick shape" during diastole. Restriction in motion or total immobility of the posterior leaflet of the mitral valve. Thus, in the parasternal short-axis view, we can detect the fusion of commissures and the leaflet thickening. [28].

Scales of the severity of valve stenosis: We also have various ways of measuring that are essential for all patients, and these measurements include:

Mitral valve area can be calculated using a "continuous wave Doppler by pressure half-time (P1/2 *t*)." "Bernoulli

equation" is one of the methods that can be used to estimate the systolic pressure of the pulmonary artery and the Rt ventricle (RVSP) from the velocity of tricuspid regurgitation. [29].

By using the modal Doppler, the mean pressure gradient across the mitral valve can be classified as: "mild (5), moderate (5–10), and severe (>10)" [30].

Chest X-Ray

The radiologic aspect differs depending on the evolutive stage, and it helps to visualize the enlargement of the heart chamber volume and the modifications in the pulmonary circulation.

It includes:

- Enlarged heart volume, especially of the left atria, could appear from the first stages.
- The chest X-ray reveals Kerley lines. These lines represent a sign seen on chest radiographs with interstitial pulmonary edema, and they are linear pulmonary opacities.
- Pulmonary edema is the most common pulmonary manifestation of mitral stenosis [31].

Septal lines may represent interstitial fibrosis and deposition of hemosiderin "brown induration" [31].

Trans-Esophageal Echocardiogram (TEE)

While transthoracic echocardiography (TTE) is the best diagnostic tool for exploring mitral valve abnormalities, transesophageal echocardiography (TEE) is an important adjunct in selected patients when valvular morphology and left atrium (e.g., to identify atrial thrombus) need to be visualized with further details.

Laboratory Test

- CBC: Leukocytosis may indicate an ongoing infection.
- Liver chemistries may show elevations due to congestive hepatopathy.
- CRP shows the presence of inflammation in rheumatic heart disease.

Cardiac Catheterization

This procedure is the most invasive and risky, but also the most accurate.

Cardiac catheterization is used to measure the mitral valve's aria using the "Gorlin equation" and to measure the pressure in the pulmonary artery.

Thus, this method will lead us to a severity classification of mitral stenosis.

Mitral valve "Aria" (cm^2):

- Large: >1.5.
- Medium: 1–1.5.
- Severe 1.

Pulmonary artery pressure (mmHg):

- Large: 30.
- Medium: 30–50.
- Severe: > 50.

Prognosis

The development of mitral stenosis is a process that is progressive in nature and takes about 20–40 years after the onset of "Rheumatic fever." It takes nearly a decade for the symptoms to become disabling once they appear. Those who develop symptoms had a poor prognosis before surgery, with "5-year survival rates" of sixty two percent among those in "NYHA Class III" and only fifteen percent among those in "Class IV." The clinical outcomes have improved, especially in those undergoing release of valvular-obstruction whether surgically or percutaneously on the basis of currently present guidelines. At the same time, the complications have become less frequent. The mortality level of the patient who is not following a treatment plan is related to the complications' development, such as cardiac failure, pulmonary congestion, systemic and pulmonary embolism, and severe infections.

Complication

- Atrial fibrillation (A-fib).
- Pulmonary hypertension.
- Pulmonary edema.
- Infective endocarditis, with an estimated risk of 0.17 per 1000 patients.
- Thrombi formation in the Lt atrium (due to A-fib) that may later cause systemic embolization.

Treatment

The treatment schema for mitral stenosis includes 3 important parts, which are:

1. Non-pharmacological treatment.
2. Medical treatment.
3. Surgical treatment:
   - Percutaneous balloon valvuloplasty/percutaneous mitral commissurotomy (PMC).
   - Surgical valvotomy/valve replacement.
   - Balloon-expandable valve implantation.

Non-pharmacological Treatment

Severe and moderate mitral stenosis patients should avoid intense physical effort.

At the same time, it recommended a hyposodic diet for all patients if pulmonary congestion is observed.

Medical Treatment

For asymptomatic patients, medical treatment is not recommended.

The medical treatment could be useful for arrhythmia prevention, especially atrial fibrillation, embolism prevention, reducing the occurrence of rheumatic fever again, providing infective endocarditis prophylactic treatment, and cardiac failure treatment. Symptoms that occur at the onset of pulmonary congestion are managed with diuretic drugs. Thus, hypo-sodium diets can provide additional benefits.

Beta-blockers and calcium channel blockers are useful for decreasing the heart rate, leading to improved exercise tolerance by prolonging the diastole. [32].

Patients with A-fib should be given a long-term oral anticoagulant (warfarin is currently the best option). When giving this drug, it is crucial to monitor the patient with international normalized ratio (INR) to achieve a target of 2.5. IV "beta-blocker or calcium channel blocker therapy" (such as diltiazem or verapamil) is used to manage the fast-ventricular rate caused by A-fib in an acute clinical scenario. Long-term control could be achieved with use of oral "beta-blockers, calcium channel blockers, amiodarone, or digoxin" [33].

The Prevention of Rheumatic Fever

- Primary prophylaxis:
  - Moldamin (benzathine penicillin G) IM, doses: children 27 kg 600,000 UI/patients >27 kg 12,000 UI.
  - Penicillin.
  - Erythromycin.
- The treatment of the symptoms:
  - Rheumatic fever with carditis → Prednisone.
  - Rheumatic fever without carditis → Aspirin.
- Secondary prophylaxis:
  - Secondary prevention of rheumatic fever can be done by using the following medications:

- Benzathine penicillin G: injected intramuscular with the following doses [34]:
    For children, 27 kg: 600000 U.
    For patients >27 kg: 12000000 U every 4 weeks.
- Penicillin V: 250 mg, oral administration.
- Sulfadiazine: oral administration.
    - For children under 27 kg: 0.5 qd.
    - Patients heavier than 27 kg: 1 g qd.

Surgical Treatment

Percutaneous mitral balloon valvuloplasty (PMBV) or percutaneous mitral commissurotomy (PMC) [35]:

PMBV is an invasive procedure that can relieve symptoms by increasing the mitral valve area and decreasing the mitral valve gradient. [36].

It is indicated for

- Symptomatic patients (NYHA Class > II).
- Asymptomatic with pulmonary hypertension with moderate or severe stenosis. [36].

PMN is the first method to be used for patients with uncomplicated mitral stenosis. With PMC, after a transseptal puncture, a catheter is inserted in the Lt atrium, then a balloon is put through the valve and inflated within the stenosed opening. As a result, the mitral leaflets separate. An increment of 2–2.5 cm^2 in the size then ensues. [37].

PMC has some good advantages over a surgical valvotomy, such as the avoidance of thoracotomy and general anesthesia.

The contraindications of the PMC are as follows:

- Lt atrium harboring a thrombus.
- Mitral regurgitation that is moderate to severe.
- Morphology of the valve being considered unfavorable.

The complications of a PMC are represented by

- Embolization.
- Ventricular rupture.
- Mitral regurgitation.
- Atrial septal defect.
- Stroke.

Surgical Valvotomy and Valve Replacement

In cases where "Ballon Valvuloplasty" is inappropriate (i.e., when the valvular morphology is deemed unfavorable) or contraindicated, valvular replacement surgery is recommended when affected individuals have moderate-to-severe mitral stenosis and are symptomatic [37]. Nowadays, using new techniques, we are getting good long-term results, even in severely affected valves (stenotic or regurgitant). Metallic prosthetic or bioprosthetic valves are used to replace valves that cannot be repaired.

Balloon-Expandable Valve Implantation

High levels of morbidity and mortality appear to occur after this procedure despite the fact that it is a feasible approach. The results of "direct transarterial implantation of a balloon-expandable valve in the mitral position" in a study that included six patients who were symptomatic with severe mitral annular calcification has supported this statement and encouraged further refinement of the approach. Although no outflow obstruction was encountered, some patients (three) developed severe "periprosthetic regurgitation," and three other patients died in hospital (noncardiac causes, 1 patient; cardiogenic shock, 2 patients).

Multiple-Choice Questions

1. Which of the following murmurs increases with standing?
    A. Pulmonary stenosis.
    B. Hypertrophic cardiomyopathy.
    C. Tricuspid regurgitation.
    D. Aortic insufficiency.
    E. Mitral regurgitation.
2. X-ray of patients with mitral stenosis may demonstrate all of the following features except
    A. Lt bronchus elevation.
    B. Shadow appearance.
    C. On lateral X-ray, there will be retrosternal shadow Obliteration.
    D. Esophageal kink in barium swallow studies.
3. Regarding MS, the following are correct concerning EXCEPT:
    A. Most commonly caused by rheumatic heart disease .
    B. Most commonly present as syncope.
    C. Pregnancy, atrial fibrillation, and anemia may cause deterioration in patients' condition .
    D. The second most prevalent symptom is hemoptysis.
    E. Atrial fibrillation almost always occurs when the defect is not corrected.

Answers

1. B.
    Explanation: Hypertrophic cardiomyopathy (HCM). Ventricular filling and venous return decrease with standing. Thus, murmurs intensity is decreased with all cases except for HCM. Giving the patient amyl nitrite will also decrease the murmur by the same mechanism of venous return reduction.

2. C.

> **Explanation**: On lateral X-ray, there will be retrosternal shadow obliteration.

When the left atrium is enlarged, it may compress on the esophagus and cause dysphagia—known as a cardio-esophageal syndrome. Obliteration of the retrosternal airspace is seen in any cause of an anterior mediastinal mass.

3. B.

> **Explanation**: Most commonly present as syncope. Syncope is mainly attributed to tachy- or brady-arrhythmias or arrhythmias related to medication and electrolyte abnormalities when it occurs in patients with structural heart disease. Outflow obstruction of the Lt ventricle (including HOCM or aortic stenosis) or the Rt ventricle (including pulmonary hypertension or pulmonary embolism) can end in developing syncope.

References

1. Walls R, Hockberger R, Gausche-Hill M. Rosen's-emergency medicine. Elsevier Health Sciences; 2018.
2. Patient Information: Glossary [Internet]. Heartsurgeonscom 2022 [cited 14 August 2022]. http://heartsurgeons.com/glossary.html
3. Jilaihawi H, Kar S. Mitral valve. Endovasc Hybrid Therap Struct Heart Aortic Dis. 2013:226–52.
4. Del Rio JM, Grecu L, Nicoara A. Right ventricular function in left heart disease. Semin Cardiothorac Vasc Anesth. 2019;23(1):88–107.
5. Rupeiks I. Computer-aided medical instruction using an interactive graphics model of the normal and congenitally defective heart. IEEE Trans Biomed Eng. 1972;BME-19(2):88–96.
6. Full text of "dental_DropBooks" [Internet]. Archive.org. 2022 [cited 14 August 2022]. https://archive.org/stream/dental_DropBooks_131/Nutrition_and_Oral_Medicine_DropBooks_App_djvu.txt
7. Rodrigues I, Branco L, Patricio L, Bemardes L, Abreu J, Cacela D, Galrinho A, Ferreira R. Long-term follow up after successful percutaneous balloon mitral valvuloplasty. J Heart Valve Dis. 2017;26(6):659–66.
8. Imran TF, Awtry EH. Severe mitral stenosis. N Engl J Med. 2018;379(3):e6.
9. Maeder MT, Weber L, Buser M, Gerhard M, Haager PK, Maisano F, Rickli H. Pulmonary hypertension in aortic and mitral valve disease. Front Cardiovasc Med. 2018;5:40.
10. Banovic M, DaCosta M. Degenerative mitral stenosis: from pathophysiology to challenging interventional treatment. How Problem Cardiol. 2019;44(1):10–35.
11. Cavalcante J, Rodriguez L, Kapadia S, Tuzcu E, Stewart W. Role of echocardiography in percutaneous mitral valve interventions. JACC Cardiovasc Imaging. 2012;5(7):733–46.
12. Blanken CPS, Farag ES, Boekholdt SM, Leiner T, Kluin J, Nederveen AJ, van Ooij P. Planken RN. Advanced cardiac MRI techniques for evaluation of left-sided valvular heart disease, J Magn Reson Imaging 2018: 48 (2) .318-329
13. Wunderlich NC, Beigel R, Ho SY, Nietlispach F, Cheng R, Agricola E, Siegel RJ. Imaging for mitral interventions: methods and efficacy. JACC Cardiovasc Imaging. 2018;11(6):872–901.
14. Oct AA, Gillitand YE, Lavie CJ, Ramee SJ, Parrino PE, Bates M, Shah S, Cash ME, Dinshaw H, Qamruddin S. Echocardiographic assessment of degenerative mitral stenosis: a diagnostic challenge of an emerging cardiac disease. Curr Probl Cardiol. 2017;42(3):71–100.
15. Shah SN, Sharma S. Mitral Stenosis. [Updated 2022 Jul 8]. In: StatPearls [Internet]. Treasure Island (FL): StatPearls Publishing; 2022 Jan-. https://www.ncbi.nlm.nih.gov/books/NBK430742/
16. Kulick D. Catheter balloon commissurotomy in adults part II: mitral and other stenoses. Curr Probl Cardiol. 1990;15(8):398–470.
17. Yousef S, Arnaoutakis G, Gada H, Smith A, Sanon S, Sultan I. Transcatheter mitral valve therapies: state of the art. J Card Surg. 2021;37(1):225–33.
18. Shah S, Sharma S. Mitral Stenosis [Internet]. Statpearls.com. 2022 [cited 14 August 2022]. https://www.statpearls.com/articlelibrary/viewarticle/25199
19. Karády J, Ntalas I, Prendergast B, Blauth C, Niederer S, Maurovich-Horvat P, Rajani R. Transcatheter mitral valve replacement in mitral annulus calcification. "The art of computer simulation". J Cardiovasc Comput Tomogr. 2018;12(2):153–7.
20. Hollenberg SM. Valvular heart disease in adults: etiologies, classification, and diagnosis. FP Essent. 2017;457:11–6.
21. Hemlata GP, Tewari S, Chatterjee A. Anesthetic considerations for balloon mitral valvuloplasty in pregnant patients with severe mitral stenosis: a case report and review of literature. J Clin Diagn Res. 2017;11(9):UD01 - UD03.
22. Hart MA, Shroff GR. Infective endocarditis causing mitral valve stenosis - a rare but deadly complication: a case report. J Med Case Rep. 2017:110.
23. Pradhan RR, Jha A, Nepal G, Sharma M. Rheumatic heart disease with multiple systemic emboli: a rare occurrence in a single subject. Cureus. 2018;10(7):c2964.
24. Mitral stenosis electrocardiogram - wikidoc [Internet]. Wikidoc.org. 2022 [cited 14 August 2022]. https://www.wikidoc.org/index.php/Mitral_stenosis_electrocardiogram
25. El Sabbagh A, Eleid MF, Foley TA, et al. Direct transatrial implantation of balloon- expandable valve for mitral stenosis with severe annular calcifications: early experience and lessons learned. Eur J Cardiothorac Surg. 2018;53(1):162–9.
26. Tanel RE. ECGs in the ED. Pediatr Emerg Care. 2006;22(11):732–3. https://doi.org/10.1097/PEC.0b013e31802b67c9.
27. Russell EA, Walsh WF, Reid CM, Tran L, Brown A, Bennetts JS, Baker RA, Tam R, Maguire GP. Outcomes after mitral valve surgery for rheumatic heart disease. Heart Asia. 2017;9(2):e010916.
28. Baumgartber H, Hung J, Bermejo J. Echocardiographic assessment of valve stenosis: EAE/ASE recommendations for clinical practice. J Am Soc Echocardiogr. 2009;22:1–23.
29. Lung B, Cormier B, Ducimetiere P, et al. Immediate result of percutaneous mitral commissurotomy A predictive model on a series of 1514 patients. Circulation. 1996;94:2124–30.
30. Omran A, Arifi A, Mohamed A. Echocardiography in mitral stenosis. J Saudi Heart Assoc. 2011;23(1):51–8.
31. Woolley K, Stark P. Pulmonary parenchymal manifestations of mitral valve disease. Radiographics. 1999;19(4):965–72.
32. Wilkins GT, Weyman AE, Abascal VM. Percutaneous balloon dilatation of the mitral valve: an analysis of echocardiographic variables related to outcome and the mechanism of dilatation. Br Heart J. 1988;60:299–308.
33. Pérez-Riera AR, de Abreu LC, Barbosa-Barros R, Grindler J, Fernandes-Cardoso A, Baranchuk A. P-wave dispersion: an update. Indian Pacing Electrophysiol J. 2016;16(4):126–33.
34. Maganti K, Rigolin VH, Sarano ME, Bonow RO. Valvular heart disease: diagnosis and management. Mayo Clin Proc. 2010;85(5):483–500.
35. Pérez-Riera AR, de Abreu LC, Barbosa-Barros R, Grindler J, Fernandes-Cardoso A, Baranchuk A. P-wave dispersion: update. Indian Pacing Electrophysiol J. 2016;16(4):126–33.
36. Mitral regurgitation https://radiopaedia.org/articles/mitral stenosis Accessed on December 7, 2016
37. Velusamy M, Mullens ML, Harrell JE, Talley JD. The chest x-ray in mitral stenosis. J Ark Med Soc. 1995;91(12):604–5.

Rhabdomyoma

Mustafa Najah Al-Obaidi, Ahmed Dheyaa Al-Obaidi,
Shkaib Ahmad, Abeer Mundher Ali,
and Sara Shihab Ahmad

Abstract

Rhabdomyomas are benign tumors of striated muscles, divided into cardiac and extracardiac types. The cardiac type is associated with tuberous sclerosis. Extracardiac is divided into further subtypes. Cardiac rhabdomyoma is a very common tumor in infants. Sporadic mutations are the main cause of cardiac rhabdomyomas. These mutations occur in tumor-suppressor genes, TSC-1 and TSC-2. Along with tuberous sclerosis, various conditions are associated with rhabdomyomas, including TOF, Epstein abnormality, and hypoplastic left heart syndrome. Macroscopically, they appear to be solid, unencapsulated lesions. Microscopically, pathognomonic spider cells can be seen. The clinical presentations rely on the location, number of tumors in the heart and their estimated sizes, the tumors obstruct the valves, thus decreasing cardiac output. Arrhythmias, whether ventricular or atrial in origin, and "Wolff-Parkinson-White syndrome" also occur commonly. Cyanosis and decreased peripheral pulses are also common findings. Prognosis depends on where the tumor is located, how large it is, and the associations that are seen with it. The presentation includes shortness of breath, heart murmurs, cerebral palsy-type sings, and altered renal functions. Cardiac rhabdomyomas can be detected on ultrasonography and MRI. The management includes the use of everolimus, which increases the regression of the tumor. Open heart surgery may be required in some cases. Complications include valvular compromise and cardiac arrhythmias.

Keywords

Rhabdomyoma · Tuberous sclerosis · Sporadic mutations
Spider cell · Valvular obstruction · Cyanosis · Everolimus
Cardiac arrhythmias · TSC · Decreased pulses

Introduction

Rhabdomyomas of the heart, benign in nature, are the tumors of striated muscles. They can be divided into two major types:

- Cardiac.
- Extracardiac.

Cardiac rhabdomyomas are hamartoma's lesions associated with tuberous sclerosis [1]. "Tuberous sclerosis" (TS) is a disorder of genetic etiology that involves multiple systems and causes the appearance on non-malignant tumors in the heart, the brain as well as other essential organs [2]. Extracardiac rhabdomyomas are further subdivided into genital, adult, and fetal subtypes. Cardiac rhabdomyomas can disturb the blood flow to the vital organs, causing arrhythmias. Cardiac rhabdomyomas grow until 30–32 weeks of gestation and then shrink naturally with time [3].

Epidemiology

Cardiac rhabdomyomas are usually detected in the prenatal period and in infants. Cardiac rhabdomyomas account for more than half of primary tumors of the heart that are occurring in children and infancy. Furthermore, in pediatrics they represent the most prevalent type of these primary tumors [2, 4]. The incidence of cardiac rhabdomyoma is 0.12% during pregnancy, 0.02–0.08% in live birth infants, and 0.002–0.25% at autopsy [5].

M. N. Al-Obaidi · A. D. Al-Obaidi · A. M. Ali · S. S. Ahmad
College Of Medicine, University of Baghdad, Baghdad, Iraq

S. Ahmad (✉)
Ghazi Khan Medical College, DG, Dera Ghazi Khan, Pakistan

Etiology

Cardiac rhabdomyoma might be caused by a genetic mutation during the development of striated muscle. It is possible for cardiac rhabdomyoma to develop spontaneously or in conjunction with other congenital disorders, most notably tuberous sclerosis [6–8]. Since, cardiac rhabdomyoma affects around half of TS patients, thus patients with cardiac rhabdomyoma usually exhibit some features that indicate the presence of TS, both radiologically and clinically, as well as a family history. Extracardiac rhabdomyoma does not occur in association with the tuberous sclerosis complex. Rarely, basal cell nevus syndrome and Trisomy 21 also show some association [5, 9–11].

Molecular/Genetics

As previously stated, tuberous sclerosis is mostly associated with cardiac rhabdomyomas. Tumor-suppressor genes that regulate the development and differentiation of developing cardiomyocytes, TSC1 and TSC2, are responsible for the condition. These genes are found on "chromosomes 9q34 and 16p13," respectively, and are responsible for the encoding of " hamartin and tuberin" proteins [12].

Pathologic Features

Gross Features

They may be found in both the atria and the ventricles, although they are more often seen in the ventricles. They are uniformly shaped, solid, tan-white, homogenous, and brighter than the surrounding healthy myocardium. Cardiac rhabdomyoma can be single or multiple in number, with diameters ranging from 1 mm to 10 cm.

Microscopic Features

Cardiac rhabdomyomas are characterized by nodules that are circumscribed, not capsulated, but can be easily distinguished from the non-affected tissues. The cells have a polygonal or a spherical shape, with a centrally located nucleus and myofibrils radiating out to the cell wall. There are eosinophilic septa in certain cells that extend from the cell membrane to the nucleus giving the cells a spidery appearance. The spider cells are the pathognomonic feature of the tumor [2, 13].

Clinical Features

Cardiac rhabdomyoma clinical features vary according to the size, location, and number of lesions. The lesions may be asymptomatic or they may induce cardiac arrhythmia, tachycardia, ventricular outflow blockage, or even mortality, according to lesions severity. When a tumor affects the myocardium or the ventricular papillary muscles in an extensive manner, congestive heart failure and poor cardiac output may result. A substantial correlation exists between cardiac rhabdomyomas and tuberous sclerosis. As a result, a medical history, full assessment, and testing for genetic abnormalities should be performed to rule out tuberous sclerosis [14, 15].

Prognosis and Predictive Factors

A full or partial regression of the tumor is expected to occur over time, and ultimately the symptoms will be resolved [5]. Because cardiac rhabdomyomas tend to spontaneously regress over time, treatment is reserved for individuals who are experiencing life-threatening obstructive symptoms or who are experiencing arrhythmias that are resistant to medical treatment [10].

Cardiac rhabdomyoma prognosis varies according to the size, location, and number of lesions, as well as whether there is an evidence of tuberous sclerosis. Tumors with more than 20 mm in diameter are recognized to produce disturbances on hemodynamic levels or cause arrhythmias, increasing the likelihood of mortality. Cardiac rhabdomyomas that block the flow of blood into or out of the heart cause regurgitation, and the prognosis is bad in these cases [16, 17].

Presentation

History: There is a shortness of breath history, that is associated sometimes with cerebral palsy symptoms and signs. Physical examination: Patients may present with heart murmurs, cerebral palsy-type signs, or altered renal functions [13].

Radiological Features

A solid hyperechoic mass may be seen in relation to the myocardium, which may be single or several in number. Small lesions may be mistaken for diffuse myocardial thickening in certain cases. They are commonly seen in close proximity to ventricles. The lesion size discovered during pregnancy might vary between 10 and 50 mm [15].

Management

Medical care: Cardiologists should follow patients diagnosed with cardiac rhabdomyoma throughout their treatment. Everolimus, an inhibitor of mTOR, had been found to significantly provide reduction of the tumor development in a number of anecdotal instances [16, 18–23].

Surgical care: It is possible that open heart surgery will be necessary. When there are serious hemodynamic disturbances or when arrhythmias need to be treated, surgery is almost always necessary to correct the problem. When lesions affect the heart valves, which might impede blood flow or induce valvular insufficiency, surgical intervention is recommended [24].

Complications

The patient may develop cardiac arrhythmias. Valvular compromise and ventricular obstruction can also occur [14, 15].

Multiple Choice Questions

1. What is the primary cardiac tumor that is considered as a most common type?
   A. Cardiac rhabdomyoma.
   B. Myxoma.
   C. Fibroma.
   D. Papillary Fibroelastoma.
2. Cardiac rhabdomyoma originates from which of the following types of tissues:
   A. A nervous tissue.
   B. The smooth muscle tissue.
   C. The striated muscle tissue.
   D. A vascular endothelium.
3. Which of the following conditions has an association with cardiac rhabdomyoma?
   A. Tuberous sclerosis.
   B. Down syndrome.
   C. Basal cell nevus syndrome.
   D. Marfan syndrome.
4. Until how many weeks of gestation does cardiac rhabdomyoma grow?
   A. 26–28 weeks
   B. 29 weeks
   C. 30–32 weeks
   D. 34–36 weeks.
5. Symptoms of cardiac rhabdomyoma arise due to:
   A. Obstruction of valves.
   B. Arrythmias.
   C. Extensive myocardial involvement.
   D. All of the above.
6. For medical care of cardiac rhabdomyoma, which drug can be prescribed?
   A. Everolimus.
   B. Hormone insulin.
   C. Bevacizumab.
   D. Carmustine.
7. When is surgery indicated for cardiac rhabdomyoma?
   A. Obstruction of blood flow.
   B. Valvular insufficiency.
   C. Decreased pulses.
   D. Both A and B.
8. What complications can occur if not treated?
   A. Cardiac arrhythmias.
   B. Valvular compromise.
   C. Ventricular obstruction.
   D. All of the above.

Answers

1. A.
   Explanations: 60% of primary cardiac tumors are cardiac rhabdomyoma.
2. C.
   Explanations: Cardiac rhabdomyomas originate from striated muscles.
3. A.
   Explanations: Cardiac rhabdomyoma affects around half of tuberous sclerosis patients.
4. C.
   Explanations: After 30–32 weeks, it starts to shrink naturally.
5. D.
   Explanations: All of the given options play a role in bringing changes to hemodynamic conditions.
6. A.
   Explanations: Everolimus is an mTOR inhibitor. It increases the regression of tumors.
7. D.
   Explanations: Both of these conditions indicate surgery because of significant hemodynamic disturbance.
8. D.
   Explanations: All the mentioned complications can occur because of the obstructive nature of the cardiac rhabdomyoma.

References

1. Neville BW, Damm DD, Allen CM, Chi AC. 12—Soft tissue tumors. In: Neville BW, Damm DD, Allen CM, Chi AC, editors. Color atlas of oral and maxillofacial diseases. Philadelphia, pa: Elsevier; 2019. p. 299–347.
2. Uzun O, Wilson DG, Vujanic GM, Parsons JM, De Giovanni JV. Cardiac tumours in children. Orphanet J Rare Dis. 2007;2(1):11.

3. Isaacs H Jr. Fetal and neonatal cardiac tumors. Pediatr Cardiol. 2004;25(3):252–73.
4. Harding CO, Pagon RA. Incidence of tuberous sclerosis in patients with cardiac rhabdomyoma. Am J Med Genet. 1990;37(4):443–6.
5. Burke A, Virmani R. Pediatric heart tumors. Cardiovasc Pathol. 2008;17(4):193–8.
6. Freedom RM, Lee KJ, MacDonald C, Taylor G. Selected aspects of cardiac tumors in infancy and childhood. Pediatr Cardiol. 2000;21(4):299–316.
7. Sarkar S, Siddiqui WJ. Cardiac rhabdomyoma. In: StatPearls. Treasure Island, FL: StatPearls Publishing; 2021.
8. Krapp M, Baschat AA, Gembruch U, Gloeckner K, Schwinger E, Reusche E. Tuberous sclerosis with intracardiac rhabdomyoma in a fetus with trisomy 21: case report and review of literature. Prenat Diagn. 1999;19(7):610–3.
9. Borkowska J, Schwartz RA, Kotulska K, Jozwiak S. Tuberous sclerosis complex: tumors and tumorigenesis. Int J Dermatol. 2011;50(1):13–20.
10. Goldblum J, Folpe A, Weiss S, Enzinger F. Enzinger and Weiss's soft tissue tumors. 6th ed. Philadelphia, PA: Elsevier; 2013.
11. Sciot R. Chapter 6 - skeletal muscle tumors. In: Folpe AL, Inwards CY, editors. Bone and soft tissue pathology. Philadelphia, PA: W.B. Saunders; 2010. p. 131–45.
12. Lee KA, Won HS, Shim JY, Lee PR, Kim A. Molecular genetic, cardiac and neurodevelopmental findings in cases of prenatally diagnosed rhabdomyoma associated with tuberous sclerosis complex. Ultrasound Obstet Gynecol. 2013;41(3):306–11. https://doi.org/10.1002/uog.11227.
13. Flood T, Veinot J. Cardiac rhabdomyoma pathology: definition, epidemiology, etiology. Medscape. https://emedicine.medscape.com/article/1612571-overview#a6. Updated 2022
14. Wacker-Gussmann A, Strasburger JF, Cuneo BF, Wiggins DL, Gotteiner NL, Wakai RT. Fetal arrhythmias associated with cardiac rhabdomyomas. Heart Rhythm. 2014;11(4):677–83.
15. D'Addario V, Pinto V, Di Naro E, Del Bianco A, Di Cagno L, Volpe P. Prenatal diagnosis and postnatal outcome of cardiac rhabdomyomas. J Perinat Med. 2002;30(2):170–5.
16. Tiberio D, Franz DN, Phillips JR. Regression of a cardiac rhabdomyoma in a patient receiving everolimus. Pediatrics. 2011;127(5):e1335–7.
17. Jacobs JP, Konstantakos AK, Holland FW 2nd, Herskowitz K, Ferrer PL, Perryman RA. Surgical treatment for cardiac rhabdomyomas in children. Ann Thorac Surg. 1994;58(5):1552–5.
18. Öztunç F, Atik SU, Güneş AO. Everolimus treatment of a newborn with rhabdomyoma causing severe arrhythmia. Cardiol Young. 2015;25(7):1411–4.
19. Wagner R, Riede FT, Seki H, Hornemann F, Syrbe S, Daehnert I, et al. Oral everolimus for treatment of a giant left ventricular rhabdomyoma in a neonate-rapid tumor regression documented by real time 3D echocardiography. Echocardiography. 2015;32(12):1876–9.
20. Goyer I, Dahdah N, Major P. Use of mTOR inhibitor everolimus in three neonates for treatment of tumors associated with tuberous sclerosis complex. Pediatr Neurol. 2015;52(4):450–3.
21. Dahdah N. Everolimus for the treatment of tuberous sclerosis complex-related cardiac rhabdomyomas in pediatric patients. J Pediatr. 2017;190:21–26.e7.
22. Chang JS, Chiou PY, Yao SH, Chou IC, Lin CY. Regression of neonatal cardiac rhabdomyoma in two months through low-dose everolimus therapy: a report of three cases. Pediatr Cardiol. 2017;38(7):1478–84.
23. Dhulipudi B, Bhakru S, Rajan S, Doraiswamy V, Koneti NR. Symptomatic improvement using everolimus in infants with cardiac rhabdomyoma. Ann Pediatr Cardiol. 2019;12(1):45–8.
24. D'Silva K, Worrell R. Rhabdomyomas treatment & management: medical care, surgical care, postoperative care medscape. https://emedicine.medscape.com/article/281592-treatment#d6

Transposition of the Great Artery

Ameer Almamoury

Abstract

The most common neonatal congenital cyanotic heart disease is ToGV. It is Characterized by atrioventricular alignments and ventriculoarterial alignments are both discordances. The clinical findings include cyanosis with the first 24 h in the life of neonate, chest X-ray reveal egg on a string appearance, narrow of mediastinum, single S2 sound. If there is mixing, there no murmur on examination. The cyanosis and the pulmonary congestion are rapidly developed if the mixing blood is inadequate. The prostaglandins should be initiated immediately if there is suspension of the TGA. The main diagnostic tool in terms of TGA is echocardiogram. The definitive treatment should start at the first week of the life by several procedure, there is no significant benefit actually from the drug. If the Rastelli operation failed, the last hope of the survival is the heart transplant which will discuss later in this chapter.

Keywords

Transposition · Great artery · Cyanosis · Atrioventricular · Stenosis · Pulmonary trunk · Malformations · Splitting · Murmur · Hump shaped · Balloon arterial septostomy · Arterial switch · Rastelli · Crisscross

Introduction

The right ventricle gives the aorta and the left ventricle gives the pulmonary artery, so result the parallel circular. Atrioventricular alignments and ventriculoarterial alignments are both discordances. The blood is pumped from the left ventricle into the pulmonary artery into the lung and the right ventricle into the aorta and systemic circulation, and the

A. Almamoury (✉)
Al Qadisiyah College of Medicine, Al Diwaniyah, Iraq
e-mail: med-16.13@qu.edu.iq

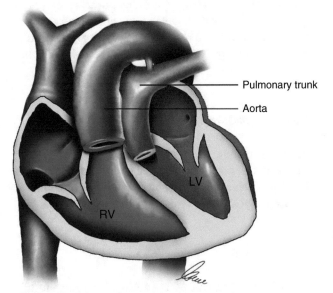

Transposition of great artery

Fig. 1 Transposition of the great artery (2-h neonate heart)

position of the pulmonary will be posteriorly and the aortic anteriorly [1]. One of the most important morphological aspects of the congenitally transposition is the coronary artery arrangement. Transposition of great vessels is highly associated with congenital cardiac malformation like ventricle septal defect, patent ductus arteriosus, and pulmonary valve disease (Fig. 1).

Pathophysiology

The physiology of the circulation is analogous. It is a cross of the heart chambers and the major vessels [2]. The consequences of the pathophysiology depend upon the functional adequacy of the subaortic morphology and the coexisting congenital malformation. One of the anomalies of the tricuspid valve is Ebstein anomalies, and the malformed valve functions normally in the early life, but the regurgitation is increase with the age [3]. It is associated with number of the valve problems and pathology caused by Ebstein like malformation.

Diagnosis

History

It is highly presented among the males compared to females population. The appearance of the clinical manifestation and presentation depends mainly on the presence of other cardiac malformation [4]. The mortality rate in infant is related directly to the congestive heart failure, heart block present shortly after birth, and also this patient announces as sudden death. The ventricle septal defect that come congenitally with the TGA is typically nonrestrictive [5]. Isolated pulmonary stenosis varies from mild to severe.

Physical Appearance

The main symptom appear is the retarded growth and development, and this symptom reserved for infant with large ventricle septal defect, cyanosis, and clopping due to pulmonary stenosis and pulmonary vascular disease reverse shunt [6].

Arterial Pulse

Bradycardia is the half of heart block or complete heart block.

Jugular Venous Pulse

Normal jugular venous pulse is presented here as in Fallot's tetralogy because of the pulmonary stenosis with a nonrestrictive ventricular septal defect. PR interval prolongation, increase the interval between the jugular wave and carotid wave [7].

Palpation

The aorta located anterior and leftward due to the presence of pulmonary hypertension and pulmonary stenosis the inverted left ventricle that occupies posterior and to the right position just behind the sternum cannot be palpated. The plan of the ventricle septum faces forward, and ventricle interventricular sulcus is closely aligned with the left sternal border [8].

Auscultation

First heart sound is soft [9]. The sign of the complete heart block has variation in intensity ejection sound in the left base. A short soft basal mid systolic murmur originates in the anterior aorta. The second heart sound is loud. The loud second heart sound at the left base is aortic not pulmonary. The aortic dominates the second sound because it is anterior. The pulmonary component is attenuated posteriorly and it is mistaken with pulmonary hypertension because of the loudness and location of the sound. The splitting is hard to detect because of the posterior position of the pulmonary trunk [10]. Systolic murmur analogous to mitral regurgitation (without inversion), the malformed tricuspid leaflet shifted medially toward the left sternal so the radiation within the left atrium toward the left edge away the axilla [11].

ECG

The major feature of the electrocardiogram is (1) disturbances of the conduction and the rhythm, (2) QRS and T wave pattern that reflect ventricular inversion, (3) modification of the P wave, QRS, and ST segment [12]. Tall peak right atrial P waves occur with pulmonary hypertension. The degree of the heart block differs from time to time in the same patient, the regular AV node does not contact infranodal right and left bundle branches so the atrial septum is misaligned with the inlet ventricular septum. The heart of the young children has long penetration of the atrioventricular bundle, this will replace with fibrous tissue which is responsible for the atrioventricular block, there are many defects detected including AV node and bundle branches. In the left side Ebstein anomaly, the supraventricular tachycardia and the atrial fibrillation not necessarily coincide with the presence of the Wolff–Parkinson–White accessory pathways [13]. One of the important diagnosis is left axial deviation. Severe pulmonary stenosis with intact septum may produce a QR complex in lead V1 and RS complex in the lead V6.

Imaging

X-Ray

The aorta is prominence in the upper left border. The classic radiological appearance is egg on string. The superior vena cava can displace to the right by dilated pulmonary trunk forming the right basal shadow, and the right ventricle has two morphological features: (1) Hump-shaped appearance and (2) Septal notch. The left atrium is giant and presented as a big ball suspended below narrow vascular pedicle [14].

Echo

The major diagnostic technique causes the echocardiography used to identify atrioventricular and atrioventricular discordance also the morphological right ventricle equipped with a mitral valve, and the relation between the great artery and their ventricle in origin determines the ventricle chamber morphology and atrioventricular valve. A morphological left ventricle is recognized by its ovoid or ellipsoid shape and its fine trabecular architecture. A fish mouth appearance in diastole is bicommissural valve [15]. The ventricle septal defect is typically nonrestrictive and perimembranous.

Management

Initial Management

Every patient and neonate suspected and confirmed diagnosis of D-TGA should be urgent transported as quickly as possible to the center and institution that have expertise in treat and manage D-TGA [16]. One of the goals of the initial management is stablize the patient and provides the patient with adequate ventilation function and good oxygenation. When the diagnosis of D-TGA is established, the prostaglandin infusion (0.05 mcq/kg per minute) is started to maintain the patency of the ductus arteriosus [17]. Patient with severe hypoxemia should performed balloon atrial septostomy to stabilize the patient. The balloon is induced across the atrial septal through cannulation of umbilical vein or femoral vein. The procedure can be repeated for one more time only, until establish the mixing. If the procedure is success, the oxygen saturation will start increase immediately, often the infusion of prostaglandin will stop at this time [18].

Surgery

Arterial Switch Procedure

Standard corrective procedure in patient with D-TGA used since 1980s. The procedure is done by the transection of the great artery and translocated to another side, mobilization of the coronary artery [19]. LeCompte maneuver used when performed the ASO procedure which place the pulmonary artery anterior to ascending aorta and used to decrease the risk of the pulmonary stenosis after operation. One of things that makes the operation difficult is the presence of Ventricle septal defect. Preoperative assessmentis essential to be done including the anatomic assessment [20].

Rastelli Procedure

In 1969, it was described for the first time in patient with D-TGA. prefer in patient with large Ventricle septal defect and LVOT obstruction, baffling and placing a conduct of the left ventricle and right ventricle [21–25]. Depend on the size of VSD if large size will oxygenate the aorta and if the restrictive VSD will enlarged to Decrease the risk of obstruction but also increase the risk of the heart block [25].

Atrial Switch Procedure

It is called also as Mustard and Senning procedure, and it is done by converting the parallel circle, so correct the condition of the hypoxemia and cyanosis, baffle into atrial direct oxygenated blood pulmonary venous into the tricuspid valve, the procedure came with long term sequelae like heart failure and arrhythmias [26–30].

Complication

Complications after arterial switch operation occurs in 5–25% of patient: pulmonary artery stenosis, which is the main indication of reintervention, area of obstruction usually common in supravalvar, also assess by transthoracic echocardiography [30, 31].

Coronary artery stenosis occurs mostly in the first three month after arterial septal operation, related to kinking lead to decrease the perfusion, end result of hemodynamically un stability, many patient may be asymptomatic, and the gold standard for detecting the stenosis is coronary angiography [32]. Intimal thickening and coronary artery disease, cardiovascular monitor, and lipid assessment are is essential in patient after ASO procedure. Neo-aortic pathology including dilation and regurgitation. Some risk factors for developing are: older age more than 1 year, presence of ventricle septal defect and previous pulmonary artery banding. Complication after Rastelli procedure is that the conduit will be replaced over time because of the stenosis issue, so one of the reasons of reintervention is the conduit replacement, arrhythmias and the heart failure, also one of complications that is established. Right side heart failure and arrhythmia are major complication after atrial switch. Obstruction of right atrial and superior vena cava junction and pulmonary venous obstruction is complication that associated with baffle [33–37].

Follow-up

Follow-up in form of; History, physical examination and testing should be take by cardiologist in every patient with D-TGA undergo procedure, follow up focused mainly on the detection and timing of complication following previous procedure, include focus and proper history asking about the episode of syncope and palpitation, chest pain and exercise tolerance [38]. On physical examination, it should include; vital signs, Cardiac auscultation, sign of heart failure also the edema in upper and lower limp, if the edema in the upper limp suggestive superior vena cava obstruction [39–43]. Routine testing and imaging done in form of ECG and routine echocardiography, assessment for atherosclerosis, and lipid profile monitoring. Antibiotic prophylaxis is not required for endocarditis [44–47].

Multiple Choice Questions

1. 2-h old boy developed cyanosis for past few minutes. The cyanosis never relieves by the oxygen hood, on the examination shows the tachypnea, single and loud second heart sound, there are no murmur. so, what is your diagnosis?
   A. Tetralogy of Fallot.
   B. Dextrocardia.
   C. Truncus arteriosus.
   D. Transposition of the great vessels.
   E. Tricuspid atresia.

2. 4-h child delivered with changed in the skin color for several minute past, afterward the patient has severe attack of cyanosis and tachypnea lead to dead of the neonate, the autopsy report reveals that the heart shape was abnormal and enlarged also, the left ventricle give the pulmonary artery and right ventricle give of aorta artery, so what the contribute the case and lead of the death in this patient:
   A. Pulmonary congestion.
   B. Arrhythmia.
   C. Cardiac arrest.
   D. Loss of the mixing blood.
   E. ARDS.

3. The 2-week neonate diagnosis with transposition of D-TGA that treated with the balloon atrial septostomy to rescue the patient, what is the definitive treatment in this patient?
   A. Beta blocker.
   B. Prostaglandin.
   C. Arterial switch operation.
   D. Catheter intervention.

4. 2-h neonate in the neonate wards after the deliver by SC in the operation room, the child remains the blue color of his skin until the moment on his examination that reveals no murmur with diffuse thrill and the single loud second heart sound, what the immediate investigation that you should obtain to confirm:
   A. X-ray.
   B. CT scan.
   C. RSB.
   D. ECHO.

5. A 1-day neonate has developed perioral discoloration, that never relieved by oxygen nasal cannula, sent for the investigation the chest X-ray show no great artery bor-

der, and the right ventricle show the hump shaped also the septal notch regarding what report in this X-ray. What is the most likely diagnosis?
   A. Coarctation of the aorta.
   B. Atrial septal defect.
   C. Aortic stenosis.
   D. Patent ductus arteriosus.
   E. Transposition of great artery.
   F. Truncus arteriosus.
   G. Ventricle septal defect.

6. The pediatric surgeon shows the case of the TGS patient 2-week age male neonate that treated with procedure as early management that save the life and adequate oxygen perfusion to the tissue, at this age the patient should undergo for the definitive repair, what the cause that surgeon prefer this age to the repair?
   A. Reduce the infection and endocarditis.
   B. Treat the hypertension progress later.
   C. Left ventricle thinning with an age.
   D. Reduce the cyanosis.

7. The 2-day neonate diagnosis with TGA .what the first line in the management this patient?
   A. Balloon arterial septostomy.
   B. Arterial baffle repair.
   C. Arterial switch operation.
   D. Rastelli operation.
   E. Prostaglandin.

8. One of the following finding on the ECG of the 2-h neonate diagnosis with TGS?
   A. Prolong QT interval.
   B. The modification on the QRS.
   C. P wave flat.
   D. ST segment prolong.

9. The mechanism behind death in the sever cyanosis in the patient with TGA?
   A. Ventricle hypertrophy.
   B. Myocarditis.
   C. Pericarditis.
   D. Septic shock.
   E. Hypoxia.
   F. Heart failure.

10. The 12 years old boy came to the center of the congenital heart disease by his parent because he was diagnosed with TGA from the first day of his life and undergo for the serial management that successfully treated him, on examination, the patient was normal and the vital sign was normal. What is the main investigator you should sent routinely on each visit to this patient?
   A. Echo.
   B. ECG.
   C. Radionuclide ventriculography.
   D. Brain CT.
   E. MRI.

Answers

1. D.

   Explanation: The most common cyanotic heart anomaly that causes tachypnea and loud single heart sound and no murmur.

2. D.

   Explanation: Cause of death is loss of shunt area of mixing, which lead to shift the deoxygenated blood from the heart to the body circulation causing severe brain hypoxia and infraction brain tissue.

3. C.

   Explanation: The definitive treatment in the TGA patient is the arterial switch operation

4. D.

   Explanation: The echocardiogram is the most accurate investigation regarding any congenital heart disease.

5. G.

   Explanation: The main feature of TGA is the hump appearance of the right ventricle.

6. C.

   Explanation: After the 2 week of time, the left ventricle become thinning and lead to potential heart failure and increase the surgical risk.

7. B.

   Explanation: The first procedure to do in the TGA patient is the balloon septostomy to maintain the mixing blood between the two-parallel circulation.

8. B.

   Explanation: The modification of the QRS, P wave and ST segment is one of the major findings in this patient

9. F.

   Explanation: The most common cause of the death in patient with TGA is the heart failure.

10. A.

    Explanation: This patient should take detailed history and proper examination also and Echo at each visiting.

References

1. Schiebler GL, Edwards JE, Burchell HB, Dushane JW, Ongley PA, Wood EH. Congenital corrected transposition of the great vessels: a study of 33 cases. Pediatrics. 1961;27(5) Suppl:849–88.
2. Williams JR. The life of Goethe. Oxford: Black well Publishers; 1998.
3. Anderson RH. Transposition introduction. Cardiol Young. 2005;15(Suppl 1):72–5.
4. Anderson RH, Weinberg PM. The clinical anatomy of transposition. Cardiol Young. 2005;15(Suppl 1):76–87.
5. Benson LN, Burns R, Schwaiger M, et al. Radionuclide angiographic evaluation of ventricular function in isolated congenitally cor. Am J Cardiol. 1986;58:319–24.
6. Ikeda U, Furuse M, Suzuki O, Kimura K, Sekiguchi H, Shimada K. Long-term survival in aged patients with corrected transposition of the great arteries. Chest. 1992;101:1382–5.
7. Lester RG, Anderson RC, Amplatz K, Adams P. Roentgenologic diagnosis of congenital corrected transposition of great vessels. Am J Roentgenol. 1960;83:985–97.
8. Perloff JK, Roberts WC. The mitral apparatus. Functional anatomy of mitral regurgitation. Circulation. 1972;46:227–39.
9. Benson LN, Burns R, Schwaiger M, et al. Radionuclide angiographic evaluation of ventricular function in isolated congenitally corrected transposition of the great arteries. Am J Cardiol. 1986;58:319–24.
10. Mckay R, Anderson RH, Smith A. The coronary arteries in hearts with discordant atrioventricular connections. J Thorac Cardiovasc Surg. 1996;111:988–97.
11. Schwartz HA, Wagner PI. Corrected transposition of the great vessels in a 55-year-old woman; diagnosis by coronary angiography. Chest. 1974;66:190–2.
12. Colli AM, De Leval M, Somerville J. Anatomically corrected malposition of the great arteries: diagnostic difficulties and surgical repair of associated lesions. Am J Cardiol. 1985;55:1367–72.
13. Graham TP Jr, Parrish MD, Boucek RJ Jr, et al. Assessment of ventricular size and function in congenitally corrected transposition of the great arteries. Am J Cardiol. 1983;51:244–51.
14. Anderson KR, Zuberbuhler JR, Anderson RH, Becker AE, Lie JT. Morphologic spectrum of Ebstein's anomaly of the heart: a review. Mayo Clin Proc. 1979;54:174–80.
15. Graham TP Jr, Bernard YD, Mellen BG, et al. Long-term outcome in congenitally corrected transposition of the great arteries: a multi institutional study. J Am Coll Cardiol. 2000;36:255–61.
16. Warnes CA. Transposition of the great arteries. Circulation. 2006;114:2699–709.
17. Huhta JC, Danielson GK, Ritter DG, Ilstrup DM. Survival in atrio ventricular discordance. Pediatr Cardiol. 1985;6:57–60.
18. Berman DA, Adicoff A. Corrected transposition of the great arteries causing complete heart block in an adult. Treatment with an artificial pacemaker. Am J Cardiol. 1969;24:125–9.
19. Huhta JC, Maloney JD, Ritter DG, Ilstrup DM, Feldt RH. Complete atrioventricular block in patients with atrioventricular discordance. Circulation. 1983;67:1374–7.
20. Walker WJ, Cooley DA, Mc ND, Moser RH. Corrected transposition of the great vessels, atrioventricular heart block, and ventricular septal defect: a clinical triad. Circulation. 1958;17:249–54.
21. Gillette PC, Busch U, Mullins CE, Mcnamara DG. Electrophysiologic studies in patients with ventricular inversion and "corrected transposition". Circulation. 1979;60:939–45.
22. Benchimol A, Sundararajan V. Congenital corrected transposition of the great vessels in a 58-year-old man. Chest. 1971;59:634–8.
23. Milici C, Bovelli D, Forlani D, et al. Images in cardiovascular medicine. An unusual case of congenitally corrected transposition of the great arteries in the elderly. Circulation. 2008;117:e485–9.
24. Pasquini L, Sanders SP, Parness I, et al. Echocardiographic and anatomic findings in atrioventricular discordance with ventriculoarterial concordance. Am J Cardiol. 1988;62:1256–62.
25. Hery E, Jimenez M, Didier D, et al. Echocardiographic and angiographic findings in superior-inferior cardiac ventricles. Am J Cardiol. 1989;63:1385–9.
26. Perloff JK. Physical examination of the heart and circulation. 4th ed. Shelton, Connecticut: People's Medical Publishing House; 2009.
27. Kraus Y, Yahini JH, Shem-Tov A, Neufeld HN. Precordial pulsations in corrected transposition of the great vessels. Diagnostic value of the electromechanical interval. Am J Cardiol. 1969;23:684–9.
28. Cumming GR. Congenital corrected transposition of the great vessels without associated intracardiac anomalies. A clinical, hemodynamic and angiographic study. Am J Cardiol. 1962;10:605–14.
29. Daliento L, Corrado D, Buja G, John N, Nava A, Thiene G. Rhythm and conduction disturbances in isolated, congenitally corrected transposition of the great arteries. Am J Cardiol. 1986;58:314–8.

30. Bharati S, Rosen K, Steinfield L, Miller RA, Lev M. The anatomic substrate for preexcitation in corrected transposition. Circulation. 1980;62:831–42.

31. Marino B, Sanders SP, Parness IA, Colan SD. Obstruction of right ventricular inflow and outflow in corrected transposition of the great arteries (S,L,L): two-dimensional echocardiographic diagnosis. J Am Coll Cardiol. 1986;8:407–11.

32. Victorica BE, Miller BL, Gessner IH. Electrocardiogram and vector cardiogram in ventricular inversion (corrected transposition). Am Heart J. 1973;86:733–44.

33. Carey LS, Ruttenberg HD. Roentgenographic features of congenital corrected transposition of the great vessels: a comparative study of 33 cases with a roentgenographic classification based on the associated malformations and hemodynamic states. Am J Roentgenol Radium Therapy, Nucl Med. 1964;92:623–51.

34. Meissner MD, Panidis IP, Eshaghpour E, Mintz GS, Ross J. Corrected transposition of the great arteries: evaluation by two- dimensional and doppler echocardiography. Am Heart J. 1986;111:599–601.

35. Lynch KP 3rd, Yan DC, Sharma S, Dhar PK, Fyfe DA. Serial echocardiographic assessment of left atrioventricular valve function in young children with ventricular inversion. Am Heart J. 1998;136:94–8.

36. Senning A. Surgical correction of transposition of the great vessels. Surgery. 1959;45:966–80.

37. Mustard WT. Successful two stage correction of transposition of the great vessels. Surgery. 1964;55:469–72.

38. Castaneda AR, Trusler GA, Paul MH, Blackstone EH, Kirklin JW. The early results of treatment of simple transposition in the current era. J Thorac Cardiovasc Surg. 1988;95:14–27.

39. Khairy P, Van Hare GF, Balaji S, et al. PACES/HRS expert consensus statement on the recognition and management of arrhythmias in adult congenital heart disease: developed in partnership between the Pediatric and Congenital Electrophysiology Society (PACES) and the Heart Rhythm Society (HRS). Endorsed by the governing bodies of PACES, HRS, the American College of Cardiology (ACC), the American Heart Association (AHA), the European Heart Rhythm Association (EHRA), the Canadian Heart Rhythm Society (CHRS), and the International Society for Adult Congenital Heart Disease (ISACHD). Heart Rhythm. 2014;11:102–65.

40. Bu'Lock FA, Tometzki AJ, Kitchiner DJ, Arnold R, Peart I, Walsh KP. Balloon expandable stents for systemic venous pathway stenosis late after Mustard's operation. Heart. 1998;79:225–9.

41. Nakanishi T, Matsumoto Y, Seguchi M, Nakazawa M, Imai Y, Momma K. Balloon angioplasty for postoperative pulmonary artery stenosis in trans- position of the great arteries. J Am Coll Cardiol. 1993;22:859–66.

42. Wu J, Deisenhofer I, Ammar S, et al. Acute and long term outcome after catheter abla-tion of supraventricular tachycardia in patients after the Mustard or Senning operation for D- transposition of the great arteries. Europace. 2013;15:886–91.

43. Poirier NC, Mee RB. Left ventricular reconditioning and anatomical correction for systemic right ventricular dysfunction. Semin Thorac Cardiovasc Surg Pediatr Card Surg Annu. 2000;3:198–215.

44. Jatene AD, Fontes VF, Paulista PP, et al. Anatomic correction of transposition of the great arteries. J Thorac Cardiovasc Surg. 1976;72:364–70.

45. Rastelli GC, McGoon DC, Wallace RB. Anatomic correction of transposition of the great arteries with ventricular septal defect and subpulmonary stenosis. J Thorac Cardiovasc Surg. 1969;58:545–52.

46. Khairy P, Van Hare GF. Catheter ablation in transposition of the great arteries with Mustard or Senning baffles. Heart Rhythm. 2009;6:283–9.

47. Zrenner B, Dong J, Schreieck J, et al. Delineation of intraatrial reentrant tachycardia circuits after Mustard operation for transposition of the great arteries using biatrial electroanatomic mapping and entrainment mapping. J Cardiovasc Electrophysiol. 2003;14:1302–10.

Wolff–Parkinson–White Syndrome

Aikaterini Kelepouri, Odysseas Kamzolas,
Andreas S. Papazoglou, Dimitrios V. Moysidis,
and Christos Tsagkaris

Abstract

Wolff–Parkinson–White (WPW) is a rare syndrome in which an accessory conduction pathway causes a form of ventricular pre-excitation. To date, the genetics and the origin of the syndrome have not been completely elucidated, despite the emergence of specific relevant mutations and the identification of its autosomal dominant pattern of inheritance in the familial type of WPW cases. The abnormal accessory electrical circuit is called the "Bundle of Kent" and causes two types of pre-excitation (A and B). The presence of two atrioventricular communications allows the development of re-entry circuits that circumvent the atrioventricular node, resulting in symptomatic supraventricular tachycardia episodes and even sudden cardiac death. The clinical appearance of the syndrome is similar to that of several tachyarrhythmias; however, specific ECG patterns are encountered in the WPW syndrome, including the characteristic delta wave, a widened QRS complex (duration > 120 ms), a shortened PR segment (duration < 120 ms), and a T wave opposite to the delta wave. The early diagnosis of the syndrome seems to be crucial since the syndrome can lead to sudden lethal arrhythmias even in asymptomatic patients. However, the reduced number of adults suffering from the WPW syndrome makes its recognition and clinical management even more challenging. Fortunately, the radiofrequency-based transcatheter ablation is considered nowadays as the gold standard treatment for carefully selected patients with recurrent arrhythmias. It treats the syndrome by ablating the accessory conduction pathway and thereby blocking the arrhythmogenic substrate in great success and low complication rates, while specific antiarrhythmic drug treatment is currently reserved for urgent manifestations of the syndrome.

Keywords

Wolff–Parkinson–White syndrome · Accessory pathway Bundle of Kent · Tachyarrhythmia · Transcatheter ablation

Introduction

Wolff–Parkinson–White (WPW) syndrome is an innate cardiac disease caused by the premature activation of the myocardium due to the abnormal presence of an accessory conduction pathway (AP), the "bundle of Kent" [1]. Plenty of physicians of multiple specialties had already referred to the WPW syndrome, from the early 1900s, when Frank Wilson and Alfred Wedd are believed to describe for the first time the electrocardiographic (ECG) characteristics of WPW [2]. However, it was just in 1930 when Wolff, Parkinson, and White thoroughly explained the syndrome characteristics, and, thereafter, the syndrome has been entitled by their names [3, 4]. In general, WPW syndrome is the most common form of pre-excitation, and it can be lethal because of the severe arrhythmias that could be generated [5].

The necessary circulation of our blood and oxygen to our organs depends on the appropriate cardiac function (i.e., cardiac rhythm and rate), which aims to promote the blood into the vessels. To that end, heart must be electrically stimulated through an electrical stimulus generated into the sinus node (SN). SN is normally located into the right atrium and is considered to be the primary pacemaker of the heart. The electrical stimulus travels from there to the atrioventricular node (AN), which is located in the Koch triangle. After arriving at the AN, the electrical impulse is delayed to ensure the blood ejection from the atria to the ventricles, and is later transmitted to the ventricles via the His-Purkinje system. In that way,

A. Kelepouri · O. Kamzolas · A. S. Papazoglou (✉)
D. V. Moysidis
Aristotle University of Thessaloniki, Thessaloniki, Greece

C. Tsagkaris
University of Crete, Herakleion, Greece

the ventricles are able to contract and thereby secure the blood circulation. However, this path is only accessible from the SN to the Purkinje fibers, while in the heart of a WPW patient there is another possible passage beside the AN for the stimulus, an AP, which could also enable the atria and ventricles to communicate. This AP is mainly known as Kent's bundle [6]. Due to the presence of Kent's bundle, the electrical signal can overpass the AN. In that way, the electrical impulse will not be delayed leading to malignant tachyarrhythmias and possibly ventricular fibrillation [1].

Epidemiology

It is difficult to estimate the exact prevalence of WPW patients since most of them seem to be asymptomatic. There is also a notable difference in the incidence of patients suffering from the WPW syndrome and those who only have the WPW pattern on the ECG. The WPW pattern is more usual than the syndrome, but both conditions are uncommon, occurring in less than 1% of the worldwide population. Specifically, the WPW's frequency is estimated approximately 0.1–0.3% or 1–3 per 1000 individuals, while in the USA almost 4 new diagnoses of the WPW syndrome are made per 100,000 individuals every year [7].

Moreover, it seems that APs could be located anywhere in the heart [8]. Their location is estimated to be the following (in descending order of frequency): (1) at the left free wall (53%), (2) posteroseptal (36%), (3) at the right free wall (8%), and (4) anteroseptal (3%). Yet, the presence of concealed APs accounts for approximately 30% of patients with apparent supraventricular tachycardias (SVT) referred for electrophysiologic studies (EPS). These patients do not have a "classic" WPW syndrome because no delta wave is present, but they do have the potential for orthodromic tachycardia. With regard to tachycardia, we should note that approximately 80% of patients with the WPW syndrome have a reciprocating tachycardia, while 10–32% of them will develop atrial fibrillation (AF), and 5% atrial flutter, whereas ventricular tachycardia seems to be uncommon [5, 9, 10].

Additionally, the age of WPW development plays also a significant role in the clinical course of the syndrome. Most

cases of the WPW syndrome are identified in early childhood and adolescence. However, 1 out of 4 WPW patients loses the pre-excitation over a 10-year period. The WPW pattern seems finally to appear equally in both sexes, while a gender-based imbalance concerns the WPW syndrome, which is more common among men according to the existing literature [1, 11].

Etiology

WPW syndrome has not been yet associated with specific genetic mutations in most patients, and, therefore, the underlying genetic etiopathology remains unknown in them. Contrary to those (random) cases, there is also a percentage of cases in which the syndrome is caused due to an autosomal dominant inherited mutation. Scientists have detected a responsible gene in some patients, named PRKAG2, which is located in the long arm of chromosome 7 and codes the gamma-2 regulatory subunit of AMP-activated protein kinase [12]. This mutation changes the kinase activity and results in the abnormal accumulation of glycogen within the myocardial cells, according to the indication of studies so far. This is known as the familial WPW syndrome, which is inherited in an autosomal dominant pattern with complete penetrance and variable degrees of expression. In addition to those two categories (random and familial), there is a percentage of 7–20% of patients developing the WPW syndrome while they suffer from congenital heart defects, with the most common of them being the Ebstein anomaly with affected tricuspid valve, or other genetic diseases [13, 14]. In Table 1, we briefly describe the potential etiology of the WPW syndrome, as retrieved from the existing literature.

Table 1 Etiology of the WPW syndrome

Random cases	→ Unknown origin
Family cases	→ PRKAG2 mutation
Comorbid congenital heart disease	→ Mostly Ebstein anomaly and Pompe disease

Pathophysiology

The WPW syndrome is caused by the existence of an abnormal accessory electrical circuit, an AP between the upper and lower chambers of the heart (the so-called bundle of Kent). This bundle is an embryonic remnant which either remains or vanishes during adult life [15]. When the bundle enables the communication between the right atrium and ventricle, it is called "pre-excitation type B," while the presence of the bundle in the left side of the heart is called "pre-excitation type A." The presence of this AP allows the electrical activity to circumvent the AV node. As a result, the signal is not delayed there and arrives earlier at the ventricles, resulting in their premature depolarization [1].

Hence, the presence of two atrioventricular communications allows the creation of re-entry circuits and tachyarrhythmias. Tachyarrhythmias can be caused in two possible ways [1]:

A. The most common way of development is the orthodromic atrioventricular reentrant tachyarrhythmia (AVRT), in which the electrical signal is transmitted from the atria to the ventricles through the natural conduction system, but it returns to the atria through the bundle of Kent due to the ability of the APs to transmit both orthodromic and antidromic signals. Some rare cases have been also described in which the cathode is happening through the bundle and the anode through the AP conduction system.

B. The second way is more straightforward: a supraventricular tachyarrhythmia is transmitted through the bundles, which cannot delay the sign in comparison with the AV node.

The aforementioned differences encountered in the electrical conduction in the WPW syndrome are also electrocardiographically apparent. In the ECG pattern of a WPW patient, there is a delta wave (formed due to the earlier depolarization of the ventricular muscle tissues), a widened QRS complex (due to the delta wave in addition to the depolarization from the natural conductive system of the heart), a shortened PR interval, and a T wave opposite to the delta one (showing the modified depolarization) [1, 6, 16] (Fig. 1).

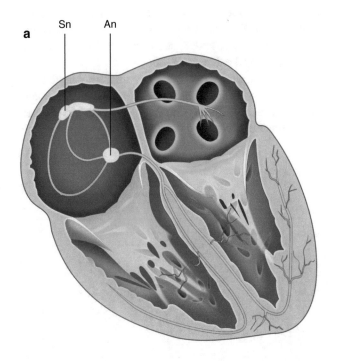
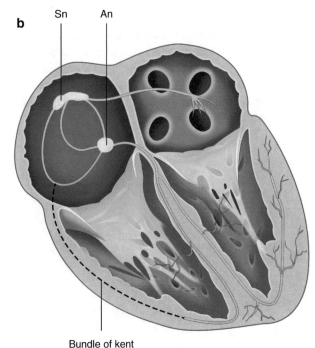
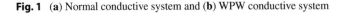

Fig. 1 (**a**) Normal conductive system and (**b**) WPW conductive system

Clinical Appearance

A WPW patient may be asymptomatic if he has not yet developed any arrhythmia (mainly atrial fibrillation and atrial flutter) and his examination may not have anything remarkable. However, the symptom onset may be abrupt, and the appearance of the symptoms is unpredictable in most cases. The symptoms are usually attributed to arrhythmias and could be one or more of the following ones [1, 17]:

- Chest pain.
- Dyspnea.
- Dizziness.
- Syncope.
- Palpitation.
- Collapse.
- Sudden cardiac death.

The syndrome may also appear as intolerance in physical activity. Moreover, a patient may suffer from polyuria after an episode of supraventricular tachycardia because of the dilated atria and the released atrial natriuretic factor. Another clinical sign usually occurring is the blood pressure disorder, which can vary from hypertension to hypotension [18].

During the physical examination, the patient may be cool, hypotensive, with crackles (on auscultation) and elevated jugular venous pressure besides the almost always increased heart rate. It is of interest to note that the physical examination becomes normal again right after the termination of the tachyarrhythmia [17].

Diagnosis

The diagnosis of the WPW syndrome is mostly made with a 12-lead ECG, with the relative clinical appearance and the family history being also of great help. The diagnosis can also be set with a Holter monitor and an electrophysiological testing [19].

The ECG patterns of WPW patients consist of the following features [6, 16, 18]:

Slurring of the initial portion of the QRS complex (delta wave).
Widened QRS complex (duration >120 ms in adults and >90 ms in children).
Shortened PR segment (duration <120 ms in adults and <90 ms in children).
T wave opposite to the delta wave (Fig. 2).

The Holter monitor shows what is exactly demonstrated by a 12-lead ECG, but the monitor is placed for a couple of days, and shows the heart function throughout the whole day [19] (Fig. 3).

Electrophysiological testing constitutes a catheterization procedure in which catheters with electrodes run through blood vessels to the heart where they can detect the abnormal electrical APs. This method also provides an additional therapeutic option, the transcatheter-based ablation, which will be later described extensively [20].

In a patient with the WPW syndrome, we can also perform laboratory blood testing to exclude other life-threatening conditions, along with echocardiography to evaluate the ventricular function [17].

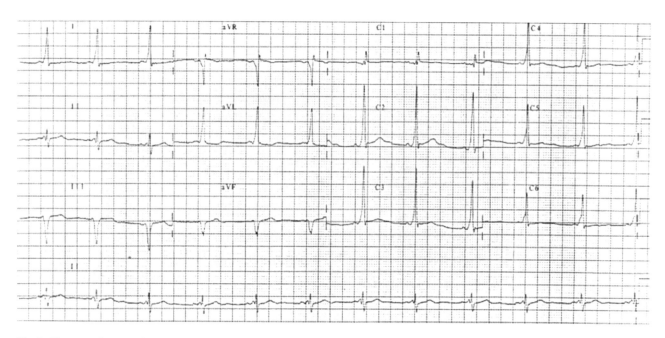

Fig. 2 Electrocardiogram of a patient with the WPW syndrome, as contributed From User Ksheka Wikimedia commons (CC By S.A.-3.0 https://creativecommons.org/licenses/by-sa/3.0/deed.en)

Fig. 3 Holter monitoring is used to assess the cardiac rhythm of a WPW patient throughout the day

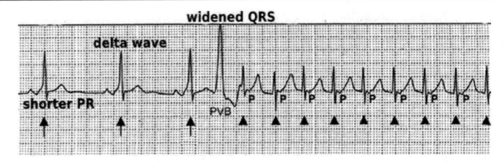

Differential Diagnosis

The differential diagnosis of WPW syndrome must include other conditions sharing similar ECG characteristics with those encountered in WPW. It is also necessary to determine if the WPW is combined with other heart anomalies and if it is a part of genetic syndromes.

Thus, the conditions that must be differentially diagnosed from the WPW syndrome are [13, 21, 22]:

- Atrial fibrillation.
- Atrial flutter.
- Atrial tachycardia.
- Atrioventricular nodal re-entry tachycardia.
- Paroxysmal supraventricular tachycardia.
- Ventricular tachycardia.
- Syncope.
- Danon disease.
- Ebstein anomaly.
- Glycogen storage diseases.

Management of a Patient with the WPW Syndrome

The treatment of the WPW syndrome has been subject to substantial changes during the last decades, with the radiofrequency-based transcatheter ablation (TCA) emerging nowadays as the gold standard treatment for patients with recurrent arrhythmias [23]. Initially, the antiarrhythmic drug treatment was the apparent management step for the clinicians. Yet it demonstrated a significant inability to induce a selective and complete conduction block over the arrhythmogenic substrate and thereby treat the WPW syndrome. Besides its inadequate efficacy, the antiarrhythmic drug treatment has also led to a proarrhythmic response in young and usually healthy populations by inducing a notable conduction delay in the reentrant circuit and thus rendering the arrhythmia incessant [23]. Hence, antiarrhythmic medication is currently reserved for urgent manifestations of the WPW syndrome. Nevertheless, the skills to correctly manage

adult patients seem to vanish along with the constantly reducing numbers of adults suffering from the syndrome. This seems to be of utmost importance for the new generations of cardiologists dealing with adult patients, and, therefore, we will provide a brief overview of the existing options to deal with the syndrome, aiming to decrease the possibility of clinical mismanagement and bolster the effective stratification and therapy of those patients.

Acute Management of a Symptomatic Patient with the WPW Syndrome

Treatment strategy in patients with the WPW syndrome generally aims to treat a symptomatic arrhythmia and reduce the risk of a life-threatening arrhythmia. Patients presenting with any symptomatic tachyarrhythmia (AF/atrial flutter, orthodromic, or antidromic AVRT), which might involve an AP, should undergo a prompt initial evaluation of their hemodynamic status. Hemodynamically stable patients can be assessed and treated in accordance with the type of the suspected arrhythmia, as presented in Table 2, while hemodynamically unstable patients should undergo urgent electrical cardioversion. We should not discount that cardioversion is further indicated in cases where the utilized pharmacotherapy is ineffective.

For hemodynamically stable patients with acute **orthodromic** AVRT, the approach is very similar to that applied to patients with other types of paroxysmal supraventricular tachycardia, where specific therapies can lengthen the AV nodal refractoriness while depressing its conduction and thereby blocking the impulse within the AV node and terminating the tachycardia. A step-wise approach is usually recommended with initial treatment with one or more vagal maneuvers (such as the Valsalva maneuver and carotid sinus massage) being preferred rather than pharmacologic therapy (Class IB) [17, 24]. If those maneuvers are ineffective, treatment with an AV nodal blocking agent (beta blockers, adenosine, and verapamil) should be instituted. Adenosine iv is preferred as the initial choice rather than verapamil IV based on its efficacy and short half-life (Class IIB), which

Table 2 Medical therapy associated with the Wolff–Parkinson–White syndrome

Arrhythmia	Treatment options	Contraindicated therapies
Orthodromic AVRT		
Acute management (termination)	**Stable patients:** **First line**: Vagal maneuvers **Second line**: IV adenosine **Third line**: IV verapamil OR IV diltiazem **Other therapies**: IV procainamide OR beta blocker **Synchronized cardioversion**: Unstable patients and if other therapies are ineffective or not feasible	
Chronic management (prevention)	**First line**: Catheter ablation of the accessory pathway **Second line**: Oral flecainide or propafenone in the absence of structural or ischemic heart disease **Third line**: Oral IA antiarrhythmic agent OR oral amiodarone	
Antidromic AVRT		
Acute management (termination)	**Stable patients (if sure of the diagnosis)**: Same progression of therapies as acute termination of orthodromic AVRT△ **Stable patients (if NOT sure of the diagnosis)**: IV procainamide **Synchronized cardioversion**: Unstable patients and if procainamide ineffective or not feasible	Adenosine, verapamil, diltiazem, beta blockers, digoxin should all be avoided if NOT certain of diagnosis
Chronic management (prevention)	**First line**: Catheter ablation of the accessory pathway **Second line**: Oral flecainide or propafenone in the absence of structural or ischemic heart disease **Other therapies**: Oral IA antiarrhythmic agent OR oral amiodarone	Digoxin, beta blockers, verapamil, diltiazem
Pre-excited atrial fibrillation or atrial flutter		
Acute management (termination)	**Stable patients:** **First line**: IV ibutilide or IV procainamide **Other therapies**: IV Flecainide, encainide, and propafenone or dofetilide; synchronized cardioversion if other therapies are ineffective or not available **Synchronized cardioversion**: Unstable patients and if other therapies are ineffective or not feasible	Amiodarone, digoxin, beta blockers, adenosine, verapamil, diltiazem
Chronic management (prevention)	**First line**: Catheter ablation of the accessory pathway **Second line**: Oral flecainide or propafenone in the absence of structural or ischemic heart disease **Third line**: Oral IA antiarrhythmic agent OR oral amiodarone	Oral digoxin

render it effective for the acute termination of the tachycardia in 80–90% of patients [25, 26]. If the tachycardia persists, IV administration of procainamide or beta blockers (e.g., metoprolol, propranolol, and esmolol) is an additional therapeutic strategy that could be utilized [27, 28].

When a WPW patient presents with acute symptomatic **antidromic** AVRT, while being hemodynamically stable, the treatment with IV procainamide is recommended to terminate the tachycardia or to slow the ventricular response and improve the patient's hemodynamic state [24]. IV administered adenosine, verapamil, and beta blockers (AV node-specific blocking drugs) should be avoided if we are not certain of the diagnosis. This is practically not feasible outside the electrophysiology laboratory, and thus a patient should be considered to have a possibly undiagnosed ventricular tachycardia, which can even degenerate into ventricular fibrillation after the administration of the aforementioned contraindicated drugs.

For patients presenting with acute pre-excited **AF or atrial flutter** pattern, we should always keep in mind that in those patients, the conduction to the ventricle often occurs either via the AV node or through the AP. Therefore, AV nodal blocking medications [non-dihydropyridine calcium channel blockers (verapamil and diltiazem), beta blockers, adenosine, digoxin, and amiodarone] are contraindicated in those patients since blocking the AV node would promote the conduction via the AP and make the ventricular rate even more rapid (Class IA). Thus, the optimal approach in those patients is to initially proceed with rhythm control medication (i.e., procainamide and ibutilide) rather than rate control (Class IIC), since sinus rhythm would make it easier to control the ventricular rate [17, 24].

Chronic Treatment to Prevent Recurrent Arrhythmias

After the stabilization of a WPW patient presenting with an acute episode of tachyarrhythmia, clinicians should consider additional therapeutic options to proceed with in an effort to prevent recurrent symptomatic arrhythmias. For almost every patient with an AP and symptomatic arrhythmic episodes (orthodromic or antidromic AVRT, and pre-excited AF or atrial flutter), the recommended long-term treatment approach is the radiofrequency-based TCA (Class IA). For those patients who are not candidates for or not willing to undergo ablation of the AP or for select patients with well-tolerated, rare arrhythmic episodes, antiarrhythmic medication is still recommended (Class IIC). The appropriate antiarrhythmic agent should be carefully selected based on the etiology of the arrhythmia and its electrophysiological properties (Table 2) to prevent future episodes and slow the ventricular response [17].

It is definitely worth mentioning that chronic preventive medication with verapamil or digoxin is contraindicated and should be avoided in **every** patient with the WPW syndrome. Flecainide and propafenone constitute the agents of choice for the prevention of recurrent orthodromic AVRT due to their favorable benefit/risk ratio [29–32], with the exception of patients with coronary artery disease history, where these drugs could decrease survival rates due to proarrhythmic effect [33]. Moreover, beta blockers could also be utilized as a second-line treatment to prevent orthodromic AVRT in low-risk patients with the WPW syndrome, but they should be avoided in patients with pre-excited AF. Additionally, amiodarone could be effective in multiple ways to suppress orthodromic AVRT, yet the frequent side effects encountered (i.e., pulmonary, thyroid, and hepatic toxicity) constitute significant concerns especially for younger patients requiring many years of preventive therapy [34–36].

With regard to the prevention of recurrent antidromic AVRT and pre-excited AF, flecainide and propafenone constitute the drugs of choice in the absence of underlying structural heart disease. In patients though with concomitant structural heart disease, amiodarone should be considered as a drug of choice by the clinicians because AV nodal blocking drugs (beta blockers, calcium channel blockers, and digoxin) should not be recommended in those patients.

Transcatheter Ablation (TCA)

Nevertheless, radiofrequency-based TCA of the AP is considered to be the treatment of choice for symptomatic patients with arrhythmias (orthodromic or antidromic AVRT) or AF and pre-excitation because of its favorable risk/benefit ratio [17]. The idea to treat the WPW syndrome through the ablation of APs is not novel, with the first successful surgical ablation being reported back in 1968 [37]. This technique remains to date as a last-resort approach (as described below), despite the applied modifications on this technique (i.e., open-heart endocardial incision or closed heart dissection and cryo-ablation) [38, 39]. However, recent research in

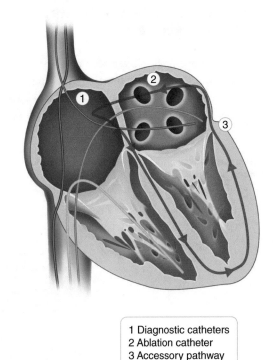

1 Diagnostic catheters
2 Ablation catheter
3 Accessory pathway

Fig. 4 Graphical presentation of the ablation of the accessory pathway in a patient with the WPW syndrome

conjunction with the experience gained in the electrophysiology laboratories, gave birth to the concept that percutaneous shock ablation of APs was feasible [40] (Fig. 4).

In the last decades, the standard energy source used to ablate APs is radiofrequency current. However, cryoablation can be used as an alternative to the radiofrequency-based one for APs with proximity to the AV node or the bundle of His [40]. TCA has been linked with especially high success rates (up to 97% in expert centers) and substantially lower complication rates (less than 1%) in a large number of studies [41–48], with those levels of safety and success being replicated in further studies considering the pediatric population, which has now evolved into the primary target of TCA [23, 49]. Nowadays, it is widely accepted that symptom control is the most frequent indication for TCA. In particular, TCA is considered as the gold-standard approach for the management of supraventricular arrhythmias in all patients with symptomatic AVRT or pre-excited AF according to the recent guidelines published by the American College of Cardiology, the American Heart Association, and the Heart Rhythm Society in 2015 [17]. Moreover, symptomatic patients who have failed TCA are usually referred for a repeat TCA attempt or consider proceeding with surgical ablation.

Management of Asymptomatic Patients with the WPW Syndrome

Although the management of asymptomatic WPW patients still remains a conundrum, for most of them, particularly those over 35–40 years of age, observation is suggested rather than TCA or pharmacological treatment (Class IIC).

However, in some asymptomatic patients, TCA of the APs is also recommended after following specific risk stratification algorithms (as presented in Fig. 5), because of the risk of sudden cardiac death (SCD) correlated with the syndrome. In particular, it is currently established that SCD might be the first manifestation of the WPW syndrome, with recent evidence supporting the link between SCD and

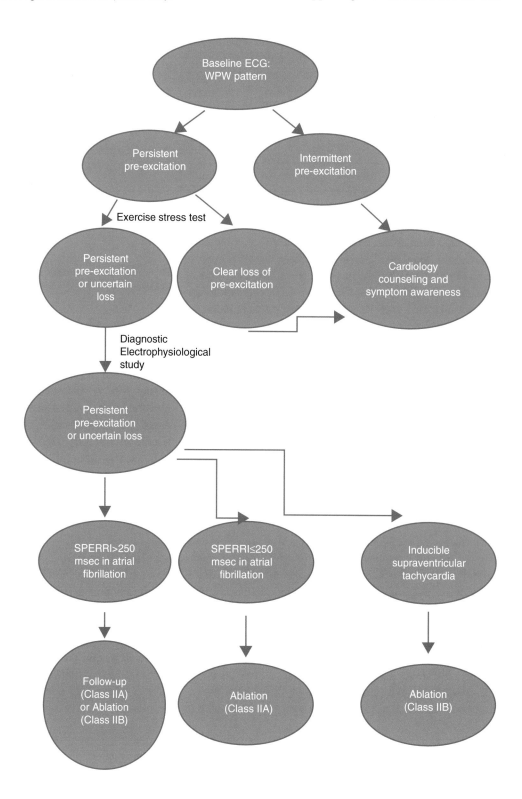

Fig. 5 Management of asymptomatic patients with the WPW syndrome

AF in the WPW syndrome [50, 51]. Nevertheless, the incidence of SCD seems to be very low regardless of age (ranging from 0.1 to 0.4% WPW patients per year in several large case series) [51], while its incidence in the asymptomatic pediatric population ranges from 0.0012 to 0.6% per year [17, 49, 52].

The main mechanism underlying SCD in WPW patients is ventricular fibrillation, occurring during an episode of AF. Therefore, identifying asymptomatic patients at significant risk for ventricular fibrillation could automatically render those patients' suitable candidates for TCA. Moreover, current literature supports the existence of some predictive indicators for the development of symptoms or SCD (high-risk asymptomatic patients with WPW) [53–55]:

- Younger age.
- Male gender.
- Short refractory period of the AP.
- Multiple APs.
- Short pre-excited RR interval (SPERRI ≤ 250 ms) during AF or during rapid atrial pacing.
- Inducible AVRT or AF during electrophysiological studies.
- Ebstein malformation.
- Some occupations (such as airline pilots or truck drivers) in which a potential symptomatic episode would put themselves or others at risk.

However, asymptomatic WPW patients (who are often young and otherwise healthy) mostly remain asymptomatic [55], and it is noteworthy that patients who remain asymptomatic over 35 years are unlikely to develop any symptoms at all [56]. Although children are at the highest risk of developing symptoms, reported rates of symptom development rise up to 20% over 3 years [57]. Therefore, the decision to refer an asymptomatic young patient with pre-excitation for TCA remains a dilemma to date since TCA could also carry potentially life-threatening complications (cardiac tamponade, complete AV block, acute inter-atrial shunting, and inappropriate sinus tachycardia) [58].To that end, a 2012 consensus statement on the management of asymptomatic young WPW patients has been published to support a risk stratification algorithm (presented in Fig. 5) utilizing both non-invasive tests and electrophysiological studies to detect asymptomatic young patients at higher risk [54].

This algorithm suggests that old enough children should undergo an exercise stress test to evaluate the persistence of pre-excitation. According to a systematic literature review published in 2019 by Raposo et al., the most relevant studies considered indeed the cut-off age ≥ 8 years old for the assessment of pre-excitation persistence, exactly as recommended in the 2012 consensus [49]. The identification of a SPERRI ≤ 250 ms seems to be the best promising indicator

for risk stratification. Thus, prophylactic non-pharmacological therapy (i.e., TCA) is nowadays recommended in asymptomatic children with 1 or multiple APs and a low SPERRI and/or a low effective anterograde period of the AP (Class II) [23]. Nevertheless, both the ambiguity regarding the usefulness/efficacy of the TCA and the various presentations of the syndrome render its treatment more of a challenge today than it was a few decades ago.

Surgical Ablation and Perioperative Management

Finally, surgical ablation of the APs could be considered as a last-resort approach once both TCA and pharmacological treatment have failed. This procedure was the standard technique used in patients with drug-refractory WPW syndrome before TCA was discovered. Despite the excellent reported outcomes of surgical ablation (long-term success rate almost 100% with an operative mortality rate <1% [59, 60], nowadays radiofrequency-based TCA is considered as the preferred therapy for the ablation of the APs. Surgical ablation remains an effective option in highly symptomatic and hemodynamically unstable, drug-refractory arrhythmias patients who had already undergone a TCA failing to treat the APs successfully [61]. It has been also reported as a safe alternative to treat the syndrome in children undergoing concomitant operation for comorbid congenital cardiac lesions [62]. Nevertheless, clinicians should always keep in mind that anesthesia (both general and regional) can unmask the WPW syndrome, and they should be very cautious with the perioperative management of a WPW patient. Perioperative circumstances (nausea, cholinergic medications, hypothermia, sympathetic blockade, laryngoscopy, and hyperventilation) can all accentuate AP travel or affect normal conduction pathways, thereby creating a proarrhythmic environment [63–66].

Sports Eligibility

Pre-participation physical evaluation usually includes an ECG examination for all athletes—irrespective of age—and thus, a WPW diagnosis is frequently made in this context. While many sudden cardiac deaths of WPW patients have been associated with exercise [67], training does not seem to alter the electrophysiological properties of WPW [68]. However, WPW syndrome accounted for almost 1% of sudden deaths in a long-term registry of athletes [68]. Hence, the European Society of Cardiology claims that all WPW athletes should undergo a comprehensive risk pre-participation assessment through an electrophysiological study [69]. In contrast, according to the 36th Bethesda

Conference, the electrophysiological assessment is recommended only in asymptomatic athletes participating in moderate- to high-level competitive sports [70]. Despite the existing disparities in the recommendations in dealing with asymptomatic WPW athletes among European and American Cardiology Societies, any adolescent with ventricular pre-excitation should prompt referral to a specialist with expertise in pediatric electrophysiology to initiate the process of risk stratification, as described in this literature review.

Conclusion

The WPW syndrome constitutes a rare and potentially lethal congenital abnormality in the cardiac conduction system, encountered quite rarely in contemporary adult populations. However, the timely recognition of the WPW pattern in an ECG of an asymptomatic individual, as well as the effective risk stratification and clinical management of both symptomatic and asymptomatic WPW patients have evolved into challenging and significant steps, with the potential to maximize patients' quality of life and minimize the risk of life-threatening arrhythmias.

Multiple Choice Questions

1. Wolff–Parkinson–White (WPW) is caused due to the presence of:
   A. Myocardial ischemia.
   B. A normal accessory pathway.
   C. Bundle of Koch.
   D. Bundle of Kent.

2. The accessory conduction pathway is more often located at the:
   A. Right free wall.
   B. Left free wall.
   C. Posteroseptal.
   D. Anteroseptal.

3. WPW is most commonly encountered as a syndrome with:
   A. Unknown origin.
   B. Familial origin.
   C. Unknown and familial origin.
   D. None of the above.

4. Individuals with the WPW syndrome are born with an extra electrical pathway between the upper chambers of the heart (atria) and the lower chambers (ventricles). This extra pathway makes which of the following more likely to occur?
   A. Heart attacks.
   B. Abnormally fast heart rhythms.
   C. High cholesterol.
   D. High blood pressure.

5. Which of the following methods is not used to diagnose the WPW syndrome:
   A. 12-lead ECG.
   B. Holter monitor.
   C. Electrophysiological testing.
   D. MRI.

6. The ECG pattern of a WPW patient consists of one of the following features:
   A. Delta wave.
   B. Shortened QRS complex.
   C. Widened PR segment.
   D. T wave generally in the same direction as the delta wave.

7. In WPW patients, antiarrhythmic drugs may be given indefinitely to prevent episodes of a fast heart rate. Which of the following treatments can eliminate the need to take antiarrhythmic drugs for a lifetime?
   A. Heart bypass surgery.
   B. Pacemaker implantation.
   C. Stent placement.
   D. Radiofrequency ablation.

8. Which of the following drugs is the drug of choice for the termination of an acute paroxysmal tachycardia when recognizing a delta wave in the ECG pattern of a hemodynamically stable patient?
   A. IV amiodarone.
   B. IV adenosine if vagal maneuvers do not succeed.
   C. Oral flecainide or propafenone.
   D. Digoxin if atrial fibrillation co-exists.

9. Which strategy is preferred for the chronic management of a WPW patient to prevent the recurrence of arrhythmic episodes?
   A. Propranolol, bisoprolol, or carvedilol.
   B. Digoxin or verapamil.
   C. Radiofrequency-based transcatheter ablation of the accessory pathway.
   D. Propafenone in a patient having previously undergone a coronary revascularization procedure.

10. Which of the following asymptomatic patients should be prioritized to be scheduled for a transcatheter ablation in your electrophysiology laboratory?
    A. A 43-year-old man with intermittent pre-excitation recognized in his ECGs.
    B. A 51-year-old woman with persistent pre-excitation and atrial fibrillation, who was referred -despite her reluctance—for an electrophysiological study, which demonstrated a SPERRI > 250 ms.
    C. A 63-year-old man who has been diagnosed with WPW 40 years ago and undergoes preoperative cardiac evaluation prior to a scheduled laparoscopic cholecystectomy.
    D. A 17 year young man willing to become an Air Force pilot.

Answers

1. D.

   Explanation: WPW syndrome is an innate cardiac disease caused by the premature activation of the myocardium due to the abnormal presence of an accessory conduction pathway, the "bundle of Kent."

2. B.

   Explanation: Accessory pathways could be located anywhere in the heart: (1) at the left free wall (53%), (2) posteroseptal (36%), (3) at the right free wall (8%), and (4) anteroseptal (3%).

3. A.

   Explanation: WPW syndrome has not been yet associated with specific genetic mutations in most patients, and, therefore, the underlying genetic etiopathology remains unknown in them.

4. B.

   Explanation: Typically, when people first experience an arrhythmia due to this syndrome, it is an episode of palpitations that begins suddenly, often during exercise. For most people, the very fast heart rate is uncomfortable and distressing. A few people faint. Wolff–Parkinson–White syndrome is a common cause of paroxysmal supraventricular tachycardia.

5. D.

   Explanation: The diagnosis of the WPW syndrome is mostly made with a 12-lead ECG, with the relative clinical appearance and the family history being also of great help. The diagnosis can also be set with a Holter monitor and an electrophysiological testing.

6. A.

   Explanation: The ECG patterns of WPW patients consist of the following features: I. Slurring of the initial portion of the QRS complex (delta wave), II. Widened QRS complex (duration >120 ms in adults and > 90 ms in children), III. Shortened PR segment (duration <120 ms in adults and < 90 ms in children), and IV. T wave opposite to the delta wave.

7. D.

   Explanation: This procedure destroys the extra electrical pathway between the atria and ventricles by delivering energy through an electrode catheter inserted in the heart. It is successful in more than 95% of people.

8. B.

   Explanation: For hemodynamically stable patients with acute orthodromic AVRT, a step-wise approach is usually recommended with initial treatment with one or more vagal maneuvers (such as the Valsalva maneuver and carotid sinus massage) being preferred rather than pharmacologic therapy (Class IB). If those maneuvers are ineffective, treatment with an AV nodal blocking agent (beta blockers, adenosine, and verapamil) should be instituted. Adenosine IV is preferred as the initial choice rather than verapamil IV based on its efficacy and short half-life (Class IIB), which render it effective for the acute termination of the tachycardia in 80–90% of patients.

9. C.

   Explanation: For almost every patient with an AP and symptomatic arrhythmic episodes (orthodromic or antidromic AVRT, and pre-excited AF or atrial flutter), the recommended long-term treatment approach is the radiofrequency-based TCA (Class IA). For those patients who are not candidates for or not willing to undergo ablation of the AP or for select patients with well-tolerated, rare arrhythmic episodes, antiarrhythmic medication is still recommended (Class IIC). However, beta blockers, verapamil, and digoxin are contraindicated in WPW patients, while flecainide and propafenone should be avoided in coronary artery disease patients.

10. D.

    Explanation: Current literature supports the existence of some predictive indicators for the development of symptoms or SCD (high-risk asymptomatic patients with WPW): younger age, male gender, short refractory period of the AP, multiple APs, short pre-excited RR interval (SPERRI≤250 ms) during AF or during rapid atrial pacing, inducible AVRT or AF during electrophysiological studies, Ebstein malformation, and some occupations (such as airline pilots) in which a potential symptomatic episode would put themselves or others at risk. Besides, patients who remain asymptomatic over 35 years are unlikely to develop any symptoms at all and patients who have intermittent pre-excitation should proceed with cardiology counseling and symptom awareness.

References

1. Chhabra L, Goyal A, Benham MD. Wolff Parkinson White Syndrome. In: StatPearls [Internet]. Treasure Island, FL: StatPearls Publishing; 2021.

2. Wedd AM. Paroxysmal tachycardia: with reference to nomotopic tachycardia and the rôle of the extrinsic cardiac nerves. Arch Intern Med. 1921;27(5):571–90.

3. Scheinman MM. History of Wolff-Parkinson-White syndrome. Pacing Clin Electrophysiol. 2005;28(2):152–6.

4. Wolff L, Parkinson J, White PD. Bundle-branch block with short P-R interval in healthy young people prone to paroxysmal tachycardia. 1930. Ann Noninvasive Electrocardiol. 2006;11(4):340–53.

5. Sethi KK, Dhall A, Chadha DS, Garg S, Malani SK, Mathew OP. WPW and preexcitation syndromes. J Assoc Physicians India. 2007;55(Suppl):10–5.

6. Wolferth CC, Wood FC. The mechanism of production of short P-R intervals and prolonged QRS complexes in patients with presumably undamaged hearts: Hypothesis of an accessory pathway of auriculoventricular conduction (bundle of kent). Am Heart J. 1933;8(3):297–311.

7. Lu C-W, Wu M-H, Chen H-C, Kao F-Y, Huang S-K. Epidemiological profile of Wolff-Parkinson-White syndrome in a general population younger than 50 years of age in an era of radiofrequency catheter ablation. Int J Cardiol. 2014;174(3):530–4.

8. Kulig J, Koplan BA. Wolff-Parkinson-White Syndrome and accessory pathways. Circulation. 2010;122(15):e480–3.

9. Duckeck W, Kuck KH. Atrial fibrillation in Wolff-Parkinson-White syndrome. Development and therapy. Herz. 1993;18(1):60–6.

10. Jamal SZ, Zaidi KA, Sheikh SA, Ahmed A, Irfan G, Qadir F. Localization of accessory pathways in Wolff Parkinson White syndrome using R/S ratios on surface Ecgs. J Ayub Med Coll Abbottabad. 2019;31(2):146–50.

11. Liu S, Yuan S, Kongstad O, Olsson SB. Gender differences in the electrophysiological characteristics of atrioventricular conduction system and their clinical implications. Scand Cardiovasc J. 2001;35(5):313–7.

12. Gollob MH, Green MS, Tang AS, Gollob T, Karibe A, Ali Hassan AS, Ahmad F, Lozado R, Shah G, Fananapazir L, Bachinski LL, Roberts R. Identification of a gene responsible for familial Wolff-Parkinson-White syndrome. N Engl J Med. 2001;344(24):1823–31.

13. Misaki T, Watanabe G, Iwa T, Watanabe Y, Mukai K, Takahashi M, Ohtake H, Yamamoto K. Surgical treatment of patients with Wolff-Parkinson-White syndrome and associated Ebstein's anomaly. J Thorac Cardiovasc Surg. 1995;110(6):1702–7.

14. Chhabra L, Goyal ABM. Wolff Parkinson White Syndrome. Treasure Island, FL: StatPearls [Internet]; 2021.

15. Dunnigan A. In: Benditt DG, Benson DW, editors. Developmental aspects and natural history of preexcitation syndromes BT - cardiac preexcitation syndromes: origins, evaluation, and treatment. Boston, MA: Springer US; 1986. p. 21–9.

16. Surawicz B, Childers R, Deal BJ, Gettes LS. AHA/ACCF/HRS Recommendations for the standardization and Interpretation of the electrocardiogram. Circulation. 2009;119(10):e235–40.

17. Page RL, Joglar JA, Caldwell MA, Calkins H, Conti JB, Deal BJ, Estes NAM 3rd, Field ME, Goldberger ZD, Hammill SC, Indik JH, Lindsay BD, Olshansky B, Russo AM, Shen W-K, Tracy CM, Al-Khatib SM. 2015 ACC/AHA/HRS Guideline for the Management of Adult Patients With Supraventricular Tachycardia: A Report of the American College of Cardiology/American Heart Association Task Force on Clinical Practice Guidelines and the Heart Rhythm Society. Circulation. 2016;133(14):e506–74.

18. Wang K, Asinger R, Hodges M. Electrocardiograms of Wolff-Parkinson-White syndrome simulating other conditions. Am Heart J. 1996;132(1 Pt 1):152–5.

19. Tseng CD, Tseng YZ, Lo HM, Chiang FT, Hsu KL, Wu TL. Holter monitoring in patients with Wolff-Parkinson-White syndrome: with special reference to intermittent pre-excitation. J Formos Med Assoc. 1992;91(1):52–6.

20. Brembilla-Perrot B. Electrophysiological evaluation of Wolff-Parkinson-White syndrome. Indian Pacing Electrophysiol J. 2002;2(4):143–52.

21. García Seara FJ, Martínez Sande JL, Cid Alvarez B, González Juanatey JR. Wolff-Parkinson-White's syndrome and Danon's disease. Med Clin. 2008;130:277.

22. Sapra A, Albers J, Bhandari P, Davis D, Ranjit E. Wolff-Parkinson-White Syndrome: a master of disguise. Cureus. 2020;12:e8672.

23. Cohen MI, Triedman JK, Cannon BC, Davis AM, Drago F, Janousek J, Klein GJ, Law IH, Morady FJ, Paul T, Perry JC, Sanatani S, Tanel RE. PACES/HRS Expert Consensus Statement on the Management of the Asymptomatic Young Patient with a Wolff-Parkinson-White (WPW, Ventricular Preexcitation) Electrocardiographic Pattern: Developed in partnership between the Pediatric and Congenital Electrophysi. Hear Rhythm. 2012;9(6):1006–24.

24. Brugada J, Katritsis DG, Arbelo E, Arribas F, Bax JJ, Blomström-Lundqvist C, Calkins H, Corrado D, Deftereos SG, Diller G-P, Gomez-Doblas JJ, Gorenek B, Grace A, Ho SY, Kaski J-C, Kuck K-H, Lambiase PD, Sacher F, Sarquella-Brugada G, Suwalski P, Zaza A. 2019 ESC Guidelines for the management of patients with supraventricular tachycardiaThe Task Force for the management of patients with supraventricular tachycardia of the European Society of Cardiology (ESC). Eur Heart J. 2020;41(5):655–720.

25. diMarco JP, Sellers TD, Lerman BB, Greenberg ML, Berne RM, Belardinelli L. Diagnostic and therapeutic use of adenosine in patients with supraventricular tachyarrhythmias. J Am Coll Cardiol. 1985;6(2):417–25.

26. Belardinelli L, Linden J, Berne RM. The cardiac effects of adenosine. Prog Cardiovasc Dis. 1989;32(1):73–97.

27. Kowey PR, Friehling TD, Marinchak RA. Electrophysiology of beta blockers in supraventricular arrhythmias. Am J Cardiol. 1987;60(6):32D–8D.

28. Jackman WM, Friday KJ, Fitzgerald DM, Yeung-Lai-Wah JA, Lazzara R. Use of intracardiac recordings to determine the site of drug action in paroxysmal supraventricular tachycardia. Am J Cardiol. 1988;62(19):8L–19L.

29. Ward DE, Jones S, Shinebourne EA. Use of flecainide acetate for refractory junctional tachycardias in children with the Wolff-Parkinson-White syndrome. Am J Cardiol. 1986;57(10):787–90.

30. Musto B, D'Onofrio A, Cavallaro C, Musto A. Electrophysiological effects and clinical efficacy of propafenone in children with recurrent paroxysmal supraventricular tachycardia. Circulation. 1988;78(4):863–9.

31. Ludmer PL, McGowan NE, Antman EM, Friedman PL. Efficacy of propafenone in Wolff-Parkinson-White syndrome: electrophysiologic findings and long-term follow-up. J Am Coll Cardiol. 1987;9(6):1357–63.

32. Kim SS, Lal R, Ruffy R. Treatment of paroxysmal reentrant supraventricular tachycardia with flecainide acetate. Am J Cardiol. 1986;58(1):80–5.

33. Echt DS, Liebson PR, Mitchell LB, Peters RW, Obias-Manno D, Barker AH, Arensberg D, Baker A, Friedman L, Greene HL. Mortality and morbidity in patients receiving encainide, flecainide, or placebo. The Cardiac Arrhythmia Suppression Trial. N Engl J Med. 1991;324(12):781–8.

34. Wellens HJ, Lie KI, Bär FW, Wesdorp JC, Dohmen HJ, Düren DR, Durrer D. Effect of amiodarone in the Wolff-Parkinson-White syndrome. Am J Cardiol. 1976;38(2):189–94.

35. Rosenbaum MB, Chiale PA, Ryba D, Elizari MV. Control of tachyarrhythmias associated with Wolff-Parkinson-White syndrome by amiodarone hydrochloride. Am J Cardiol. 1974;34(2):215–23.

36. Feld GK, Nademanee K, Weiss J, Stevenson W, Singh BN. Electrophysiologic basis for the suppression by amiodarone of orthodromic supraventricular tachycardias complicating preexcitation syndromes. J Am Coll Cardiol. 1984;3(5):1298–307.

37. Cobb FR, Blumenschein SD, Sealy WC, Boineau JP, Wagner GS, Wallace AG. Successful surgical interruption of the bundle of Kent in a patient with Wolff-Parkinson-White syndrome. Circulation. 1968;38(6):1018–29.

38. Rowland E, Robinson K, Edmondson S, Krikler DM, Bentall HH. Cryoablation of the accessory pathway in Wolff-Parkinson-White syndrome: initial results and long term follow up. Br Heart J. 1988;59(4):453–7.

39. Cox JL, Gallagher JJ, Cain ME. Experience with 118 consecutive patients undergoing operation for the Wolff-Parkinson-White syndrome. J Thorac Cardiovasc Surg. 1985;90(4):490–501.

40. Scheinman MM, Morady F, Hess DS, Gonzalez R. Catheter-induced ablation of the atrioventricular junction to control refractory supraventricular arrhythmias. JAMA. 1982;248(7):851–5.

41. Scheinman MM, Huang S. The 1998 NASPE prospective catheter ablation registry. Pacing Clin Electrophysiol. 2000;23(6):1020–8.

42. Kuck KH, Schlüter M, Geiger M, Siebels J, Duckeck W. Radiofrequency current catheter ablation of accessory atrioventricular pathways. Lancet (London, England). 1991;337(8757):1557–61.

43. Jackman WM, Wang XZ, Friday KJ, Roman CA, Moulton KP, Beckman KJ, McClelland JH, Twidale N, Hazlitt HA, Prior MI. Catheter ablation of accessory atrioventricular pathways (Wolff-Parkinson-White syndrome) by radiofrequency current. N Engl J Med. 1991;324(23):1605–11.

44. Chen SA, Tai CT. Ablation of atrioventricular accessory pathways: current technique-state of the art. Pacing Clin Electrophysiol. 2001;24(12):1795–809.

45. Ceresnak SR, Dubin AM. Wolff–Parkinson–White syndrome (WPW) and athletes: Darwin at play? J Electrocardiol. 2015;48(3):356–61.

46. Calkins H, Sousa J, el Atassi R, Rosenheck S, de Buitleir M, Kou WH, Kadish AH, Langberg JJ, Morady F. Diagnosis and cure of the Wolff-Parkinson-White syndrome or paroxysmal supraventricular tachycardias during a single electrophysiologic test. N Engl J Med. 1991;324(23):1612–8.

47. Calkins H, Langberg J, Sousa J, el Atassi R, Leon A, Kou W, Kalbfleisch S, Morady F. Radiofrequency catheter ablation of accessory atrioventricular connections in 250 patients. Abbreviated therapeutic approach to Wolff-Parkinson-White syndrome. Circulation. 1992;85(4):1337–46.

48. Aguinaga L, Primo J, Anguera I, Mont L, Valentino M, Brugada P, Brugada J. Long-term follow-up in patients with the permanent form of junctional reciprocating tachycardia treated with radiofrequency ablation. Pacing Clin Electrophysiol. 1998;21(11 Pt 1):2073–8.

49. Raposo D, António N, Andrade H, Sousa P, Pires A, Gonçalves L. Management of asymptomatic Wolff-Parkinson-White pattern in young patients: has anything changed? Pediatr Cardiol. 2019;40(5):892–900.

50. Qiu M, Lv B, Lin W, Ma J, Dong H. Sudden cardiac death due to the Wolff-Parkinson-White syndrome: a case report with genetic analysis. Medicine (Baltimore). 2018;97(51):e13248.

51. Obeyesekere M, Gula LJ, Skanes AC, Leong-Sit P, Klein GJ. Risk of sudden death in Wolff-Parkinson-White Syndrome. Circulation. 2012;125(5):659–60.

52. Etheridge SP, Escudero CA, Blaufox AD, Law IH, Dechert-Crooks BE, Stephenson EA, Dubin AM, Ceresnak SR, Motonaga KS, Skinner JR, Marcondes LD, Perry JC, Collins KK, Seslar SP, Cabrera M, Uzun O, Cannon BC, Aziz PF, Kubuš P, Tanel RE, Valdes SO, Sami S, Kertesz NJ, Maldonado J, Erickson C, Moore JP, Asakai H, Mill L, Abcede M, Spector ZZ, Menon S, Shwayder M, Bradley DJ, Cohen MI, Sanatani S. Life-threatening event risk in children with Wolff-Parkinson-White syndrome: a multicenter international study. JACC Clin Electrophysiol. 2018;4(4):433–44.

53. Kay GN, Epstein AE, Dailey SM, Plumb VJ. Role of radiofrequency ablation in the management of supraventricular arrhythmias: experience in 760 consecutive patients. J Cardiovasc Electrophysiol. 1993;4(4):371–89.

54. Crossen KJ, Lindsay BD, Cain ME. Reliability of retrograde atrial activation patterns during ventricular pacing for localizing accessory pathways. J Am Coll Cardiol. 1987;9(6):1279–87.

55. Chen X, Borggrefe M, Shenasa M, Haverkamp W, Hindricks G, Breithardt G. Characteristics of local electrogram predicting successful transcatheter radiofrequency ablation of left-sided accessory pathways. J Am Coll Cardiol. 1992;20(3):656–65.

56. Wellens HJ. Should catheter ablation be performed in asymptomatic patients with Wolff-Parkinson-White syndrome? When to perform catheter ablation in asymptomatic patients with a Wolff-Parkinson-White electrocardiogram. Circulation. 2005;112(14):2201–7. discussion 2216

57. Sellers TDJ, Bashore TM, Gallagher JJ. Digitalis in the pre-excitation syndrome. Analysis during atrial fibrillation. Circulation. 1977;56(2):260–7.

58. Obeyesekere MN, Sy RW, Modi S. When can ablation be considered a reasonable option in young asymptomatic patients with a Wolff–Parkinson–White ECG? Expert Rev Cardiovasc Ther. 2012;10(12):1451–3.

59. Johnson DC, Nunn GR, Richards DA, Uther JB, Ross DL. Surgical therapy for supraventricular tachycardia, a potentially curable disorder. J Thorac Cardiovasc Surg. 1987;93(6):913–8.

60. Hamdan MH, Page RL, Wasmund SL, Sheehan CJ, Zagrodzky JD, Ramaswamy K, Joglar JA, Adamson MM, Barron BA, Smith ML. Selective parasympathetic denervation following posteroseptal ablation for either atrioventricular nodal reentrant tachycardia or accessory pathways. Am J Cardiol. 2000;85(7):875–8. A9

61. Holman WL, Kay GN, Plumb VJ, Epstein AE. Operative results after unsuccessful radiofrequency ablation for Wolff-Parkinson-White syndrome. Am J Cardiol. 1992;70(18):1490–1.

62. Misaki T, Watanabe G, Iwa T, Matsunaga Y, Ohotake H, Tsubota M, Takahashi M, Yamamoto K, Watanabe Y. Surgical treatment of patients with Wolff-Parkinson-White syndrome and associated acquired valvular heart disease. J Thorac Cardiovasc Surg. 1994;108(1):68–72.

63. Wellens HJ. The wide QRS tachycardia. Ann Int Med. 1986;104:879.

64. Mandel WJ, Laks MM, Obayashi K, Hayakawa H, Daley W. The Wolff-Parkinson-White syndrome: pharmacologic effects of procaine amide. Am Heart J. 1975;90(6):744–54.

65. Kang KT, Potts JE, Radbill AE, La Page MJ, Papagiannis J, Garnreiter JM, Kubus P, Kantoch MJ, Von Bergen NH, Fournier A, Côté J-M, Paul T, Anderson CC, Cannon BC, Miyake CY, Blaufox AD, Etheridge SP, Sanatani S. Permanent junctional reciprocating tachycardia in children: a multicenter experience. Heart Rhythm. 2014;11(8):1426–32.

66. Dorostkar PC, Silka MJ, Morady F, Dick M 2nd. Clinical course of persistent junctional reciprocating tachycardia. J Am Coll Cardiol. 1999;33(2):366–75.

67. Wiedermann CJ, Becker AE, Hopferwieser T, Mühlberger V, Knapp E. Sudden death in a young competitive athlete with Wolff-Parkinson-White syndrome. Eur Heart J. 1987;8(6):651–5.

68. Mezzani A, Giovannini T, Michelucci A, Padeletti L, Resina A, Cupelli V, Musante R. Effects of training on the electrophysiologic properties of atrium and accessory pathway in athletes with Wolff-Parkinson-White syndrome. Cardiology. 1990;77(4):295–302.

69. Corrado D, Pelliccia A, Bjørnstad HH, Vanhees L, Biffi A, Borjesson M, Panhuyzen-Goedkoop N, Deligiannis A, Solberg E, Dugmore D, Mellwig KP, Assanelli D, Delise P, van Buuren F, Anastasakis A, Heidbuchel H, Hoffmann E, Fagard R, Priori SG, Basso C, Arbustini E, Blomstrom-Lundqvist C, WJ MK, Thiene G. Cardiovascular pre-participation screening of young competitive athletes for prevention of sudden death: proposal for a common European protocol. Consensus Statement of the Study Group of Sport Cardiology of the Working Group of Cardiac Rehabilitation an. Eur Heart J. 2005;26(5):516–24.

70. Pelliccia A, Zipes DP, Maron BJ. Bethesda Conference #36 and the European Society of Cardiology Consensus Recommendations revisited a comparison of U.S. and European criteria for eligibility and disqualification of competitive athletes with cardiovascular abnormalities. J Am Coll Cardiol. 2008;52(24):1990–6.

Laparoscopic Surgery of Congenital Heart

Morad Al Mostafa

Abstract

There have been many developments in the field of congenital heart surgery and with the accumulation of expertise and the development of medical tools and treatment methods it is possible for a child with congenital heart disease to live a valuable life. This chapter discusses the medical approaches for the surgical correction of congenital heart disease, surgical methods of congenital heart disease repair, benefits, and the complication of heart surgeries. We have been familiar with the latest scientific research, articles and studies related to congenital heart disease surgeries, the risks of these surgeries, and the efficiency of these surgeries in improving the lives of children with these diseases. The chapter is also talked about robotically assisted heart surgery which is a new approach to minimally invasive heart surgery. The benefits, risk, and complications of this new method were discussed. Laparoscopic surgery, which requires smaller incisions instead of the larger incisions required in open surgery, has becoming more prevalent. Many studies about mortality, morbidity, and outcomes after laparoscopic surgery in children with and without congenital heart disease were discussed in this chapter and showed that children with congenital heart disease are more susceptible to hemodynamic effects of gas insufflation in laparoscopic surgery, and these consequences may counteract any benefits given by the less invasive method.

Keywords

Congenital heart disease · Septostomy · Laparoscopic Minimally invasive · Tetralogy of Fallot · Complications Heart surgeries · Open-heart surgery · Ventricular septal defect · Repair · Fontan procedure · Shunt

Introduction

The flow of blood through the heart is disrupted by congenital heart abnormalities. Congenital cardiac abnormalities come in various severity. They might range from minor defect that may be readily corrected or do not require treatment at all to major defect with life-threatening symptoms that require prompt medical care.

Congenital anomaly of the heart is the most common birth disorder. Over the last few decades, the identification and treatment of these complicated abnormalities have dramatically improved. As a result, virtually all children with complex heart abnormalities have valuable life.

How Are Congenital Heart Defects Treated?

A congenital heart defect is treated through congenital heart defect correction surgery.

Open-heart surgery includes surgical procedure where the chest is opened surgically to perform surgery on heart valves, muscles, or arteries. In typical open-heart surgery, the heart is stopped and the surgeon performs the procedure while a heart-lung machine performs the job. Compared to open-heart surgery, catheter operations simpler than surgical treatments since they just involve a needle incision in the skin to introduce the catheter into a vein or artery.

Improvements in surgical methods, as well as collected expertise in the treatment of CHD patients, have resulted in a significant reduction in overall mortality, as well as improved CHD patient long-term survival. But on the other hand, the vast spectrum of cardiac defects, the presence of recurrent lesions, and the individuality of each case all provide distinct challenges in the monitoring and management of this growing community of people with CHD. A significant number of people reach adulthood without having their CHD corrected surgically due to multiples factors despite the early identification and surgical treatment of congenital heart disease (CHD).

M. Al Mostafa (✉)
Jordan University of Science and Technology, Ar-Ramtha, Jordan

G. Tagarakis et al. (eds.), *Clinical and Surgical Aspects of Congenital Heart Diseases*,
https://doi.org/10.1007/978-3-031-23062-2_29

Patent Ductus Arteriosus Repair

The patent ductus arteriosus can be corrected without the need for surgery. The procedure can be done as open surgery, video-assisted thoracoscopic surgery, and catheter closure. Typically, the operation is performed in an X-ray-equipped laboratory to close the connection that remains patent after birth. During this procedure, the surgeon makes a small cut in the groin and a catheter is passed through the femoral vein. A coil-like metal device is advanced through the infant's ductus arteriosus artery by the catheter to correct the problems and block the blood flow [1].

Pulmonary Valve Stenosis Repair

Severe symptoms necessitate treatment. In congenital pulmonary valve stenosis, the surgeon will do valvectomy, where an incision in the pulmonary valve is made to open it and the old pulmonary valve is removed and a new valve is attached.

In transcatheter pulmonary valve replacement, a catheter with a new, balloon-expandable replacement pulmonary valve at its end is placed into a large blood vessel in the groin or chest and directed to the heart.

Coarctation of Aorta Repair

Coarctation is a non-shunt, obstructive lesion. There is obstruction in the distal part of aortic arch (just distal to subclavian artery), blood flow to the lower extremities is restricted due to the constriction, which will cause the heart to pump at a higher pressure in order to perfuse the lower extremities. Coarctation of the aorta is generally treated by a thoracotomy. Coarctation of the aorta can be repaired by balloon angioplasty or surgery. The surgical treatment includes removing the constricted region and suturing the remaining two ends together.

A third method for correcting this problem is to allow blood to bypass the constricted segment by connecting a tube to the normal portions of the aorta on each side of the constricted segment.

A fourth method for correcting this problem is a subclavian flap. An incision is made in the thin portion of the aorta. Then a patch from the left subclavian is used to widen the aorta's constricted section.

Atrial Septal Defect (ASD) Repair

The atrial septum is a muscular wall that separates the heart's two upper chambers (left and right atria). A tiny hole in the wall is present in every child at birth, the opening is no longer required after delivery, and it generally closes within weeks or months. Atrial septal defect happens when the hole between left and right atria dose not close. Oxygen-rich blood and oxygen-poor blood will be mixed up in this defect.

ASD can be closed without open-heart surgery in some cases. Atrial septal defects can be closed with a transcatheter procedure where catheters are driven into the heart chambers. To assess the size atrial septal defect, a balloon-tipped catheter is positioned in the middle of it and inflated. Atrial septal defect then closed using a device. The blood pressure between the right and left atria will maintain the device in place. In around 3 months, heart tissue will develop over the device.

ASD might be treated with open-heart surgery where the septum can be stitched or patched.

Ventricular Septal Defect (VSD) Repair

A VSD is a hole in the ventricular septum. By the age of one, the majority of small VSDs will close on their own and do not require treatment. However, VSDs that are still open after the child reaches the age of ten need to be closed.

Surgery is still the gold standard, surgical intervention is needed when VSD is associated with heart failure unresponsive to medical therapy, pulmonic stenosis, and pulmonary hypertension. A patch is stitched over the hole then heart tissue will develop over the patch, and the hole will be entirely filled with normal heart lining tissue by 6 months after surgery. The surgeon may choose to close the hole with stitches rather than a patch, or to utilize child's own pericardium. Some children may benefit from a minimally invasive technique using cardiac catheterization to correct their ventricular septal defect [2].

There are five approaches for ventricular septal defect repair:

- Right atrial which is the most often utilized.
- Transpulmonary.
- Transaortic.
- Right ventricular.
- Left ventricular.

A method has been developed to repair ventricular septal defect done as a keyhole procedure that include inserting a tiny blocking device (known as an occluder) into the heart through a blood vessel. To close the hole, the occluder is pushed into place with guide wires. The keyhole procedure cannot be used in very young children and in specific kinds of ventricular septal defects.

Tetralogy of Fallot Repair

It usually includes four defects in the heart:

1. Pulmonary stenosis or right ventricular outflow tract (RVOT) obstruction.
2. VSD.
3. Overriding of aorta.
4. RV hypertrophy.

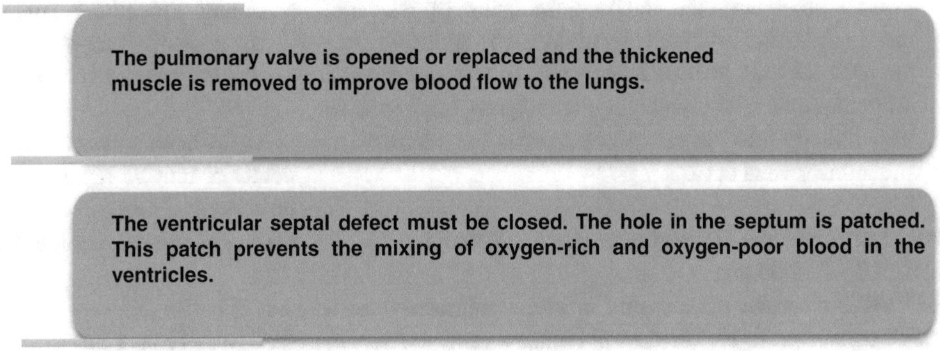

Fig. 1 Tetralogy of Fallot repair

The pulmonary valve is opened or replaced and the thickened muscle is removed to improve blood flow to the lungs.

The ventricular septal defect must be closed. The hole in the septum is patched. This patch prevents the mixing of oxygen-rich and oxygen-poor blood in the ventricles.

Open-heart surgery is needed to correct the four defects to allow the heart to work normally, either shortly after birth or later in infancy and it is usually performed between the ages of 6 months and 2 years.

The surgery involves (Fig. 1):

Transposition of the Great Vessels Repair

Normally, the aorta arises from the left ventricle, and the pulmonary artery arises from the right ventricle. In transposition of the great vessels, the aorta and pulmonary artery are connected to the wrong ventricles. There must be some mixing in order for patient to survive; because he will not survive more than few minutes if there is no communication, the communication has to be at the atria level (patent foramen ovale or atrial septal defect). Other cardiac defects might temporarily decrease the problems caused by this defect.

There is a variety of surgical techniques to correct transposition of the major arteries. The treatment of major vessel transposition needs open-heart surgery. If feasible, this procedure is conducted as soon as possible following birth. An arterial switch is the most frequent and preferred method of repairing transposition of the great arteries. The aorta and the pulmonary artery are separated. The pulmonary artery is connected to the right ventricle, as it should be. The aorta and coronary arteries are attached to the left ventricle [3].

Truncus Arteriosus Repair

Is a common trunk arising from right and left ventricles so it means that there is VSD, there is no truncus without ventricular septal defect? This common trunk is divided into the pulmonary artery and the aorta. There will be complete mixing of oxygen-rich blood and oxygen-poor blood, and the blood will pass depending on the pulmonary and systemic vascular resistance.

The surgical correction is usually done within the first few days or weeks of the baby's life. The pulmonary arteries are isolated from the aortic trunk, and ventricular septal defect is closed. The right ventricle and the pulmonary arteries are then linked together. As patient become older, they will need one or two further procedures.

Tricuspid Atresia Repair

The tricuspid valve is found between the right atrium and right ventricles. Tricuspid atresia happens when the valve is missing, narrow, or developed abnormally.

Atresia means the valve did not form so no communication between right atrium and right ventricles and this means that the blood cannot go to the lungs. Because of that patients with tricuspid atresia have to have communication at the atrial level to allow blood to pass from right atrium to left atrium, where there will be mixing of blood that return from the body with blood returning from the lungs. The lungs received blood via 2 options: either ventricular septal defect because blood in the right atrium will mix with the blood in the left atrium complete mixing or across patent ductus arteriosus to pulmonary artery. In order to keep the patent ductus arteriosus open, prostaglandin E is given to the infant shortly after the delivery, but this will only work for a limited period of time and the child will eventually need surgery.

To correct this problem, the child will need more than one surgical procedure. The purpose of surgery is to allow sufficient blood flow through the heart and into the lungs.

There are some procedures that can be done in tricuspid atresia:

- Atrial septostomy to enlarge the opening between left and right atria.
- Shunting to make a bypass from the aorta to pulmonary arteries. The shunt is created during the first 4–8 weeks of life.
- Pulmonary artery band placement.
- Glenn procedure, it's done between the ages of 3 and 6 months. The initial shunt is removed, and the pulmonary artery is connected to one of the major veins that returns blood to the heart (the superior vena cava). This permits blood that is deficient in oxygen to travel directly to the lungs.

- Fontan procedure, the standard treatment of tricuspid atresia, it is not performed on children with tricuspid atresia until they are at least 2 years old. In this surgery, the surgeon constructs a pathway for oxygen-poor blood to pass directly into the pulmonary arteries from a blood to the inferior vena cava.

Total Anomalous Pulmonary Venous Return (TAPVR) Correction

TAPVR is a cardiac abnormality in which pulmonary veins aren't connected right. The four pulmonary veins connect to the heart by anomalous route instead of the left atrium as they should, and this means that oxygen-rich blood goes to the wrong chamber.

Corrective surgery is the definitive treatment. Obstructed total anomalous pulmonary venous return is a surgical emergency, while non-obstructed total anomalous pulmonary venous return is corrected by an elective surgery a few days after the diagnosis.

TAPVR repairing is done by open-heart surgery. In supracardiac and infracardiac TAPVR, an anastomosis between the pulmonary venous confluence and the left atrium is created and the vertical vein is divided and ligated. The goal of surgery is to create a communication between pulmonary veins and left atrium and to close any aberrant connections.

Hypoplastic Left Heart Repair

This is a severe and critical cardiac defect caused by an underdeveloped left heart structure. The left side of the heart is unable to effectively pump oxygen-rich blood to the body. If not treated, it kills the majority of newborns who are born with it. Babies with hypoplastic left hearts do not have other cardiac defects. The oxygen-rich blood bypasses the left side of the heart in the first few days of life via the patent ductus arteriosus and the patent foramen ovale.

Multiple operations, performed in a specific schedule, are required soon after birth to improve blood flow to the body and bypass the heart's poorly performing left side. These procedures aid in the restoration of heart function.

Three heart surgeries are required.

- Norwood Procedure: The first procedure, performed during the first 2 weeks of life. This is a challenging procedure where a "new" aorta is made and connected to the right ventricle. The surgeon inserts a tube from the aorta or the right ventricle to pulmonary arteries. The right ventricle becomes the body's primary chamber that pump blood to the lungs and the rest of the body.
- Bi-directional Glenn Shunt Procedure: When the baby is 4–6 months old, this procedure is generally undertaken. This operation establishes a direct link between the pulmonary artery and the superior vena cava.

- Fontan Procedure: This operation is performed between the ages of 18 months and 3 years. The pulmonary artery and the inferior vena cava are connected.

Open-heart surgery may be necessary if a child's cardiac defect cannot be repaired with a catheter. The problem can be completely repaired with a single procedure or may need many operations over months or years.

In Open-Heart Surgery the Surgeon May

- Close holes in the heart by stitches or patch.
- Repair or replace heart valves and Widen arteries.

Topics Related to Surgery

- Blood transfusions are commonly required in heart surgery. The amount of blood required depends on the operation.
- Care of child at ICU.
- Care of child after discharge at home.
- School-aged children don't go to school for several weeks following surgery.
- The incision in the chest should be maintained clean and dry.
- Swimming is usually banned following surgery for at least a few weeks. Children can generally participate in regular household activities, but they should avoid hard play or sports.
- If child has a fever, chest pain, general weakness, difficulty in breathing, or redness, swelling at the incision site, the doctor must be notified.

Types of monitoring and support in the ICU include the following:

- Central venous line: to give medications, fluids and to monitor the pressure in veins.
- Arterial line: A catheter to measure blood pressure continuously.
- Arterial Blood Gas (ABG).
- Oxygen saturation.
- Mechanical ventilator.
- Continuous Positive Airway Pressure (CPAP): to maintain the lungs expanded without the use of a mechanical ventilator.
- Nasal cannula.
- Chest tube: to drain fluid and air formed by the surgery.
- Foley catheter.
- Pacing wires: Small wires that are inserted after open-heart surgery to diagnose and treat arrhythmias.

Robotically Assisted Heart Surgery: New Approaches to Minimally Invasive Heart Surgery

Robotically assisted atrial septal defect surgery is a type of minimally invasive cardiac surgery that uses an endoscopic, closed chest approach to do heart surgery. a series of keyhole-sized cuts is made on the side of chest and surgeon will insert guided robotic arms that hold small instruments into these incisions. Another incision will be used to insert a small video camera that will offer a magnified image of the operating site.

Robotically assisted atrial septal defect (ASD) and patent foramen ovale (PFO) repair procedures employ small incisions in the right side of the chest. The patient is placed on heart-lung bypass utilizing a peripheral catheter in order to do the procedure using a completely endoscopic robotic approach.

The surgeon's hands move the endoscopic instruments used to extract patch of pericardial tissue to repair the defect between the right and left atrium in cases of atrial septal defect or patent foramen ovale.

A study, robotically assisted totally endoscopic atrial septal defect repair, was conducted to explore whether extended cardiopulmonary bypass and aortic occlusion durations affect intraoperative and postoperative results based on a single-center experience and to address learning curve concerns of completely endoscopic atrial septal defect repair. The results of this study demonstrate that endoscopic atrial septal defect repair may be done safely, and longer cardiopulmonary bypass periods had no effect on the intraoperative or postoperative outcomes [4].

Another study, early results of robotically assisted congenital cardiac surgery, found that robotic technology may be used to safely and successfully conduct congenital cardiac operations and can be an alternative to traditional, minimally invasive and endoscopic approaches [5].

What Are the Benefits of Robotically Assisted Surgery?

Some of the advantages of robotically assisted surgery over traditional surgery are as follows:

- Less invasive.
- Incisions are smaller resulting in less scarring.

Traditional cardiac surgery involves making an incision through the breastbone in the middle of chest. The incision measures 6–8 in.

- Less bleeding and less discomfort.

- Having to stay in the hospital for a shorter period of time (usually 3–4 days).
- Painkillers are being used less often.
- Infection rate is decreased.
- Recovery time is shorter, after robotically assisted surgery, the patient can return to regular activities and work earlier.

Problems are infrequent, and effective training and close observation of the patient reduce the chance of complication. Risks and complications include:

- Pulmonary edema.
- Allergic reactions to the administered substances and reactions to anesthetics.
- Arteriovenous fistulas in the vascular puncture.
- Bleeding.
- Fever, headache, migraine.
- Infection.
- Gas embolism.
- Arrhythmia.
- Stroke and heart attack.

Robotically assisted heart surgeries:

- Repair of mitral valve.
- Repair of tricuspid valve.
- Correction of atrial fibrillation when other robotic surgery is required.
- Atrial septal defect repair.
- Patent foramen ovale repair.
- Cardiac tumors removal.

A study that looked into the possibility and safety of totally endoscopic repair of an atrial septal defect through small incisions on the chest without the use of a robotically assisted surgical system found that it is possible to do totally endoscopically repair of atrial septal defect safely without the use of a robotically assisted surgical system [6].

In a study of totally thoracoscopic closure of ventricular septal defect without a robotically assisted surgical system where total thoracoscopic VSD closure was performed on 119 patients, it was found to be safe and successful [7].

Laparoscopic surgery, which requires 3–12 mm incisions instead of the larger incisions required in open surgery, has becoming more prevalent. In order to visualize the operating site during laparoscopy, the surgical area must be insufflated with carbon dioxide.

Pathophysiology of pneumoperitoneum:

- Carbon dioxide insufflation results in compression of the inferior vena cava, which will decrease the venous return and will decrease the cardiac output, resulting in tachycardia, and an increase in the peripheral vascular resistance.

- Decreased tidal volume (TV) and functional residual capacity (FRC), decreased compliance, and respiratory acidosis.
- Shifting blood from the outer renal cortex to the juxtamedullary zone, the glomerular filtration rate will decrease resulting in activation of renin–angiotensin–aldosterone system and decreased urine output.

Because infants with congenital heart disease are more susceptible to hemodynamic effects of gas insufflation, these physiologic consequences of insufflation may counteract any benefits given by the less invasive method.

A study of mortality and morbidity after laparoscopic surgery in children with and without congenital heart disease showed that children who had a major or severe CHD had considerably greater mortality and morbidity than children who did not have a CHD. 30-day postoperative complications were considerably greater in children with mild CHD than in children without CHD. These results might be attributable to one of three factors: surgery's stress, the impacts of laparoscopic surgery, or the pathophysiology of their CHD [8].

In a study aims to determine the outcomes of children with congenital heart disease who underwent laparoscopic procedures. The results show that there are no major contraindications to conducting laparoscopic procedures in children with congenital heart disease [9].

Multiple Choice Questions: At Least Ten MCQs

1. Regarding coarctation of aorta repair, which of the following methods is used:
   A. Surgical removal of the constricted region and suturing the remaining two ends together.
   B. Bypassing the constricted segment by connecting a tube to the normal portions of the aorta on each side of the constricted segment.
   C. Subclavian flap.
   D. All the above.
2. Regarding atrial septal defect (ASD) repair, one of the following is false:
   A. ASD cannot be closed without open-heart surgery.
   B. Atrial septal defects can be closed with a transcatheter procedure.
   C. A balloon-tipped catheter is positioned in the middle of the defect and inflated to assess the size of it.
   D. None of the above.
3. Tetralogy of Fallot surgery is usually performed at age:
   A. 4 years
   B. At birth.

C. Between the ages of 6 months and 2 years.
D. First month.
4. The preferred method of repairing transposition of great arteries is:
   A. Atrial switch.
   B. Redirecting the pulmonary and systemic venous return to result in a physiologically normal state.
   C. Arterial switch.
   D. Opening up the atrial septum by a balloon (balloon atrial septostomy).
5. Regarding tricuspid atresia repair, Glenn procedure is done at age:
   A. Between the ages of 3 and 6 months.
   B. 2 years
   C. At birth.
   D. None of the above.
6. The first procedure to be done in hypoplastic left heart repair is:
   A. Bi-directional Glenn shunt procedure.
   B. Norwood procedure.
   C. Fontan procedure.
   D. None of the above.
7. One of the following is advantages of robotically assisted surgery over traditional surgery:
   A. More bleeding.
   B. Having to stay in the hospital for a shorter period of time (usually 3 to 4 days).
   C. Painkillers are being used more.
   D. Infection rate is increased.
8. One of the following is not a consequence of pneumoperitoneum:
   A. Compression of the inferior vena cava.
   B. Decrease cardiac output.
   C. Increased tidal volume.
   D. Respiratory acidosis.
9. Regarding hypoplastic left heart repair, Fontan procedure is performed at age:
   A. 4 to 6 months old
   B. Between the ages of 18 months and 3 years.
   C. During the first 2 weeks of life.
   D. None of the above.
10. One of the following is false:
    A. Infants with congenital heart disease are more susceptible to hemodynamic effects of gas insufflation.
    B. In pneumoperitoneum, the glomerular filtration rate will decrease resulting in activation of renin–angiotensin–aldosterone system and decreased urine output.
    C. Children cannot generally participate in regular household activities after cardiac surgery.
    D. All the above.

Answers

1. D.

    Explanation: Coarctation of the aorta is generally treated by a thoracotomy. Coarctation of the aorta can be repaired by balloon angioplasty or surgery. The surgical treatment includes removing the constricted region and suturing the remaining two ends together. A third method for correcting this problem is to allow blood to bypass the constricted segment by connecting a tube to the normal portions of the aorta on each side of the constricted segment.

    A fourth method for correcting this problem is a subclavian flap. An incision is made in the thin portion of the aorta. Then a patch from the left subclavian is used to widen the aorta's constricted section.

2. A.

    Explanation: ASD can be closed without open-heart surgery in some cases. Atrial septal defects can be closed with a transcatheter procedure where catheters are driven into the heart chambers. To assess the size atrial septal defect, a balloon-tipped catheter is positioned in the middle of it and inflated. Atrial septal defect then closed using a device. The blood pressure between the right and left atria will maintain the device in place. In around three months, heart tissue will develop over the device.

    ASD might be treated with open-heart surgery where the septum can be stitched or patched.

3. C.

    Explanation: 3. Open-heart surgery is needed to correct the four defects to allow the heart to work normally, either shortly after birth or later in infancy and it is usually performed between the ages of 6 months and 2 years.

4. C.

    Explanation: There is a variety of surgical techniques to correct transposition of the major arteries. The treatment of major vessel transposition needs open-heart surgery. If feasible, this procedure is conducted as soon as possible following birth. An arterial switch is the most frequent and preferred method of repairing transposition of the great arteries.

5. A.

    Explanation: Glenn procedure, it's done between the ages of 3 and 6 months. The initial shunt is removed, and the pulmonary artery is connected to one of the major veins that returns blood to the heart (the superior vena cava). This permits blood that is deficient in oxygen to travel directly to the lungs.

6. B.

    Explanation: Norwood procedure: The first procedure, performed during the first 2 weeks of life. This is a challenging procedure where a "new" aorta is made and connected to the right ventricle. The surgeon inserts a tube from the aorta or the right ventricle to pulmonary arteries. The right ventricle becomes the body's primary chamber that pump blood to the lungs and the rest of the body.

7. B.

    Explanation: The advantages of robotically assisted surgery over traditional surgery are less invasive, incisions are smaller resulting in less scarring, less bleeding and less discomfort, having to stay in the hospital for a shorter period of time (usually 3 to 4 days), painkillers are being used less often, infection rate is decreased, recovery time is shorter.

8. C.

    Explanation: Pathophysiology of pneumoperitoneum:

    - Carbon dioxide insufflation result in compression of the inferior vena cava, which will decrease the venous return and will decrease the cardiac output, resulting in tachycardia, and an increase in the peripheral vascular resistance.
    - Decreased tidal volume (TV) and functional residual capacity (FRC), decreased compliance, and respiratory acidosis.
    - Shifting blood from the outer renal cortex to the juxtamedullary zone, the glomerular filtration rate will decrease resulting in activation of renin–angiotensin–aldosterone system and decreased urine output.

9. B.

    Explanation: Fontan procedure is performed between the ages of 18 months and 3 years. The pulmonary artery and the inferior vena cava are connected.

10. C.

    Explanation: Swimming is usually banned following surgery for at least a few weeks. Children can generally participate in regular household activities, but they should avoid hard play or sports.

References

1. Chu DI, et al. Outcomes of laparoscopic and open surgery in children with and without congenital heart disease. J Pediatr Surg. 2018;53(10):1980–8.
2. Chu DI, et al. Mortality and morbidity after laparoscopic surgery in children with and without congenital heart disease. J Pediatr. 2017;185:88–93.
3. Herrick NL, et al. Laparoscopic surgery requiring abdominal insufflation in patients with congenital heart disease. J Cardiothorac Vasc Anesth. 2022;36(3):707–12.
4. Pilkington M, Craig Egan J. Noncardiac surgery in the congenital heart patient. Semin Pediatr Surg. 2019;28(1):11–7.
5. Waje ND, et al. Anaesthetic challenges and transesophageal echocardiography-guided perioperative management in a patient with uncorrected adult congenital heart disease presenting for emergency laparoscopic hysterectomy. Turk J Anaesthesiol Reanim. 2021;49(2):169.

6. Jooste E, et al Anesthesia for adults with congenital heart disease undergoing noncardiac surgery. Nussmeier N, Yeon S (ur.) UpToDate. 2019

7. Chang S-L, et al. A case of congenital long QT syndrome, type 8, undergoing laparoscopic hysterectomy with general anesthesia. Taiwan J Obstet Gynecol. 2019;58(4):552–6.

8. Gupta A, et al. Laparoscopic cholecystectomy in a patient with Glenn shunt-aided with erector spine block. Turkish J Anaesthesiol Reanim. 2021;49(4):338–42.

9. Srinivas VY, Rao SG, Sudarshan MB. Anaesthetic management of a parturient with single ventricle posted for laparoscopic surgery. J Evol Med Dent Sci. 2019;8(4):281–3.

Perfusion in Congenital Heart Surgery

Nida Hashmi, Ahmed Dheyaa Al-Obaidi,
Abeer Mundher Ali, and Sara Shihab Ahmad

Abstract

Cardiopulmonary bypass (CPB) technology enables the performance of cardiac surgical procedures in a stable, bloodless operative field. It is equipped with a circuit named as the extracorporeal circuit which provides physiological support. Classically, blood is drained out from heart and lungs and carried into a reservoir by the venous cannulation and tubing then it will be given back again to the cannulated arterial system by a pump and artificial lung (oxygenator or gas-exchanger) as fully oxygenated. Therefore, an ideal CPB circuit is composed from pumps, tubing, cannulae, reservoir, oxygenator, heat exchanger, and an arterial line filter. Up to date, there are complete machines for CPB that will include monitoring system for oxygen saturation, temperature, pressure, hemoglobin, electrolytes, and blood gases. In addition to specific measures, we should place also for safety a sensor for oxygen, detectors for bubbles, and a reservoir alert for detection of presence of low levels.

Keywords

Cardiopulmonary bypass · Perfusion in surgery
Congenital surgery · Heart-lung machine · Congenital heart surgery · Hemodialysis · Extracorporeal circulation
Oxygenator · Advance perfusion techniques
Congenital disease

Introduction

Dr John Gibbon is widely regarded as the pioneer of contemporary cardiopulmonary perfusion surgery. Extracorporeal circulation (ECC) is a term that refers to the process of continuously withdrawing and returning a patient's blood through plastic tubing in an artificial organ function that is not part of the body's blood circulation. In an ECC, a variety of artificial organs are employed to complement a patient's failing organs. Artificial lungs (oxygenators), artificial hearts (blood pumps), artificial livers, and artificial kidneys (hemodialysis) are already available to therapeutic use. An ECC was designed to treat patients with specific curable illnesses by combining sterile tubes and artificial organs so that the patient's condition becomes operable. One of the forms of the extracorporeal circulation is (CPB) also termed as the cardiopulmonary bypass which defined as surgical operation that can allow blood to flow and oxygenation to be preserved throughout the body by temporarily performing the function of both the lungs and the heart, thereby providing respiratory and cardiac support in addition to management of temperature which makes performing a surgery on the great vessels and the heart is possible [1, 2]

The Parts of the Cardiopulmonary Bypass Circuit

(a) *Oxygenating membrane*: The oxygenator is used to supplement infused blood with oxygen and to eliminate carbon dioxide from venous blood. CPB using bubble oxygenators enabled cardiac surgery, however membrane oxygenators have typically substituted bubble oxygenators for nowadays. Membrane oxygenators are made of microporous polypropylene fibers hollow from inside as the internal diameter ranges from 100 to 200 μm. While the blood phase passing outside the fiber, on the other hand, the gas phase flows within, hence unraveling the gas and blood phases. They considered to have a lower risk of air embolism and provide more accurate blood gas management. Recent designs incorporate an embolic filter, obviating the need for an extra arterial filter. There is another oxygenator form that has

N. Hashmi (✉)
Karachi Medical and Dental College, Karachi, Pakistan

A. D. Al-Obaidi · A. M. Ali · S. S. Ahmad
College of Medicine, University of Baghdad, Baghdad, Iraq

gained popularity lately known as the heparin coated blood oxygenator. It is considered to cause lower systemic inflammation and reduce likelihood clotting to the blood in the circuit of CPB. An exchange of heat known also as heat exchanger is incorporated inside and adjacent to the oxygenator to minimize the emission of gaseous emboli caused by changes in the temperature degrees of the saturated blood [3]. To choose an oxygenator, the maximum predicted pump flows for neonates and infants are employed. The oxygenators are normally approved for a maximum of 6 h of operation, and exceeding this limit results in a significant drop in performance [3–7].

(b) *Venous reservoir*: They gather the blood that has been drained from the heart. The most typical type of reservoir is an open reservoir. They enable for passive venous air evacuation in addition to the suggestion of suction applying to aid the drainage. They incorporate a separate defoaming and cardiotomy circuit for the suctioned blood processing. Whenever they are utilized, a secure amount of the blood is maintained in reservoir which help to prevent air from entering the arterial circuit. The closed reservoirs tend to have a restricted capacity for blood volume yet provide reduced the contact area between blood and the artificial surfaces. This feature results in lower inflammatory activity, decreases postoperative transfusions, and improves sterility. However, closed reservoirs require a separate circuit for suctioned blood processing [8]. The venous reservoir is made up of two components: a venous filter that collects venous blood, and the cardiotomy. Additionally, it requires extra systems for venous bag air elimination, the cardiotomy blood is filtered independently by distinct flowing pathways in cardiotomy venous reservoir (CVR), which should be prepared to accommodate the blood volume of the patient in events of a scheduled or unanticipated low-flow or cardiac arrest. The device to remove air is critical. The preponderance of air in the venous blood flow channels and cardiotomy is collected at the intakes of their respective filtration systems, which are alternately located immediately above also known as the top feeders or just below which called as the bottom feeders. Both of them have a low-profile extension tube that assists in maintaining a constant flow of liquid which works as a gravity siphon drain. Cardiotomy and venous filters are frequently covered with a chemical to aid in the reduction of foam generation and the removal of foam formed on the filter. When blood is more critical than usual and a high reservoir level is discovered throughout bypass, a greater reservoir level should maintain by the perfusionist to provide

help in the process of defoaming. This will provide a longer transit time through the reservoir, which help in elimination of gaseous microemboli [7, 9, 10].

(c) *Cardiotomy filter*: Cardiotomy filter is elevated and situated in the back of venous reservoir. This will allow the blood of the cardiotomy to flow in a passive way into the venous reservoir. In the presence of any chance that the integrated CVR may flood due to circulatory arrest or low pump flow, a backup cardiotomy reservoir is supplied. This can be utilized temporarily for blood volume storage. Another cardiotomy filter provides extra filtration, or prefiltering, of expelled blood, so increasing the efficacy of the first cardiotomy filter. Defoaming chemicals are frequently used to maintain the integrity of cardiotomy and venous filters [4, 6, 11, 12].

(d) *Heat exchangers*: In the lack of an exterior source providing heat to control the temperature of the body, patients under ECC will develop hypothermia. As a result, majority of CPB systems include a type of heat exchanger in order to warm the blood of the patient. Each oxygenator incorporates a heat exchanger through which blood travels prior to the gas exchange. The heat exchangers could be placed in number of positions throughout the circuit, the most typical being located on proximal part of the oxygenator. Venous-side or proximal heat exchanger is thought to reduce the risk of outgassing of the solution induced due to fast rewarming of the blood following CPB hypothermia, that might produce massive bubbles of gas [6]. The difference in the temperature of the input (venous) and output (arterial) blood is determined. Typically, the temperature of venous blood and water inlets is less than $10°C$. Reduced gradients during rewarming may result in more uniform warming, assisting in the prevention of after-drop. Lowering the temperature can extend the length of a bypass scenario due to the longer rewarming times. Thus, temperature gradients should have close monitoring [12].

(e) *Arterial Line Filters (ALF)*: The arterial line filters minimize particle and gaseous emboli considerably and supposed to be utilized in circuits of CPB. According to certain research, 20-m filtration screen is better than 40-m filtration screen in terms of reducing cerebral emboli. Several investigations had revealed that arterial line filtration has a protective impact on neurologic outcomes [6]. Microporous membrane wrapping technology has the potential to act as both an oxygenator and an arterial filter. However, it is not well verified yet. The arterial line filters are known to have a large surface area and are certified for flows well along certain shear force and turbulence limitations [4, 10, 12–16].

Pumping

There are 2 rollers mounted on spinning arm compressing a span of tubing in order to create a forward flow. This activity could result in tube debris and hemolysis which both become more prevalent with passing time. As a result, operation that might take long duration is discouraged to use roller pumps. The impellers/stacked cones of a centrifugal pump are contained within the housing. When the inlet valves are rapidly rotated, a negative pressure is being generated at one of them and positive pressure at the other one, driving the blood to flow forwardly. They are dependent on the afterload, which means that when the systemic vascular resistance (SVR) of the patient grows, the generated cardiac output decreases until the pump flow being raised. In prolonged situations, the centrifugal pumps might enhance, renal function, platelet preservation, and neurological outcomes [8]. Appropriate flow is heavily dependent on the right placement of the roller head occlusion (which also impacts the degree of blood damage and hemolysis) and a precise knowledge of the pump head revolution rate and tubing size is required as any inaccurate accounting for any of these variables might result in excessive or insufficient pump flow [2].

Heater-Cooler System

As the ability to effectively control a patient's temperature while on bypass and patients may be greatly harmed by inadequate water flow. An independent heater-cooler system is employed. They are mobile, reliable, economical, and easy to maintain. Recently they have reduced significantly in size as a result they became quieter. And others are easy to operate as connected to remote-controlled systems [11, 17].

Cannulae

These tubes are conduits by which patients are linked to their CPB machines. To avoid kinking, they are made of polyvinylchloride (PVC) and strengthened with wire [8]. In congenital heart disease patients, the superior and inferior vena cava are by far the most common locations for venous cannulation. Another site is ascending aorta atriocaval cannulation which is generally the most widely used method now [18–20].

Venous cannulae: They are used to drain systemic blood which is deoxygenated into the CPB machine. Cannulation can be via a central or a peripheral approach. Central cannulation is usually done by means of cavoatrial (dual-stage) or bicaval cannulation (single stage). The first approach is used for most closed-heart procedures, it includes cannulation of the right atrium. The used cannula has two ends.

Proximal area is broader, whereas distal area is narrower. Blood from the superior vena cava and the coronary sinus flows into the proximal section, which contains side perforations. Since the right atrium is far bigger than the cannulae, blocking its side holes is extremely unlikely. Its distal end is inserted into the inferior vena cava, where it receives its oxygen-rich blood supply. When it comes to bicaval cannulation (cannulation of both the superior and inferior vena cava), a Y-piece is used to connect the two cannulations. Patients undergoing congenital cardiac surgery are more likely to require bicaval cannulation due to the more frequent occurrence of intracardiac work. Another factor to consider when selecting a cannula is its diameter and the form of its tip [21]. A venous cannula with a larger internal diameter is likely to have lower pressure and a greater flow capacity. Despite their inflexibility, metal tips have the advantage of having the highest I/O ratios. Tip flexibility and conical shape may help in insertion into the cavae despite the reduced (I/O) ratios of silicone compared to metal. Estimated flow on the bypass, surgical needs, and surgeon judgment all influence venous cannula size [6, 8, 22].

Arterial Cannulae: These return oxygenated blood from the CPB to the systemic circulation. It is usually done by distal ascending-aorta cannulation. This site provides ease of insertion and improved venous drainage with equally adequate arterial perfusion. The size of used cannulae is selected by consulting with the perfusionist team to choose the size that is sufficient for enough flow in the circuit. Large cannulae will require aortotomy which is difficult to close and those that are too small will impede flow. Furthermore, high pressure gradients or jets of flow caused by tiny cannulae may enhance the risk of dissection. Metal or plastic can be used to make the cannula's tip, which can also be angled, tapered, or straight. Some of the arterial cannulae have diffusion tips which secure a multidirectional flow thus reducing the created jets. As a result, surgical outcomes will be affected by the cannula's length and if it is compressible (being restricted or prone to kinking by the purse strings). The tip of various arterial cannulae can be used to monitor central aortic pressure before and after bypass [4, 20, 23–25].

Primers for Congenital Surgery

Priming is the process by which the perfusion can accomplish two things: the first is the CPB circuit which becomes de-aired and the second is that priming causes hemodilution that enhances flows while the patient is hypothermic. It is done by means of priming solutions (the prime) which consist of a mixture of crystalloids and colloids [8]. Using solutions with a "high colloid osmotic pressure" such as albumin decreases fluid overload. Albumin-based primers were found to be more suitable for neonates than crystalloid-based primers. Furthermore, mixing FFP with the CPB priming solutions has been proved to reduce postoperative blood loss in neonates undergoing complex repairs or have cyanotic diseases. FFP is useful in the sense that it prevents coagulation abnormalities that might be encountered. Hence, ideal priming in neonates would be done by a mixture of albumin or FFP and RBCs in adequate proportions to maintain a hematocrit range between 28 and 30% in normothermia [26, 27]. Volume of the prime is determined depending on the diagnosis, body surface area, scheduled operation, and anticipated maximal bypass pump flow. However, one critical point to address is to avoid excessive priming, since a high level of hemodilution caused by a priming volume greater than the projected blood volume of the infant leads in a considerable decrease in platelet count and coagulation factors. Further, prime volume was found to be independently linked to perioperative transfusion requirements in pediatric patients with congenital heart disease. This is further amplified in neonates [28, 29]. The minimal prime volume that is considered to be safe is defined as the minimum amount that completely fills both the venous and arterial limbs of the CPB circuit and maintains sufficient volume in the venous reservoir to prevent air from entering into the arterial side of the circuit during CPB initiation [30]. Prior to the patient's arrival, the perfusionist can test the heart-lung machine and operating room equipment by priming the circuit. Once the perfusionist identifies what the hematocrit will be right before the treatment, blood priming can start. The oxygenator is the ideal route to circulate the venous reservoir. During priming, the arterial and venous lines should be maintained shut until the main components have indeed been de-aired properly and thus priming has been successfully taken place [17, 23].

The Role of Heparin

One of the most important complications encountered during CPB is coagulopathy [31]. Heparin is used during CPB to avoid blood from clotting within the CPB circuit. It accomplishes that by facilitating antithrombin III action. The use of unfractionated heparin is favored as it has a rapid onset, low cost, safety and it can be rapidly neutralized by protamine. Heparin dosing for initiation and maintenance of CPB is 300–400 U kg^{-1} in addition to further doses required to maintain an activated clotting time (ACT) more than 480 s [32]. A whole blood anticoagulation test should be performed prior to and at regular intervals throughout CPB. This is accomplished by the use of ACT, which is widely regarded as the gold standard for monitoring anticoagulation for CPB. Bolus administration of unfractionated

heparin based upon weight in kgs is reasonable for achieving adequate anticoagulation, Nevertheless, the response to heparin varies from among individuals and requires continued monitoring during CPB, independent of the bolus dose used [33].

Blood and Gas Management

Neonates have a faster metabolic rate and a greater oxygen need, necessitating a higher pump flow rate during CPB. When measuring blood gases during CPB, increased PaO_2 reflects a high rate of dissolved oxygen transport, however, does not mean improved oxygen delivery. Conversely, it has been observed that elevated PaO_2 levels are detrimental in preterm and near-term newborns. Although there is no guideline for the optimal PaO_2 during bypass surgery, avoiding excessive PaO_2 during newborn surgery is reasonable [27].

Carbon Dioxide Management

CO_2 is created during CPB as a result of two physiologic process, one is as a byproduct of normal aerobic metabolism and the other is during buffering of lactate produced by cells with anaerobic metabolism. As a result, monitoring carbon dioxide removal is critical for determining the sufficiency of oxygen delivery and perfusion of tissues. The American Society of Extracorporeal Technology considers this practice (i.e., monitoring of CO_2 removal) to be a recommended practice guideline, while the "Australian New Zealand College of Perfusion" considers it to be a standard of practice. This monitoring is often accomplished via capnometry examination of gases exiting the oxygenator's exhaust port. Carbon dioxide partial pressure (pCO_2) can be determined by taking sequential samples from the CPB circuit's lines both arterial and venous. Modern monitoring system has succeeded in creating devices that provide sustained, on-line monitoring of both. Nevertheless, due to the non-linear relationship between CO_2 amount and tension, these parameters cannot be utilized to calculate VCO_2 in a consistent manner. Infrared (IR) spectrography is now known to be a better technique for CO_2 monitoring. CO_2 monitoring has clinical utility which extends beyond ensuring that the patient maintains an adequate $PaCO_2$ throughout the CPB process. Increased values of $ePCO_2$ and hence VCO_2 can be observed after the cross-clamp is released, during the phases of rewarming after deep hypothermia and as a result of the heart being reperfused. Other causes might be due to increasing VO2 (aerobic CO_2) and reduced solubility of CO_2. In many institutions, the frequent use of temperature-lowering approach has been replaced by using moderate hypothermia or even normothermia. Yet, temperatures of 28 °C in the CPB circuit may be still employed in congenital cardiac surgery and other highly demanding surgeries. Changes in CO_2 solubility in the presence of deep hypothermia result in comparable changes in pH, which have an effect on cerebral blood flow. The pH-stat technique involves the injection of exogenous CO_2 to compensate for its low values during hypothermia. The presence of increased $ePCO_2$ readings is seldom due to an oxygenator failure, which is manifested more frequently as inadequate blood oxygenation [34].

pH and Blood Gas Management

While conducting hypothermic CPB, blood gas management can be assessed using either a "pH-stat" or an "alpha-stat" technique. The principle behind the pH stat is to keep the pH consistent at all given temperatures. CO_2 must be supplied into the oxygenator all through hypothermic CPB to maintain constant levels of pH and pCO_2. On the other hand, when using alpha-stat technique, the pH is kept at 37° C regardless of the patient's temperature. Alpha-stat works to sustain normal levels of pH levels intracellulary by monitoring the natural shift of the oxyhemoglobin dissociation curve. Because in-line blood gas analysis offers instantaneous detection of changes in air/oxygen/carbon dioxide parameters, it is a useful technique for determining optimal blood gas management. Numerous investigations have concluded that the pH-stat method is superior during neonatal cardiac bypass. While cooling, this technique promotes cerebral blood flow and tissue oxygenation. Additionally, data suggest that pH-stat control improves outcomes following pediatric heart surgery by reducing ventilation periods and intensive care unit stays [35].

Multiple Choice Questions

1. Extracorporeal circulation (ECC) is a term that refers to the process of continuously withdrawing and returning a patient's blood through plastic tubing in order to perform an artificial organ function outside of the body's blood circulation. In an ECC, a variety of "artificial organs" are employed to complement a patient's failing organs. Artificial hearts (blood pump), artificial lungs (oxygenator), artificial kidneys (hemodialysis), and artificial livers are only a few examples of therapies that are now available. The following is a list of the oxygenator components that should be included in the perfusion during cardiopulmonary bypass surgery:
   A. Cannula ALF and tube.
   B. Cardiotomy filter and venous reservoir and filter, ALF, tubing pack, heat exchanger.
   C. Venous filter, ALF, and pump.
   D. Cannula and venous reservoir.

2. Using the preceding topic, how much pressure must be reduced in each cannula during perfusion surgery in order for the high flow capacity be maintained?
   A. Arterial pressure: 100 mmHg and venous pressure: 35–40 mmHg.
   B. Arterial pressure: 110 mmHg and venous pressure: 40–45 mmHg.
   C. Arterial pressure: 105 mmHg and venous pressure: 45–50 mmHg.
   D. Arterial pressure: 120 mmHg and venous pressure: 55–60 mmHg.

3. During cardiopulmonary bypass, arterialized blood is coupled with an arresting agent and other additives obtained from a source downwards the oxygenator. Any additive concentration can be changed to maximize advantage. The delivery area may be cool or warm, and the temperature fluctuates throughout the arrest time. They are used seldom in congenital cardiac surgery. Which form of cardioplegia is this?
   A. Continuous cardioplegia.
   B. Cardioplegia system without the recirculation.
   C. Cardioplegia system with the recirculation.
   D. None.

Answers
1. B.
2. A.
3. A.

References

1. Menahem S, Poulakis Z, Prior M. Children subjected to cardiac surgery for congenital heart disease. Part 1–emotional and psychological outcomes. Interact Cardiovasc Thorac Surg. 2008;7(4):600–4.
2. DiNardo J, Shukla A, McGowan F (2011) Anesthesia for congenital heart surgery. Smith's Anesthesia for Infants and Children. 605–673
3. Davies H Cardiopulmonary bypass machine—CPB [Internet]. Ebmecouk 2022 [cited 28 February 2022]. https://www.ebme.co.uk/articles/clinical-engineering/cardiopulmonary-bypass-machine-cpb
4. Stark JF, De Leval MR, Tsang VT, editors. Surgery for congenital heart defects. London: John Wiley & Sons; 2006.
5. Liu A, Sun Z, Liu Q, Zhu N, Wang S. Pumping O2 with no N2: an overview of hollow fiber membrane oxygenators with integrated arterial filters. Curr Top Med Chem. 2020;20(1):78–85. https://doi.org/10.2174/1568026619666191210161013).
6. Groom R, Fitzgerald D, Gutsche J, Ramakrishna H (2022) Extracorporeal devices including extracorporeal membrane oxygenation
7. Stammers AH, Miller R, Francis SG, Fuzesi L, Nostro A, Tesdahl E. Goal-directed perfusion methodology for determining oxygenator performance during clinical cardiopulmonary bypass. J Extra Corpor Technol. 2017;49(2):81–92.
8. Sarkar M, Prabhu V. Basics of cardiopulmonary bypass. Indian J Anaesth. 2017 Sep;61(9):760.
9. Alkan T, et al. Benefits of pulsatile perfusion on vital organ recovery during and after pediatric open heart surgery. ASAIO J. 2007;53(6):651–4.

10. Schuldes M, Riley JB, Francis SG, Clingan S. Effect of normobaric versus hypobaric oxygenation on gaseous microemboli removal in a diffusion membrane oxygenator: an in vitro comparison. J Extra Corpor Technol. 2016;48(3):129–36.

11. Sturmer D, Beaty C, Clingan S, Jenkins E, Peters W, Si MS. Recent innovations in perfusion and cardiopulmonary bypass for neonatal and infant cardiac surgery. Transl Pediatr. 2018;7(2):139–50. https://doi.org/10.21037/tp.2018.03.05.

12. Guimarães DP, Caneo LF, Matte G, et al. Impact of vacuum-assisted venous drainage on forward flow in simulated pediatric cardiopulmonary bypass circuits utilizing a centrifugal arterial pump head. Braz J Cardiovasc Surg. 2020;35(2):134–40. https://doi.org/10.21470/1678-9741-2019-0311.

13. Stehouwer MC, de Vroege R, Hoohenkerk GJF, et al. Carbon dioxide flush of an integrated minimized perfusion circuit prior to priming prevents spontaneous air release into the arterial line during clinical use. Artif Organs. 2017;41(11):997–1003. https://doi.org/10.1111/aor.12909).

14. Reagor JA, Holt DW. Removal of gross air embolization from cardiopulmonary bypass circuits with integrated arterial line filters: a comparison of circuit designs. J Extra Corpor Technol. 2016;48(1):19–22.

15. Stehouwer MC, Boers C, de Vroege R, Kelder C, J, Yilmaz A, Bruins P. Clinical evaluation of the air removal characteristics of an oxygenator with integrated arterial filter in a minimized extracorporeal circuit. Int J Artif Organs. 2011;34(4):374–82. https://doi.org/10.5301/IJAO.2011.774.

16. Ginther RM Jr, Gorney R, Cruz R. A clinical evaluation of the Maquet Quadrox-i neonatal oxygenator with integrated arterial filter. Perfusion. 2013;28(3):194–9.

17. Drury NE, Horsburgh A, Bi R, Willetts RG, Jones TJ. Cardioplegia practice in paediatric cardiac surgery: a UK & Ireland survey. Perfusion. 2019;34(2):125–9. https://doi.org/10.1177/0267659118794343.

18. Ler A, Sazzad F, Ong GS, Kofidis T. Comparison of outcomes of the use of Del Nido and St. Thomas cardioplegia in adult and paediatric cardiac surgery: a systematic review and meta-analysis. Perfusion. 2020;35(8):724–35.

19. Ad N, Holmes SD, Massimiano PS, Rongione AJ, Fornaresio LM, Fitzgerald D. The use of del Nido cardioplegia in adult cardiac surgery: a prospective randomized trial. J Thorac Cardiovasc Surg. 2018;155(3):1011–8.

20. Guyton RA, Mora CT, Finlayson DC, Rigatti RL, editors. Cardiopulmonary bypass: principles and techniques of extracorporeal circulation. New York: Springer Science & Business Media; 2012.

21. Saczkowski R, Maklin M, Mesana T, Boodhwani M, Ruel M. Centrifugal pump and roller pump in adult cardiac surgery:

a meta-analysis of randomized controlled trials. Artif Organs. 2012;36(8):668–76.

22. Boburg RS, Rosenberger P, Kling S, Jost W, Schlensak C, Magunia H. Selective lower body perfusion during aortic arch surgery in neonates and small children. Perfusion. 2020;35(7):621–5.

23. Kim SY, Cho S, Choi E, Kim WH. Effects of mini-volume priming during cardiopulmonary bypass on clinical outcomes in low-bodyweight neonates: less transfusion and postoperative extracorporeal membrane oxygenation support. Artif Organs. 2016;40(1):73–9.

24. El-Sherief AH, Wu CC, Schoenhagen P, Little BP, Cheng A, Abbara S, Roselli EE. Basics of cardiopulmonary bypass: normal and abnormal postoperative CT appearances. Radiographics. 2013;33(1):63–72.

25. Bond E, Valadon C, Slaughter M (2019) Cannulation for cardiopulmonary bypass. In: Cardiac Surgery Procedures. IntechOpen

26. Pouard P, Bojan M. Neonatal cardiopulmonary bypass. Sem Thorac Cardiovasc Surg Pediatr Card Surg Annu. 2013;16(1):59–61.

27. Oliver WC Jr, Beynen FM, Nuttall GA, Schroeder DR, Ereth MH, Dearani JA, Puga FJ. Blood loss in infants and children for open heart operations: albumin 5% versus fresh-frozen plasma in the prime. Ann Thorac Surg. 2003;75(5):1506–12.

28. Dieu A, Rosal Martins M, Eeckhoudt S, Matta A, Kahn D, Khalifa C, Rubay J, Poncelet A, Haenecour A, Derycke E, Thiry D. Fresh frozen plasma versus crystalloid priming of cardiopulmonary bypass circuit in pediatric surgery: a randomized clinical trial. Anesthesiology. 2020;132(1):95–106.

29. Richmond ME, Charette K, Chen JM, Quaegebeur JM, Bacha E. The effect of cardiopulmonary bypass prime volume on the need for blood transfusion after pediatric cardiac surgery. J Thorac Cardiovasc Surg. 2013;145(4):1058–64.

30. Georgiou C, Irons J (2015) Priming solutions for cardiopulmonary bypass circuits. Cardiopulmonary Bypass, pp. 42–50

31. Bartoszko J, Karkouti K. Managing the coagulopathy associated with cardiopulmonary bypass. J Thromb Haemost. 2021;19(3):617–32.

32. O'Carroll-Kuehn BU, Meeran H. Management of coagulation during cardiopulmonary bypass. Contin Educ Anaesth Crit Care Pain. 2007;7(6):195–8.

33. Shore-Lesserson L, Baker RA, Ferraris V, et al. STS/SCA/AmSECT clinical practice guidelines: anticoagulation during cardiopulmonary bypass. J Extra Corpor Technol. 2018;50(1):5–18.

34. Ranucci M, Carboni G, Cotza M, De Somer F. Carbon dioxide production during cardiopulmonary bypass: pathophysiology, measure and clinical relevance. Perfusion. 2017;32(1):4–12.

35. Griffin DA. Blood gas strategies and management during pediatric cardiopulmonary bypass. ASAIO J. 2005;51(5):657–8.

Printed in the United States
by Baker & Taylor Publisher Services